Current Topics in Pathology

Continuation of Ergebnisse der Pathologie

67

Carcinogenesis

Contributors

P. Höhn, E. Kunze, K. Nomura
C. Witting, W. Schlake

Editor

E. Grundmann

With 112 Figures

Springer-Verlag Berlin Heidelberg New York 1979

E. Grundmann, Professor Dr., Pathologisches Institut der Universität, Westring 17,
D–4400 Münster/Westf., Germany

ISBN-13: 978-3-642-67294-1 e-ISBN-13: 978-3-642-67292-7
DOI: 10.1007/978-3-642-67292-7

Library of Congress Cataloging in Publication Data. Main entry under title: Carcinogenesis. (Current topics in pathology; 67). Bibliography: p. Includes index. 1. Carcinogenesis. 2. Oncology, Experimental. I. Höhn, P. II. Grundmann, Ekkehard. III. Title. IV. Series. [DNLM: 1. Neoplasms–Etiology. W1 CU821H v. 67 / QZ202.3 C264] RB1.E6 vol. 67 [RC268.5] 616.07'08s [616.9'94'071]
79–10558

Softcover reprint of the hardcover 1st edition 1979

2122/3130 – 543210

Contents

Indexed in ISR

List of Contributors

Höhn, Prof. Dr. P.	Pathologisches Institut der Universität, Postfach 3960, Langenbeckstr. 1, 6500 Mainz, Fed. Rep. of Germany
Kunze, Priv. Doz. Dr. E.	Pathologisches Institut der Universität, Goßlerstr. 10, 3400 Göttingen, Fed. Rep. of Germany
Nomura, Dr. K.	Pathologisches Institut der Universität, Westring 17, 4400 Münster, Fed. Rep. of Germany
Schlake, Dr. med. W.	Pathologisches Institut der Universität, Westring 17, 4400 Münster, Fed. Rep. of Germany
Witting, Priv. Doz. Dr. Ch.	Pathologisches Institut der Universität, Westring 17, 4400 Münster, Fed. Rep. of Germany

Histogenesis of Carcinoma in the Glandular Stomach of the Rat After B I Resection *

W. SCHLAKE and K. NOMURA

---

* Supported by Landesamt für Forschung, Ministerium für Wissenschaft und Forschung Nordrhein-Westfalen

Introduction

The present concepts of etiology and pathogenesis of gastric carcinoma are still far from definite (*Wanke,* 1971; *Wiendl,* 1975). The significance and biologic behavior of possible precancerous histologic findings are equally unclear (*Oehlert,* 1978; *Oehlert* et al., 1975; *Grundmann,* 1975; *Grundmann* and *Schlake,* 1978). Definition and appraisal of true precancerous lesions are the prerequisites of early diagnosis which offers the only chance of improving the poor diagnosis of gastric carcinoma (*Rösch* and *Elster,* 1977; *Wiendl,* 1975; *Wanke,* 1971).

Actual histologic precursor stages are readily found in those conditions properly called "precancerous" (*Hamperl,* 1974). They occur in the stomach with the characteristic chronic gastritis of patients with pernicious anemia. The changes are located in the area surrounding large gastric polyps and, after partial resection, in the gastric remnant where carcinomas have been described with increasing frequency in recent years (*Domellöf* et al., 1977; *Gschnitzer,* 1977; *Clemençon* et al., 1976; *Peitsch* and *Burkhardt,* 1976; *Morgenstern* et al., 1973; *Saegesser* and *Jämes,* 1972; *Stalsberg* and *Taksdal,* 1971; *Kobayashi* et al., 1970).

The term "carcinoma in the resected stomach" (i.e., gastric stump carcinoma) is used under the following conditions:

1. The primary surgical intervention must have been for a benign gastric lesion (histologically confirmed) such as gastroduodenal ulcer, developmental disorders, or trauma.

2. The interval between primary surgery and the manifestation of a carcinoma must be no less than 5 years.

Some authors (*Morgenstern* et al., 1973) wished also to include those cases who, after primary surgery for gastric carcinoma, developed "gastric stump carcinoma" after as long an interval as 20 years or more. We think that these new manifestations should rather be considered as independent primary tumors.

Systematic morphologic investigations of resected stomachs are uncommon (*Konjetzny,* 1938; *Boller,* 1947; *Rosenow* and *McDonald,* 1944; *Becker,* 1969). The question whether the resection might create morphologic conditions that would favor or provoke subsequent cancerous degeneration was not studied or discussed in detail. Equally unknown is whether carcinomas in the resected stomach, in particular those near the anastomosis, might show any morphologic features differing from those of "normal" gastric carcinoma, and possibly related to the grave patho-anatomical changes necessarily induced by the surgical procedure. The first indications towards such morphologic peculiarities of anastomotic tissue were made by *Konjetzny* (1938). Like many authors after him (*Siurala,* 1965; *Henning,* 1966; *Kuru,* 1966; *Siurala,* 1974; *Strickland* and *Mackay,* 1973), *Konjetzny* saw chronic atrophic gastritis as the cruical etiologic factor for gastric carcinogenesis, and held this same factor responsible for carcinogenesis in the resected stomach. He had observed, predominantly in the area surrounding the stoma, chronic gastritis of a partly atrophic, partly hypertrophic character with adenomatous hyperplasia and cystic dilatation of glands. The anastomotic area was held to be specifically endangered because of the contact between the glandular epithelia of different types with polyps and pseudopolyps and because these epithelia showed destruction as well as regeneration (*Boller,* 1947).

Further morphologic studies of gastrointestinal stoma were carrried out by *Rosenow* and *McDonald* (1944). Morphologic findings in 60 resection cases were followed over various periods (from 14 days up to 27 years). The results of other studies published by *Becker* (1969) have essentially substantiated the first extensive light microscopic descriptions by *Konjetzny* (1938).

The problems of carcinogenesis and related morphologic phenomena may also be studied in experimental assays specially designed to imitate human conditions in an appropriate animal model. *Dahm* and *Werner* were the first to try this approach in 1973: The classic model of chemical carcinogenesis in the rat glandular stomach by N-methyl-N'-nitro-N-nitrosoguanidine (MNNG) (*Sugimura* and *Fujimura,* 1967; *Saito* et al., 1970; *Bralow,* 1972; *Kobori* et al., 1976; *Uchida* et al., 1976) was modified by a preceding surgical intervention, i.e., gastroduodenostomy (Billroth-I) or gastrojejunostomy (Billroth-II). The authors intended to prove that

1. Carcinogenesis in the operated stomach occurred earlier than in non-resected animals.

2. Carcinomas preferably developed at the site of the gastrointestinal anastomosis.

Schlag et al. (1977a) modified this model by effecting gastroenterostomy without resection under otherwise identical conditions. In all their cases, observation revealed glandular proliferation near the anastomotic site, but no carcinomas. They concluded that resection itself, i.e., reduction of gastric surface, must be chiefly responsible for carcinogenesis. However, quite similar epithelial changes may be open to different interpretation, and the comparison of results obtained by different methods might, therefore, seem questionable. In both studies postoperative monitoring was done for about 35 weeks.

Another group (*Rumpf* et al., 1978) compared the results of chemical carcinogenesis in the rat stomach after (a) vagotomy and (b) Billroth-II resection. Carcinoma incidence was markedly higher in Billroth-II-resected rats than in non-resected or vagotomized controls that were equally exposed to the carcinogen. The lesions were chiefly localized in the anastomosis area.

These results, indicating a higher susceptibility of the anastomotic site to carcinogenesis, opened the way for new studies focused on histologic prestages or precancerous lesions. The advantage of this kind of assay is seen in the fixed site where experimental gastric carcinomas are bound to arise. Our present study takes up the open question of experimental carcinoma histogenesis in analogy to human gastric stump carcinoma. Since the interval between first operation and subsequent manifestation of carcinoma in the human resected stomach is an average 20 years in most publications, our follow-up in the experimental model had to cover as long a postoperative period as possible.

Partial resection of the stomach offers the double advantage of increased prevalence of chemically induced carcinoma (*Dahm* and *Werner,* 1973) and of precancerous histologic reactions at a strictly circumscribed site (*Schlag* et al., 1977a; *Rumpf* et al., 1978). Consequently, our histogenetic study might help to differentiate the effect of the carcinogen (MNNG) from that of the partial resection. The latter is seen as a cocarcinogenic factor that directs the influence of MNNG to the anastomotic area. Another question of relevance to the pathogenesis of human gastric carcinoma is whether the sequelae of resection themselves would exert a carcinogenic influence, i.e., whether carcinomas arise in the anastomosis under experimental conditions without previous administration of MNNG. This problem has not been studied in an animal model until now.

Finally, our experimental model with a high tumor incidence offered an opportunity to study the effect of concomitant immunosuppression. Since the local immune response against malignant tumors is predominantly of a cellular type (*McCluskey* and *Bhan,* 1977; *Howell* et al., 1974), we chose anti-lymphocyte-globulin (ALG) as an immunosuppressive agent. The susceptibility of oncogenesis to anti-lymphocyte serum (ALS) or ALG has been the topic of many studies (*Baroni* et al., 1973; *Trainin* and *Linker-Israeli,* 1970; *Rabbat* and *Jeejeebhoy,* 1970; *Cerilli* and *Treat,* 1969). Nonetheless, the results regarding the effect of ALG are rather controversial, the mechanism of its action on chemical carcinogenesis is not fully explained. According to *Taub* and *Deutsch* (1977), ALG affects carcinogenesis via modulation of the immune defense system; according to *Shearer* et al. (1977) the type and nature of chemically induced tumors have an important influence on the effect of ALG. The effect of ALG on gastric carcinoma in particular, has not been investigated so far. Our results will be presented in a separate publication.

The histologic description of precancerous lesions and actual tumors is supplemented by data about histochemical enzyme reactions. Several enzymes, e.g., unspecific esterase and acid phosphatase, have been measured at higher levels in regenerating and proliferating tissue and in closing wounds (*Schmidt,* 1968; *Raekallo,* 1961, 1965a, b). The concentration of other enzymes, such as β-glucuronidase, was different in both normal and tumor tissue. Occasionally, such enzymes occurred suddenly in tumor tissue of an animal whose healthy tissue was normally free of them (*Kondstaal* et al., 1975; *McGinty* et al., 1973; *Brown,* 1978). In human gastric mucosa, duodenal brush border enzymes could be demonstrated in areas of intestinal metaplasia (*Wattenberg,* 1959; *Planteydt* and *Willighagen,* 1960). No similar findings were ascertained in the rat (*Kobori* et al., 1976; *Uchida* et al., 1976). Systematic enzyme histochemical studies on this subject have not been published.

The prerequisite for understanding precancerous changes is familiarity with the pattern of proliferation kinetics under various experimental conditions. Previous histo-autoradiographic studies of cell turnover in the stomach have shown that more than 90% of labeled cells are found in the depths of the gastric pits and in the upper part of the gland necks (*Willems* et al., 1970; *Teir* and *Räsänen,* 1961; *Stevens* and *Leblond,* 1953; *Hunt,* 1957). Human findings (*Eastwood,* 1977) were paralleld by similar results in rats (*Willems* et al., 1972).

Cell proliferation may be influenced by many factors (*McDonald* et al., 1964) such as radioactive irradiation (*Sherman* and *Quastler,* 1960), cytotoxic drugs (*Trier*, 1962), carcinogenic substances (*Oehlert,* 1973), or by other diseases of the gastrointestinal tract in general (*Padykula* et al., 1961). Investigations revealed not only changes in cell proliferation, but also the enlargement and displacement of the proliferative zone proper as happens, e.g., in chronic gastritis with subsequent mucosal atrophy (*Eder,* 1969). Extensive proliferation kinetic studies of cell repair and discontinuity in squamous epithelia of skin or tongue revealed an increase of DNA-synthesizing cells within traumatized areas. This proliferation starts near the edge and advances towards the wound as the assay proceeds (*Oehlert,* 1969). Proliferation kinetics in the resected rat stomach under carcinogen influence have not been studied until now.

In accordance with the above conditions and methodologic prerequisites, our study was focused on the following questions:

1. Are there any specific histologic precursors or prestages to experimental anastomosis carcinoma?
2. Are these prestages more readily identified in an earlier phase by histochemical methods than by conventional histology?
3. What is the pathogenetic significance of atrophic gastritis?
4. What is the role of mucosal proliferation in anastomotic areas?
5. Is gastric resection, i.e., Billroth I surgery, in itself a carcinogenic factor?

II. Materials and Methods

1. Animals

400 male SPF-Wistar rats (Wistar-Han, colony-bred) were obtained from Zentralinstitut für Versuchtierzucht/Hannover. Their body weight was between 160 and 200 g, the median weight being 175 g.

2. Maintenance

The animals were fed the standard maintenance diet Altromin of Altromin-GmbH/Lage; they were kept under conventional conditions in fully climatized rooms at a constant 21°C with a controlled day-and-night schedule of 12 h. Humidity was 50%. Tap water was given ad libitum.

3. Preparation for Surgery

After an adjustment period of 10 days the animals were prepared by stopping feeding 24 h before surgery; free access to drinking water was maintained.

4. Gastric Surgery

Anesthesia was carried out by intraperitoneal injection of 5-ethyl-5(1-methylbutyl) barbituric acid in its sodium salt (Nembutal/Abbott) at a dose of 0.25 mg/10 g body weight. Surgery was performed in analogy to the Billroth I-technique used in human surgery (partial resection of the pylorus with end-to-end inferior gastroduodenostomy). Fifty percent of the glandular stomach was resected, including the pylorus and a small cuff of the duodenum. Reduction of the gastric lumen was effected by means of 6–8 interrupted sutures connecting successively all the layers of the gastric wall (suture material: Mersilene 4/0, atraumatic, from Ethicon/Hamburg). A complete serosal anastomosis between the residual lumen of the glandular stomach and the proximal duodenum, was carried out with 10–12 interrupted sutures through all layers of the wall.

From a total of 400 animals, 20 were used for testing and training surgical techniques. These all died postoperatively during the first 12 days, mainly from insufficient sutures, postoperative atonicity, and pneumonia. Of the remaining 380 animals, 24 were left unoperated as controls. Twelve of these were killed at the beginning, the other 12 at the end of the assay. The remaining 356 animals were operated at four biweekly intervals.

The first set contained 18 animals, none of which survived the 14th day following surgery. The second set comprised 144 animals, of which 74 were alive 2 weeks after surgery (51%). The third set contained 110 animals, of which 66 survived more than 14 days (60%). In the fourth set of 102 resected animals, 91 survived the 14th day postoperatively (90%). The survival expectancy of resected animals was shown to equal that of nonresected controls if they were able to survive the first 2 weeks after surgery.

Of 356 animals operated during the main assay, 231 were entered into a specific trial. A small number of animals died during the further course of the assay, but this was several months after resection and mostly from pneumonia.

5. Postoperative Phase

Starting the 3rd day after resection, the animals were fed slowly increasing amounts of their standard diet plus drinking water ad lib. After the 6th day, the animals were fed the same diet as in the preoperative phase. For 2 weeks after surgery the rats were kept singly, then in groups of three per cage. Their general health status was monitored daily, body weight was controlled each 4th week until the 50th week of the assay.

6. Test Groups

All animals surviving resection were maintained without further treatment for 5 weeks, and then divided into four test groups (Table 1). The number of animals for each group was determined after the general schedule of the assay, with an added 10%–15% of "risk animals" in order to ensure that a sufficient number would be available for evaluation at the end of the long-term assay.

Group I	=	Billroth I resection only (OP group); 42 rats, 36 animals were evaluated
Group II	=	Billroth I resection + exposure to carcinogen 5 weeks after surgery (OP + early MNNG group), 72 rats, 70 animals were evaluated
Group III	=	Billroth I resection + carcinogen exposure one year after surgery (OP + late MNNG group); 20 rats, 15 animals were evaluated
Group IV	=	Billroth I resection + ALG administration + carcinogen exposure (OP + ALG + MNNG); 97 rats, 90 animals were evaluated. The results will be published separately (*Schlake* et al., in press).

7. Carcinogen Exposure

With the beginning of the 6th week after surgery (1st week of the assay) we started to expose the animals of group II (and IV) to the carcinogen N-methyl-N'-nitro-N-nitrosoguanidine (MNNG). A matrix solution of the carcinogen in tap water was prepared at 2 g/l and preserved lightproof of 4°C. The matrix solution was diluted with tap water to a concentration of 50 mg/l MNNG in the animals' drinking water during the first 4 weeks, and 100 mg/l during the following weeks of the assay. The solution was freshly prepared twice a week, the carcinogen-containing water was given ad libitum. Group I was given only pure tap water, and so were, at this stage, the animals of group III. These rats were exposed to the carcinogenic substance as late as 52 weeks after surgery; concentrations and schedule were the same as in the early exposed group II.

8. Killing

The schedule for sacrificing the animals was fixed from the start to the 50th week of the assay (Table 1). For comparison of the groups among themselves, 10 or 15 animals were picked at random from each and sacrificed by an overdose of Nembutal. For follow-up control, two animals from each group were killed at consecutively shorter intervals.

In group III (OP + late MNNG), 15 animals were sacrificed after the 104th week of the assay. In that week we were also able to additionally sacrifice three rats from group I and six of group II (plus 13 of group IV). All animals dying during the assay were also autopsied in order to ascertain the cause of death.

9. Preparation for Light Microscopy

After the usual fixation in 4% buffered formaldehyde for a minimum of 3 days, the resected stomach was cut according to a previously fixed schema and embedded in paraffin. Typical portions of all stomach segments were taken fresh and subjected to

Table 1. Schedule of the assay: no. of animals, duration of treatment, no. and time of killing, spontaneous deaths. Significant groups and dates are marked with dotted areas

Group \ Week	0	1	5	9	13	17	21	25	29	33	37	41	45	50	52	56	77		104	sacrif.	died	total
I OP		2	2		2	2		15						10					3	36	6	42
II OP+MNNG early			2	2	2	2	2	15	2	15	2	10		10					6	70	2	72
III OP+MNNG late																			15	15	5	20

50 mg/l N-methyl-N'-nitro-N-nitrosoguanidine (MNNG); 100 mg/l MNNG

special preparation for enzyme histochemical investigation. Paraffin sections were stained either with hematoxyline eosin, or PAS, or Alcian blue at pH 2.5 and pH 1.0, and with a combination of PAS and Alcian blue..

10. Histoautoradiography

For histoautoradiographic investigation, one half of the animals were given 1 Ci/kg body weight [^{3}H] thymidine i.p. ([6-^{3}H] thymidine, the Radiochemical Centre, Amersham/UK, spec. activity 5000 mCi/mmol). The radioactive assay lasted 60 min. In parallel to the sections for histologic investigation, paraffin sections of 3–4 μ were prepared for autoradiography. The autoradiograms were made with dipping technique (*Schultze,* 1968), with Ilford K2 jelly, and with exposure over 4 weeks at 4°C. Nuclei were stained with hemalum for 10 min.

11. Enzyme Histochemistry

Demonstration of enzyme histochemical reactions was prepared by deep freezing representative portions of all tissues in Isopentan (Riedel de Haen) precooled to –140°C with liquid nitrogen. Deep frozen tissues were then stored at –80°C until definitive work-up which was always carried out within 4 weeks of deep freezing. Staining of enzyme reactions was done in 8 μ thick sections made with a cryostate (Slee) at –20°C.

The following enzymes were demonstrated in their reaction products:

a) Alkaline phosphatase (E.C. 3.1.3.1)
Method after *Burstone* and *Keyes* (1957), *Burstone* (1962) modified after *Lojda* et al. (1967)

b) Leucinaminopeptidase (E.C. 3.4.11.2)
Method after *Nachlas* et al. (1960)

c) Acid phosphatase (E.C. 3.1.3.2)
Method after *Burstone* (1958), *Lojda* et al. (1976)

d) Unspecific esterase (E.C. 3.1.1.1.)
   Method after *Davis* and *Ornstein* (1959), *Lojda* et al. (1974)
e) β-Glucuronidase (E.C. 3.2.1.31)
   Method after *Hayashi* et al. (1964), *Lojda* et al. (1974)
f) Succinate dehydrogenase (E.C. 1.3.99.1)
   Method after *Thomas* and *Pearse* (1961), modified after *Pearse* (1972), using Menadion for additional activator (*Jakobsen* and *Jørgenson,* 1973).

In each procedure control sections inactivated by heat (*Lojda* et al., 1976) were prepared for excluding unspecific staining; some sections without substrate were also incubated.

With regard to the semipermeable membrane technique, and in order to avoid unspecific background staining during incubation, we added $10^{-3}M$ sodium fluoride (Merck) to the medium for analysis of acid phosphatase (*Meijer,* 1972), and $2 \times 10^{-2}M$ sodium fluoride to the medium for unspecific esterase (*Meijer* and *Vloedman,* 1973). We checked unspecific background staining of membranes and sections for glucuronidase by adding $10^{-2}M$ saccharolactone (Calbiochem) which is a specific inhibitor (*Meijer* and *Vloedman,* 1973).

III. Results

1. Carcinogenesis in the Rat Stomach After B I Resection, Macroscopic and Microscopic Findings

a) Anastomosis Bulge

This was a typical finding in all groups of the assay. The bulge occurred in or near the gastrointestinal anastomosis, protruding like a mucosal prolapse into the duodenal lumen in particularly well-marked cases. The mucosal bulge was found either spreading over the front or back side of the anastomosis (Fig. 1), or encircling the junction.

The original mucosal folds of the gastric remnant usually meet the mucosal bulge of the gastroenteroanastomosis at almost a right angle. Residual sutures were occasionally found in these bulges during the course of the assay. The upper crest of the bulge was sometimes of a more intense red color, but there were no erosive or ulcerative lesions in this area. Histologically, the anastomotic bulge was composed of gastric mucosa (corpus type) in the great majority of cases. A minority of anastomotic bulges was composed of gastric and duodenal mucosa; in some isolated cases we found a small bulge of only duodenal mucosa.

The correct array of strata in the wall was always disturbed in anastomotic areas (i.e., in gastroenteroanastomosis and reducing suture at the lesser curvature). Below the mucosa, the wall was completely pervaded by granulating and sclerosing tissue. The mucosa of the anastomosis was tightly fixed to the underlying stratum by scarred tissue; there was no movable submucosal layer near or below the perianastomotic mucosa. Parts of gastric or duodenal mucosa that had been displaced into deeper layers,

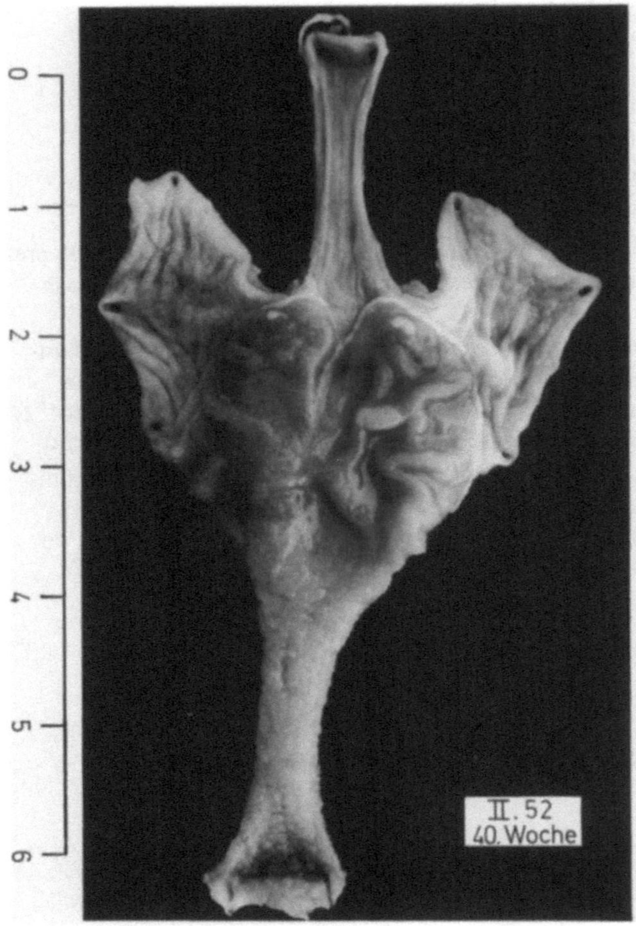

Fig. 1. Development of mucosal bulge at the posterior wall of the gastroenteroanastomosis

or suture remnants causing foreign body reactions, were frequent findings in this area. Mucosal atrophy in gastroentero- or gastro-gastric anastomoses increases proportionally with time after surgery. It is caused by the reduction of parietal and chief cells and found only in the anastomosed mucosal tissue.

The reduction of specific gastric glands coincides with hyperplasia of the foveolar epithelium in both types of anastomosis. In a gastroenteroanastomosis we see proliferation of mucus-forming surface epithelia, accompanied by an increase in the number of mucus-forming gland neck cells. The two cellular components are separated from the gland neck region by a zone of undifferentiated cells of varying width. At that time the gland neck region has lost its original character and the three typical layers of the mucosa have also almost completely lost their normal array in this area.

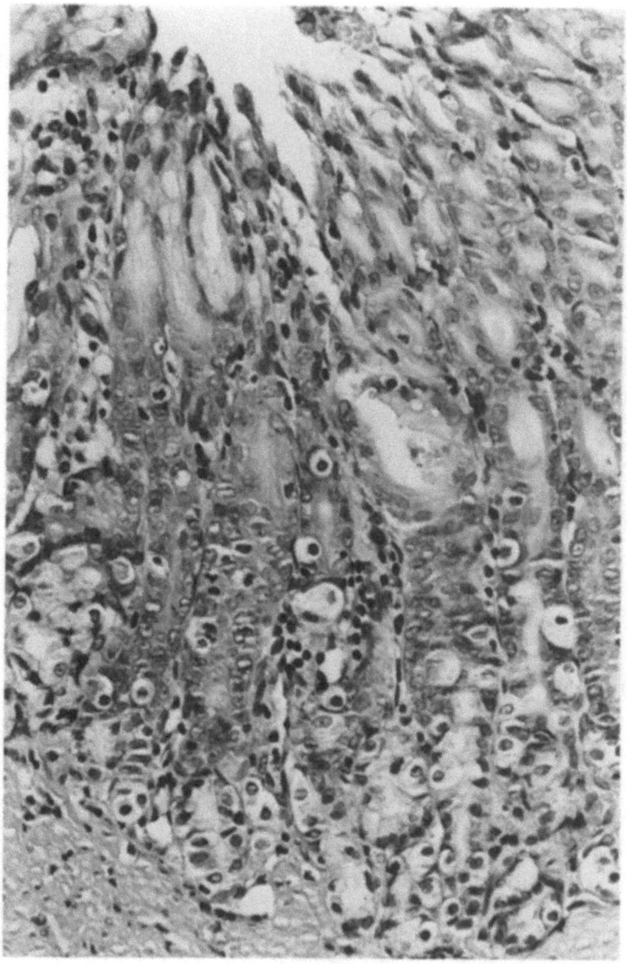

Fig. 2. Dysplastic gland tubules (grade II) in corpus mucosa close to the anastomosis. Scanty lymphocytic infiltration. HE × 288

As were epithelial changes, chronic inflammation was strictly localized in the anastomotic bulge or within anastomosed mucosal tissue. Chronic inflammatory infiltration was also found in the vicinity of residual sutures.

From the 6th week after surgery, we observed atypical epithelial cells among the proliferation of undifferentiated gland neck cells and among basal gastric pits. We called these findings "dysplasia," i.e., atypical mucosa limited to the epithelial zone, distinguishing the three grades of light, moderate, and severe dysplasia (*Grundmann*, 1975) (Figs. 2, 3, 6, 7) in analogy to the criteria for classification of human gastric mucosa (*Grundmann*, 1975; *Oehlert* et al., 1975).

Dysplasia grade I (light, Fig. 6) showed beginning dedifferentiation of surface epithelia and reduced mucus production, together with an increase in the number of active-

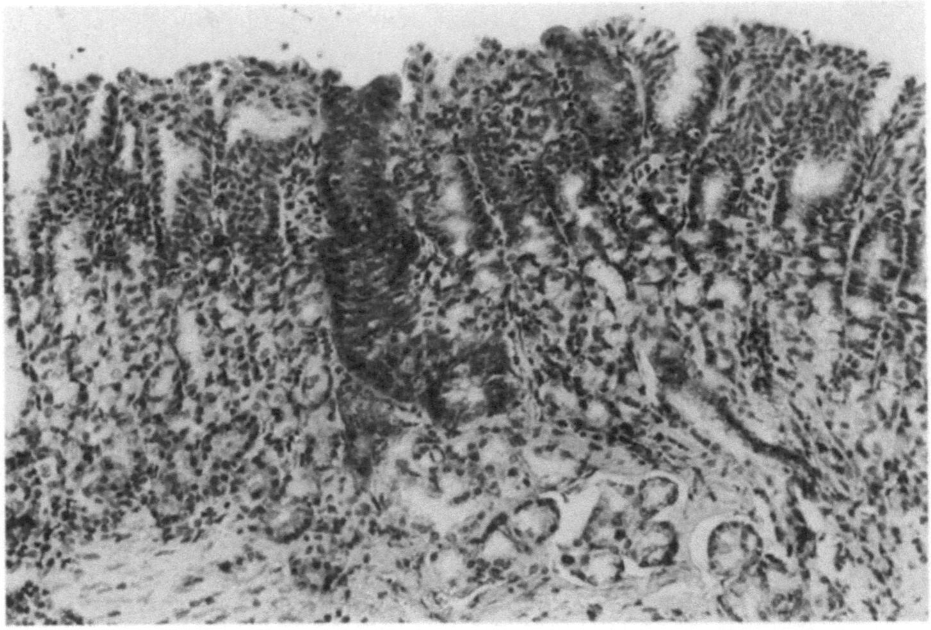

Fig. 3. Dysplastic gland tubule (grade II) in anastomotic corpus mucosa. Autoradiogram, HE X 288

ly proliferating cells. Dysplasia II (moderate, Fig. 2) was characterized by continuous reduction of epithelial differentiation at the surface, while gastric pits were transformed to glandular structures, often lined with basophil epithelia showing dark nuclei. Cells in active mitosis occurred in all areas thus changed, mucus production had ceased completely. A shift in the nucleo-cytoplasmic ratio in favor of nuclei, was accompanied by nuclear polymorphism. Basophilic epithelia were often found in a multilayered arrangement.

In dysplasia III (severe, Fig. 3) secretory epithelia were completely substituted by proliferating epithelial cells. The epithelial lining is multilayered throughout, the glands are arranged more closely. A striking feature is the strong nuclear polymorphism with frequent large nucleoli. Some atypical mitoses are seen among frequent normal mitotic patterns.

From the 25th postoperative week these dysplasias were found regularly and in all groups. At first, epithelial lesions were invariably localized in anastomosed mucosal tissue; at late as week 104 of the assay we sometimes found small dysplastic foci in areas of corpus mucosa distant from the anastomosis.

b) Polypoid Lesions of Mucosa

These lesions were found exclusively in gastroenteroanastomoses as a focal thickening of the mucosa that was not identified, macroscopically, as a polyp. In following up an

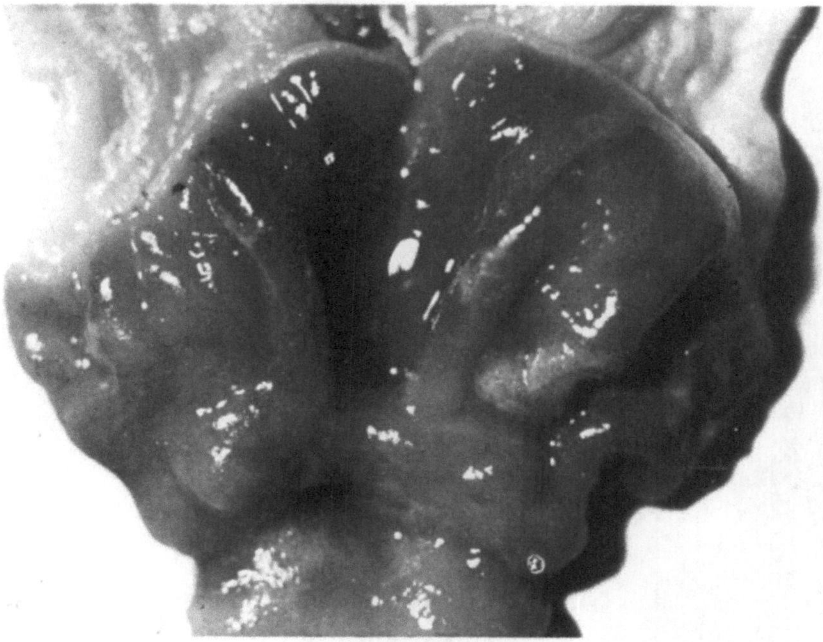

Fig. 4. Beadlike arrangement of polypoid foci near the gastroenteroanastomosis

anastomosis we often found several of these lesions, some containing a residual suture. In other cases, three or four polypoid foci were laying close together like beads on a string (Fig. 4). Histology identified these polypoid lesions mostly as focal bulgings of the mucosa; in some cases, the polypoid focus was already covering a true anastomotic polyp.

c) Anastomotic Polyps

These developed exclusively in anastomosed mucosal tissue, as well in gastroentero-anastomoses as at the angle between these and the reducing suture in the lesser curvature (Fig. 5). The largest polyp had a diameter of 5 mm. Histologically, their structure was that of adenomatous polyps (Fig. 6) containing gastric mucosa alone, gastric plus duodenal mucosa, or duodenal mucosa alone. Unspecific gland tubules of indistinct origin were found in the polyps; mitotic activity was over varying intensity, even in one and the same polyp. Their stroma showed varying density of inflammatory infiltration, mainly by plasma cells, lymphocytes, and macrophages. Some polyps contained glandular dysplasias (Fig. 7). Among the 114 animals evaluated in our assay, ten had developed polyps in the anastomotic area; seven of these polyps showed dysplastic glandular components.

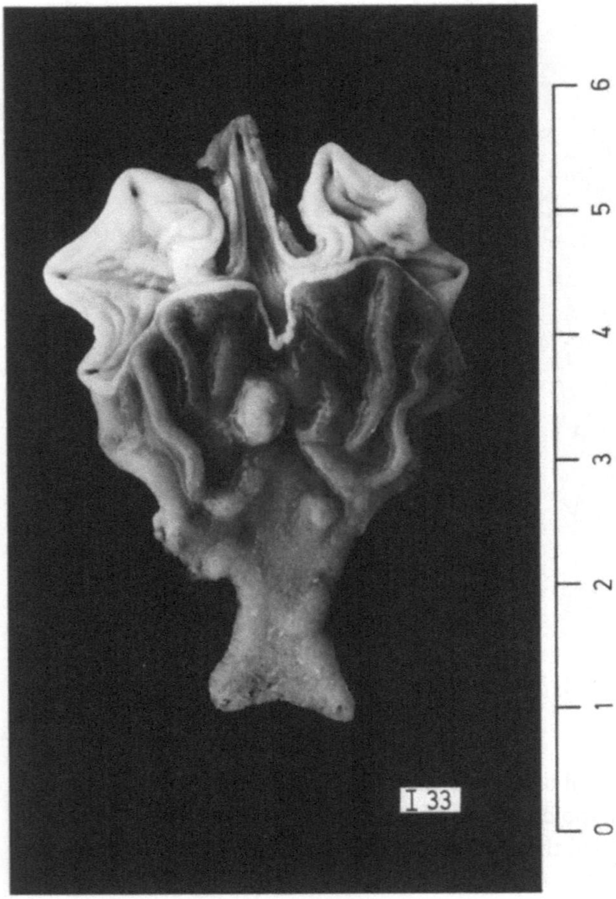

Fig. 5. Large anastomotic polyps at the angle between reducing suture of lesser curvature, and gastroenteroanastomosis

d) Adenocystic Proliferation of Glands

From the 13th week of the assay on, we observed an increasing number of adenocystic glandular proliferations arising either in the anastomosis mucosa, or from the mucosal complexes that had been transferred to deeper layers of the gastric wall by operation. Glandular proliferation was oriented either toward the gastric lumen where it reinforced the bulge or formed the basis of an anstomotic polyp, or toward the serosa. Inflammatory reactions were more numerous around glandular proliferations; the infiltrations consisted of lymphocytes, plasma cells, frequent eosinophilic granulocytes, mastocytes, and macrophages.

Adenomatous glandular proliferation initially showed an intramural spread (Fig. 8). Of 114 animals evaluated 68 had developed intramural adenocystic proliferation; in five of the 68, these had formed a nodular tumorous mass. Residual sutures were frequently

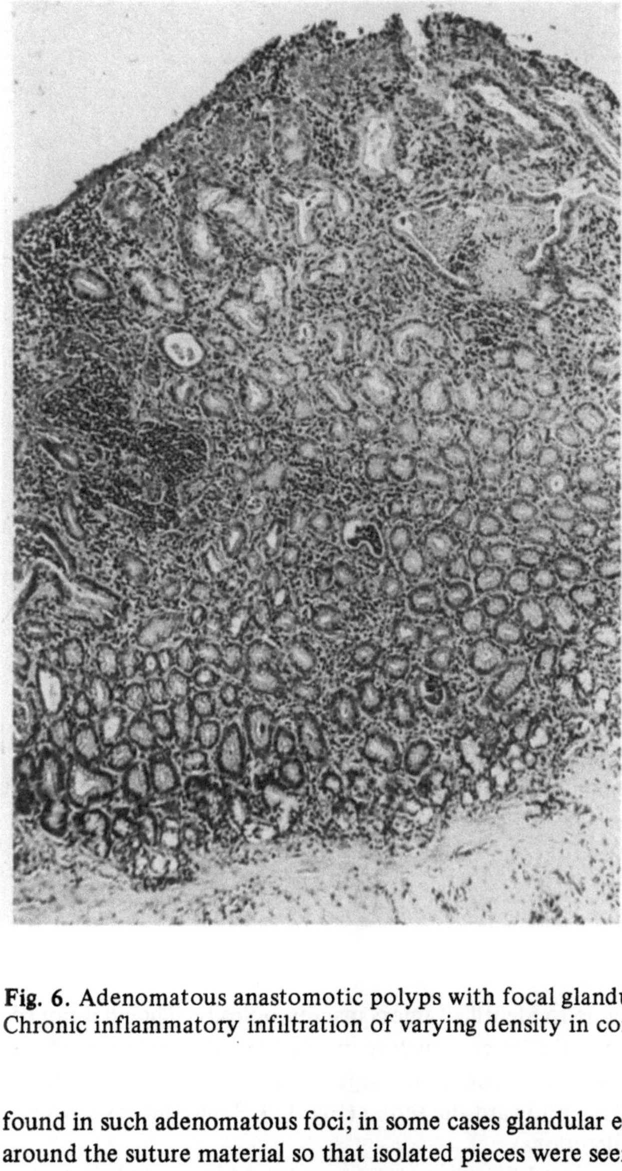

Fig. 6. Adenomatous anastomotic polyps with focal glandular dysplasia at the surface. Chronic inflammatory infiltration of varying density in connective stroma. HE X 90

found in such adenomatous foci; in some cases glandular epithelia had accumulated around the suture material so that isolated pieces were seen in the lumen of dilated gland tubules (Fig. 9). Focal foreign body reaction, chronic inflammatory infiltration, and high mitotic activity of glandular epithelia were typical and frequent findings. Adenomatous glandular proliferation was composed of different epithelial cells: there were undifferentiated, cuboid or cyclindric cells, mucin-producing cells of goblet or foveolar type, and unspecific mucoid gland cells in varying numbers. Severely dilated gland tubules, whose epithelial lining showed some mucus production, had burst and spilt their mucus over the surrounding connective tissue. Glandular dysplasia was found in some parts, especially in advanced cases of adenomatous proliferation. Cystic, often bizarre gland formation were tightly filled with cellular detritus and granulocytes. The

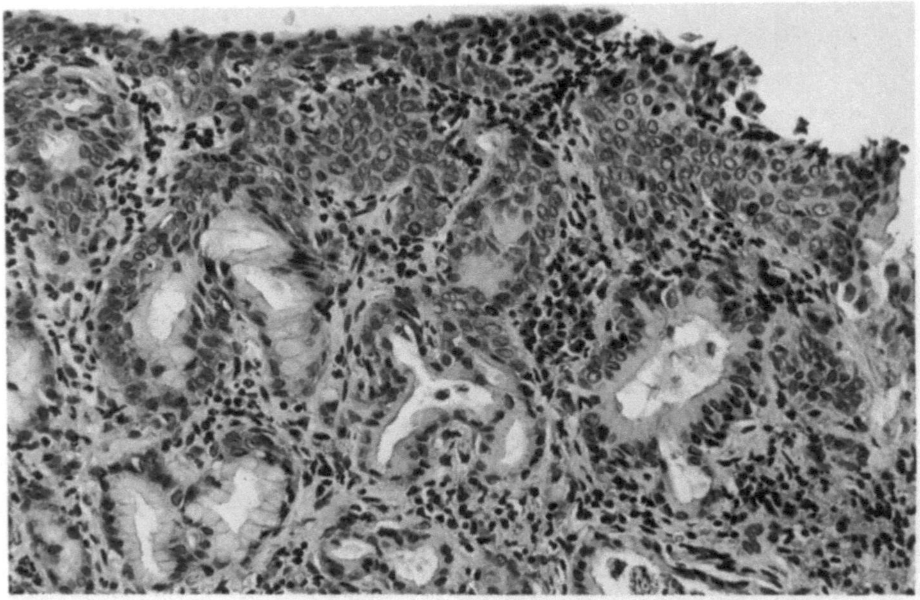

Fig. 7. Glandular dysplasia at the surface of a polyp (enlarged from Figure 6). HE × 225

surrounding stroma was infiltrated to varying degrees by plasma cells, lymphocytes, neutrophilic and eosinophilic granulocytes, mastocytes, and macrophages. These cells produced different kinds of mucus; acid and neutral mucins were found separately, or in proportions together in one and the same cell.

e) Tumors[1]

In 19 of 114 animals we were able to identify tumors macroscopically. They developed partly from the reducing suture at the lesser curvature, partly from the gastroentero-anastomosis. Their growth was either polypous and largely lumen-oriented (Fig. 10), or nodular with primary orientation toward the serosa (Fig. 11). Some tumors showed simultaneous growth in both directions.

Among the nodular serosa-oriented tumors, some were covered by serosal tissue and some had broken through the serosa and started to invade the liver, pancreas, or adjacent fatty tissue. The cut surface of these tumors showed larger or smaller cystic deformation. Some cysts were filled with viscous, transparent mucous substances. Certain tumors of serosa-oriented growth type could not be safely identified macro-

[1] The term "tumor" is used exclusively for the macroscopic appearance. Histologically, the lesions may be either carcinomas or nodular (tumorous) adenocystic glandular proliferations.

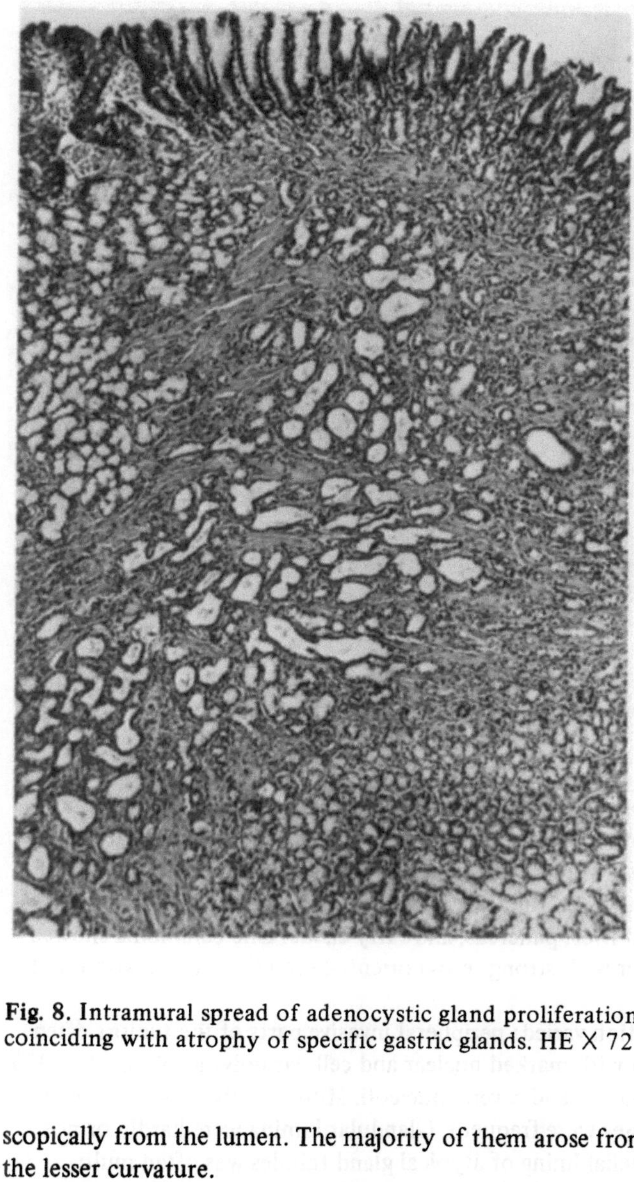

Fig. 8. Intramural spread of adenocystic gland proliferation in gastroenteroanastomosis coinciding with atrophy of specific gastric glands. HE X 72

scopically from the lumen. The majority of them arose from the reducing suture at the lesser curvature.

The polypous lumen-oriented type, arising predominantly from the gastroentero-anastomosis, tended to encircle the anastomotic site and strangle the lumen; in advanced stages, invasion was extended to adjacent organs.

Histologic analysis of these 19 tumors revealed 14 carcinomas and 10 nodular adenocystic glandular proliferations. Two carcinomas were not recognized macroscopically, so a total of 16 carcinomas was found in anastomotic areas of 114 animals. Four of these had developed in a polyp and were beginning to invade the fibrous tissue of the pedicle. Nine carcinomas showed primary serosa-oriented growth, seven of them were more or less well-differentiated adenocarcinomas, one was a medullary

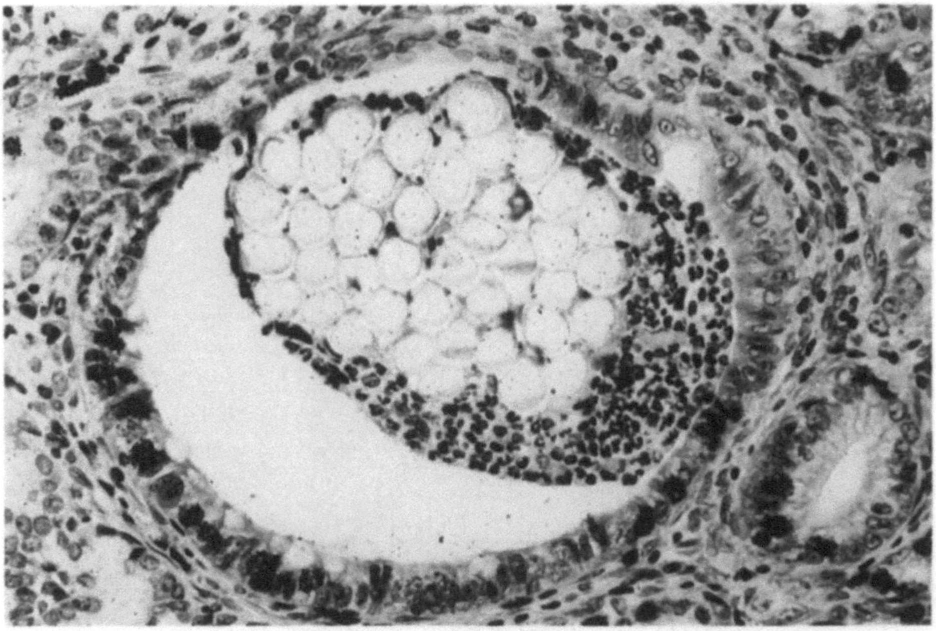

Fig. 9. Residual suture in the lumen of a dilated gland tubule. Many nuclei of glandular epithelium are labeled. Autoradiogram, HE ×360

(Fig. 12) and one was a signet ring cell carcinoma (Fig. 13). Two carcinomas had invaded the liver (Fig. 14); another had invaded liver, pancreas (Fig. 15), and fatty tissue (Fig. 16). Four carcinomas were identified as polypous adenocarcinomas, two of which displayed increased mucus production. One adenocarcinoma had invaded the liver and another had invaded liver, pancreas, and fatty tissue. One carcinoma showed substantial polypous, together with strong serosa-oriented growth, and had also invaded the liver.

The degree of differentiation varied: peripheral invasive parts of the tumors often showed lower differentiation with marked nuclear and cellular polymorphism (Fig. 17). Nuclei showed vesicular dilatation and several nucleoli. Mitotic activity was considerably increased, atypical mitoses were frequent. Glandular lumina were hardly or not at all recognizable. The epithelial lining of atypical gland tubules was often multilayered and interspersed with monocellular, mucus-producing cells.

Strongly mucus-producing areas also showed considerable formation of cysts. Excessive mucus production in these parts resulted in the bursting of many cysts lined with atypical epithelia. Mucus masses prevaded broken epithelia and entered the connective stroma (Fig. 18). Some extremely large cysts had merely rudimentary lining with atypical epithelial cells.

The well-developed stromal tissue was partly sclerosed and poorly cellular (Fig. 19) but in some parts pervaded by many inflammatory cells, mostly plasma cells (Fig. 20). PAS and Alcian blue staining, separately or combined, revealed different mucines in

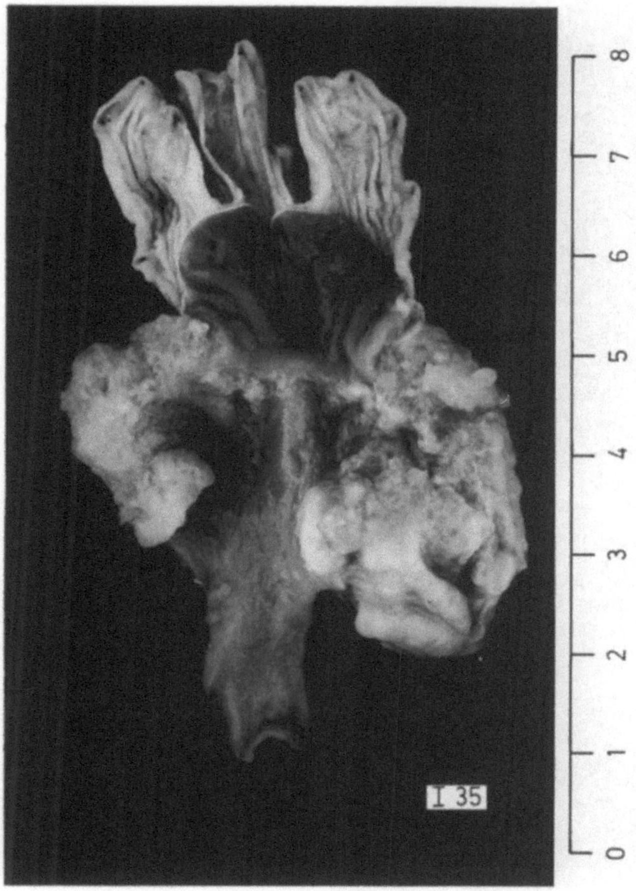

Fig. 10. Polypous carcinoma growing towards the gastric lumen, arising in the gastroenteroanastomosis

those tumor areas with excessive production: Production of acid mucins was predominant in some parts, in others, we found neutral mucins or a mixture of both. Isolated signet ring cells were sometimes identified in the tumor stroma, but there was only one carcinoma that showed a predominant signet ring cell growth type (Fig. 13).

2. Histochemical Results

Enzymatic patterns and activities of chief and parietal cells correspond to those of normal corpus mucosa. Demonstration of succinate dehydrogenase reveals the severe reduction of parietal cells in anastomosed mucosal tissue, with proportional increase of surface epithelia. In surface epithelia near the anastomosis, we found considerably increased activity of acid phosphatase, unspecific esterase, and dehydrogenases, as

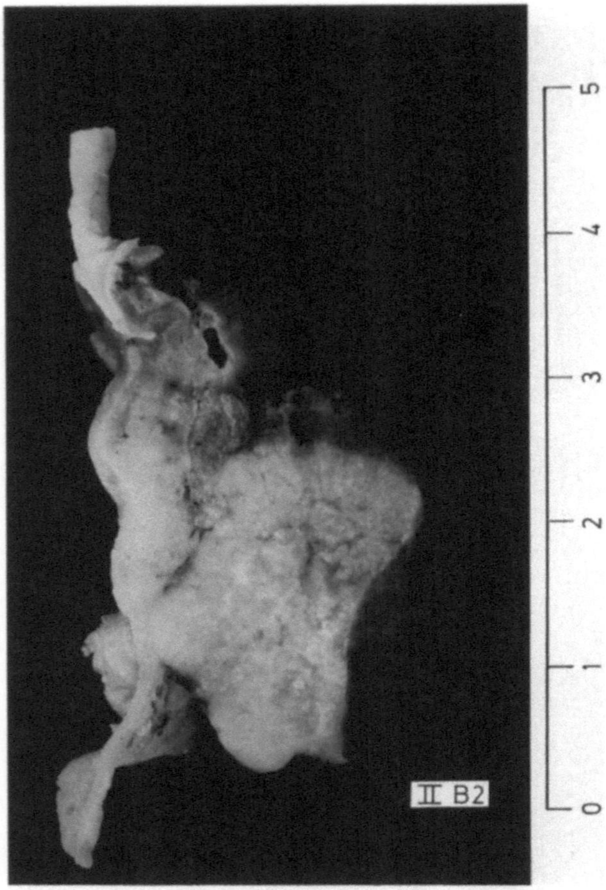

Fig. 11. Carcinoma growing chiefly in serosal orientation, from its origin in the gastro-enteroanastomosis

compared to surface epithelia distant from the anastomosis. When we compared distant corpus mucosa to the corresponding tissue in non-resected animals we were unable to identify any marked difference with regard to enzyme patterns and activity. Neither alkaline phosphatase, nor leucinaminopeptidase was ever demonstrated in these epithelia throughout the assay.

Duodenal mucosa close to the anastomosis showed reduction or complete loss of leucine aminopeptidase activity in lumen-adjacent surface epithelium of the villous apex. The activities of acid phosphatase and succinate dehydrogenase were reduced by one grade. For unspecific esterase, alkaline phosphatase, and β-glucuronidase the enzyme pattern and activity remained unchanged. In the regions of *adenocystic glandular proliferation,* all three enzymes showed parallel localization, with predominant activity of unspecific esterase in all glandular proliferations. Acid phosphatase activity was strongly granular throughout these areas, while the lesser granular activity of β-glucuronidase was visible

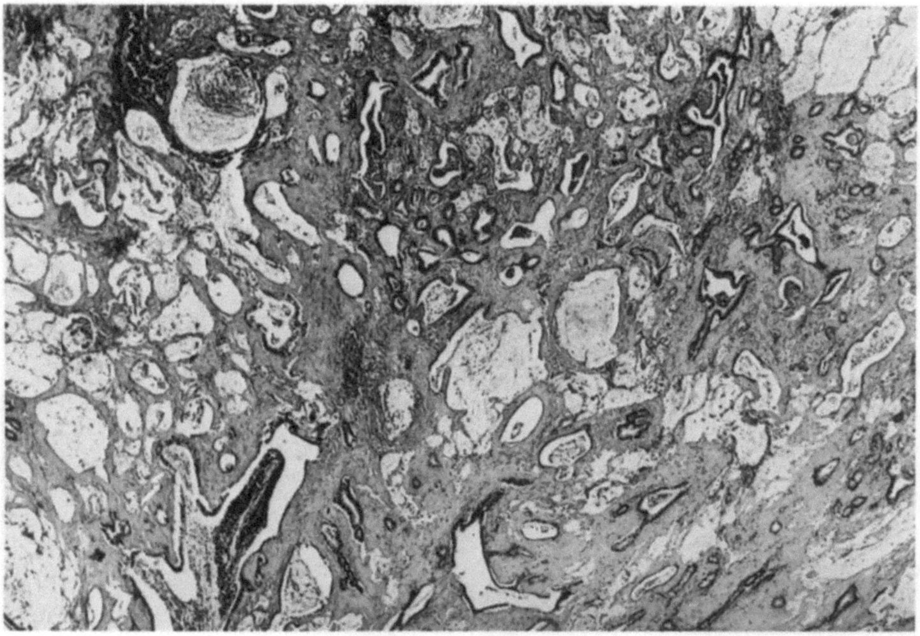

Fig. 12. Large portion of a mucus-producing adenocarcinoma (medullary carcinoma). HE X 30

only focally. In *nodular adenocystic gland proliferation,* acid phosphatase and β-glucuronidase activities were irregular, but unspecific esterase also showed uniform and strong activity in these areas. Succinate dehydrogenase showed only feeble signs of activity; alkaline phosphatase and leucinaminopeptidase were always negative.

Carcinomatous tissues showed varied activity of acid phosphatase, all possible grades demonstrable. Reaction products were always granular, sometimes scattered all over the cytoplasm. Very dense agglomerations of macrophages with highest acid phosphatase activity were seen in the tumor stroma. Unspecific esterase activity was equally and strongly positive everywhere in carcinomatous tissues. In necrotic tumor areas, results of unspecific esterase reactions could be identified over a long time; macrophages of tumor stroma showed a particularly active response.

The behavior of β-glucuronidase was nearly the same as that of the other enzymes, but its reaction products provoked, on the whole, a less colorful granular reaction in the epithelium. Macrophages, however, were always characterized by their high enzyme contents. Succinate dehydrogenase activity was rather low in tumor epithelia; alkaline phosphatase or leucinaminopeptidase were negative in carcinomatous tissues.

3. Histoautoradiographic Results

In corpus mucosa distant from the anastomosis, ^{3}H-indices failed to signal significant differences between the assay groups at different stages of the assay (weeks 25, 33, 41,

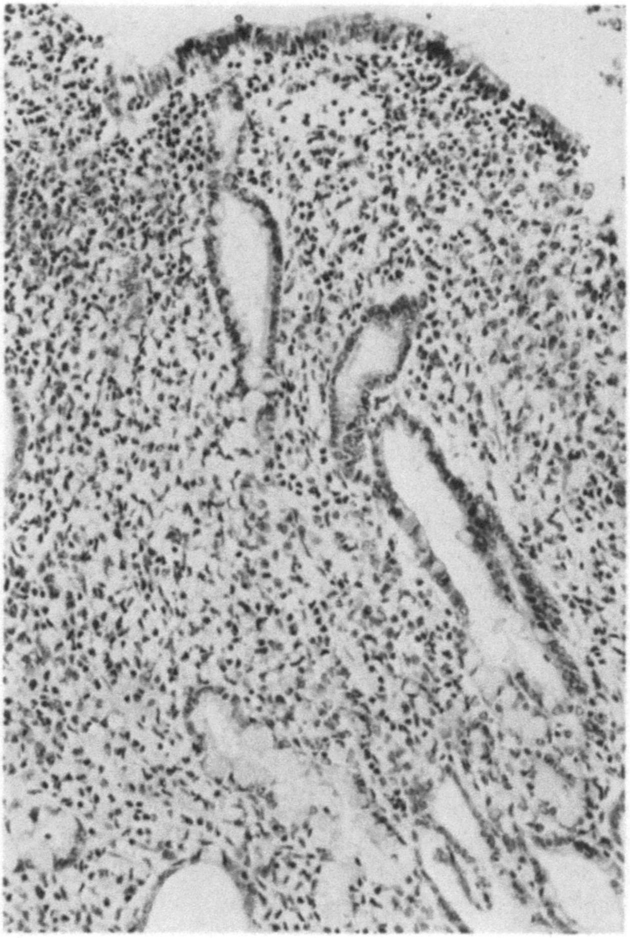

Fig. 13. Diffuse invasive spread of a signet ring cell carcinoma. HE × 184

50, and 104). The mean ^{3}H-index was a steady 2.84%. The majority of labeled cells were found in the gland neck region and in basal gastric pits (Fig. 21).

Comparison of labeling indices in the gastric mucosa of anastomoses also failed to distinguish the groups at parallel stages of the assay. We therefore decided to total the results of all groups in order to calculate a mean labeling index for each consecutive phase. Our follow-up revealed a steady rise in labeling from 5.8% in week 5 of the assay, to 10.7% in week 21. This level was approximately maintained through week 25 (11.6%), 33 (10.7%), and further until week 41 (12.4%). It then decreased to 9.8% in the 50th week. One year later, in the 104th week of the assay, the mean labeling index was 6.9% for gastric mucosa in the anastomotic site (Fig. 22). The labeling indices were taken from the entire width of these mucosal tissues since the distinction of separate layers was no longer possible (Fig. 23). Duodenal mucosa in anastomotic sites revealed

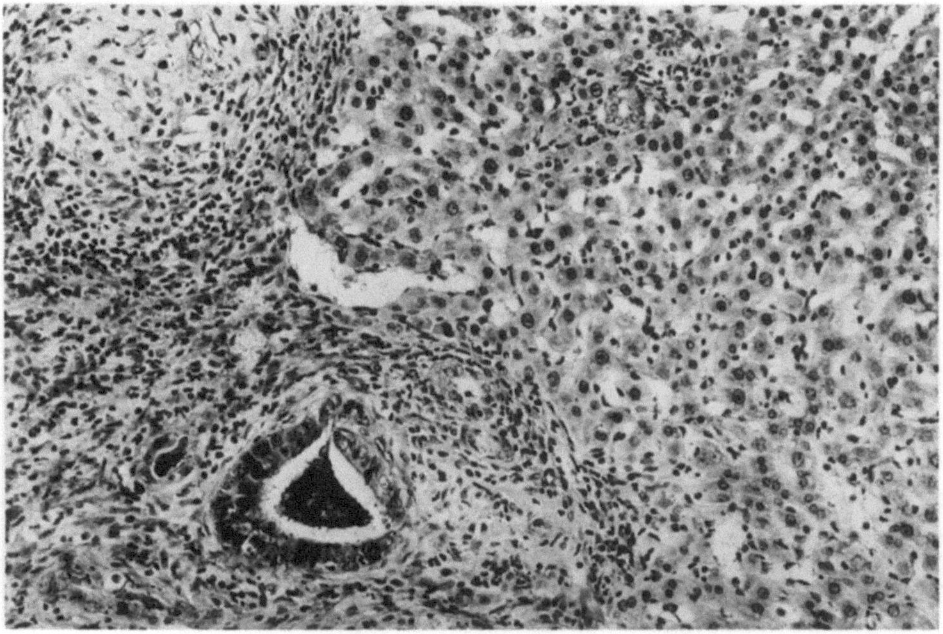

Fig. 14. Invasive growth of an anastomotic carcinoma to the liver. HE × 184

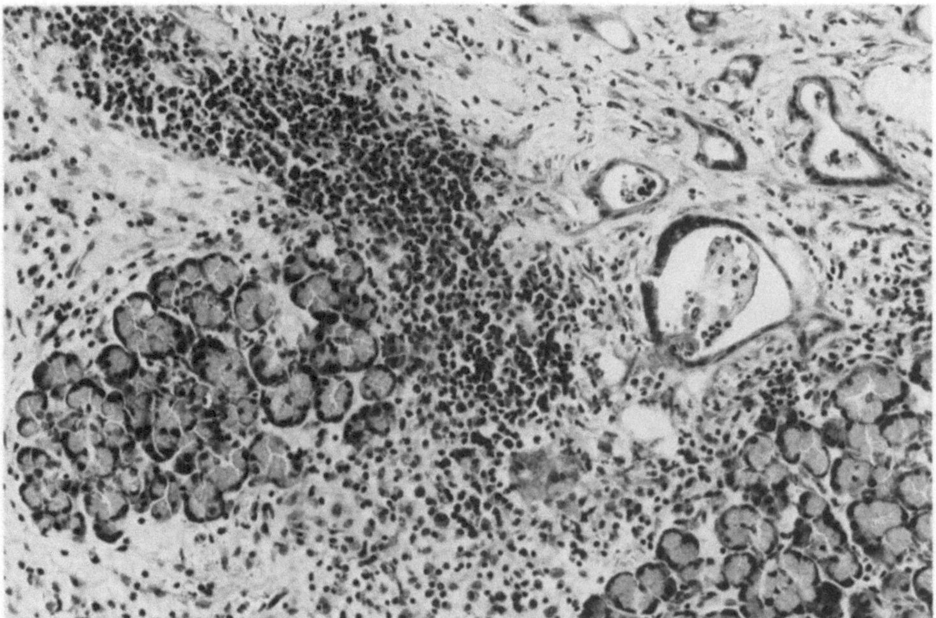

Fig. 15. Anastomotic carcinoma infiltrating the pancreas. Lymphocytic and plasma-cellular infiltration of connective stroma. HE × 184

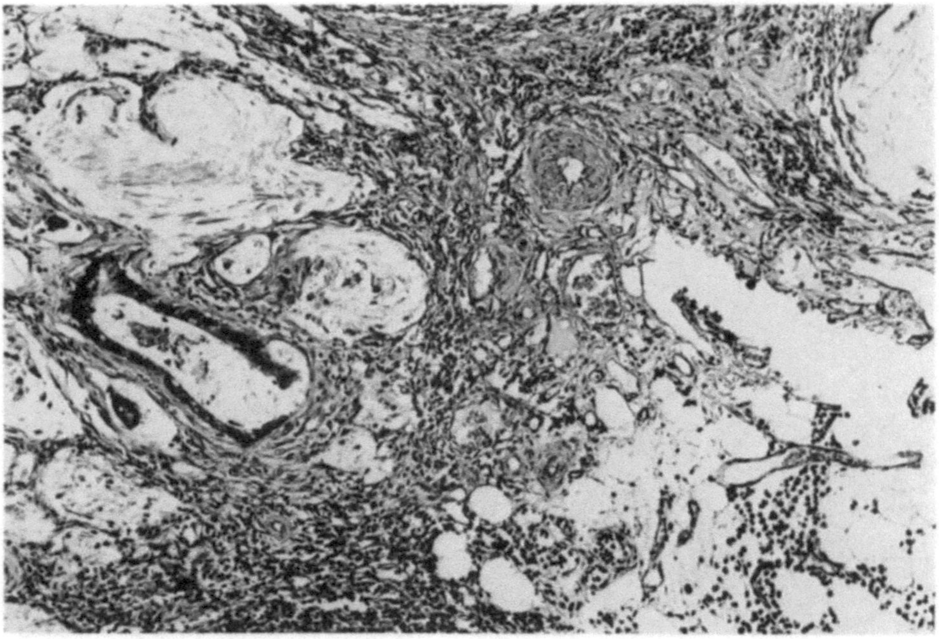

Fig. 16. Mucus-forming adenocarcinoma infiltrating the fatty tissue of the greater omentum. HE X 115

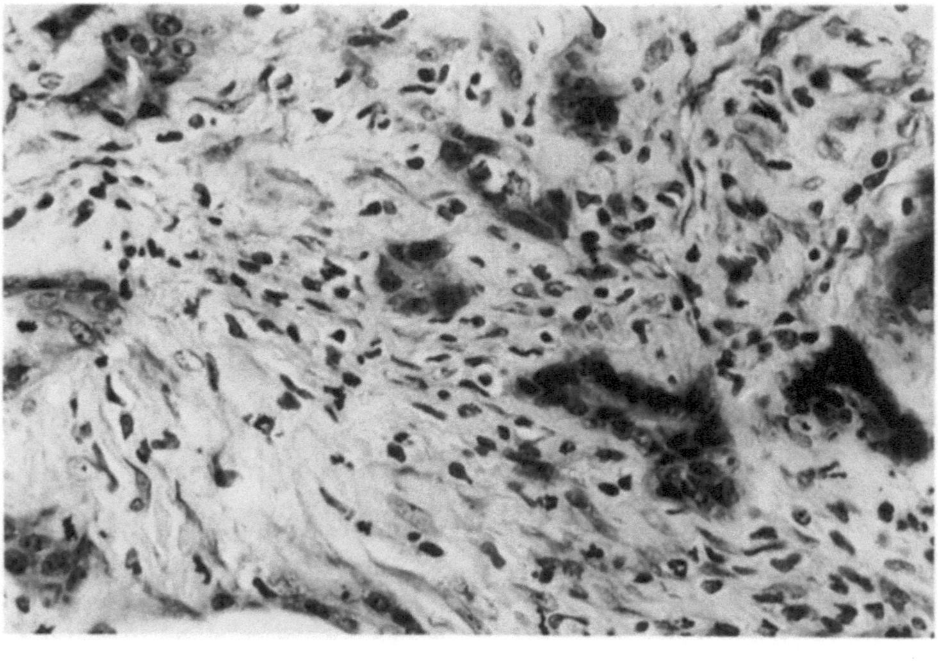

Fig. 17. Poorly differentiated adenocarcinoma of invasive growth type. Scanty stromal infiltration by lymphocytes and plasma cells. HE X 460

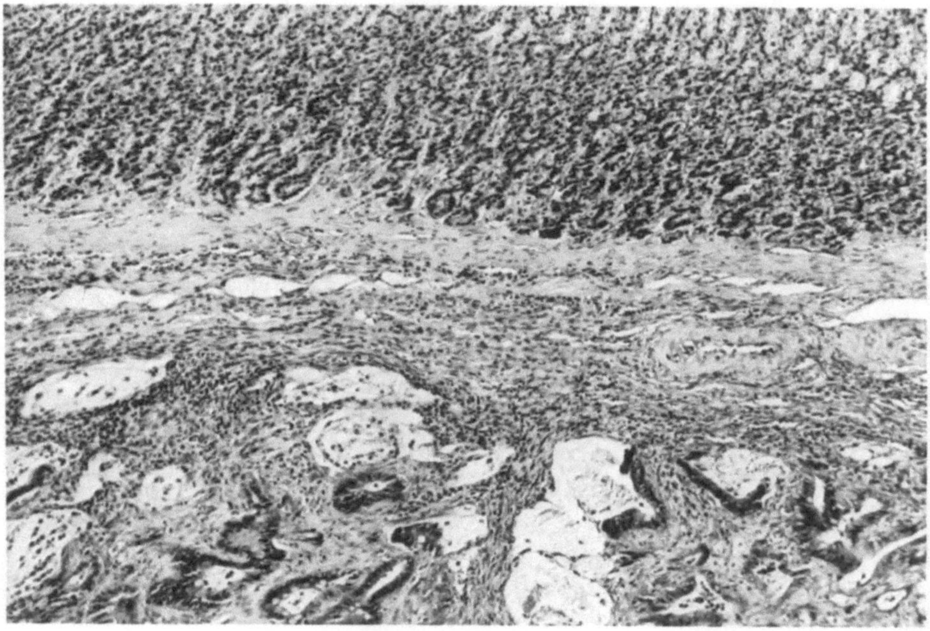

Fig. 18. Broken mucous cysts of a mucus-producing adenocarcinoma. Tumorous spread in submucosal scarred tissue near the anastomosis. HE X 90

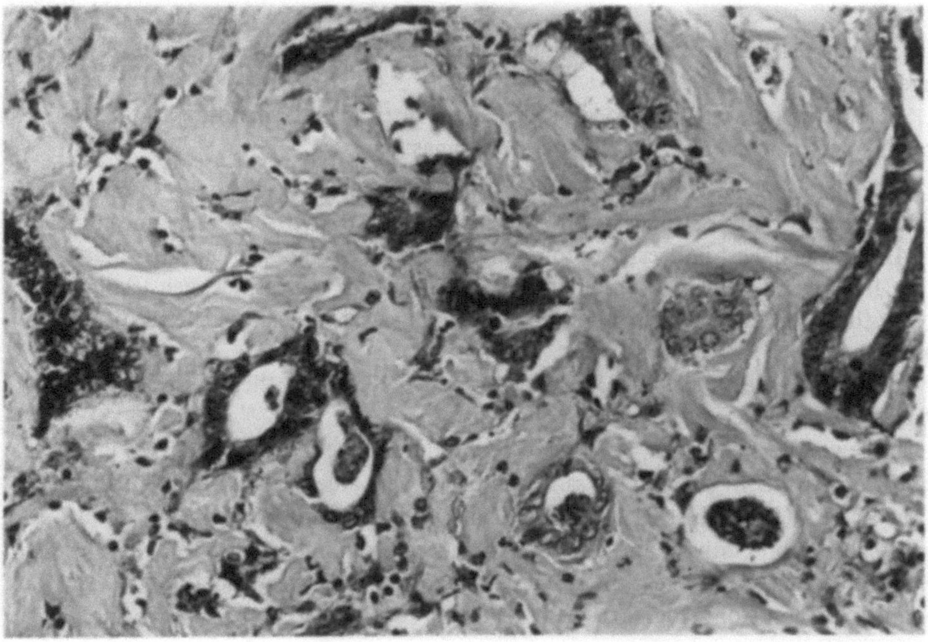

Fig. 19. Invasive growth of a poorly differentiated adenocarcinoma with severe nuclear and cellular polymorphism and stromal sclerosis. HE X 288

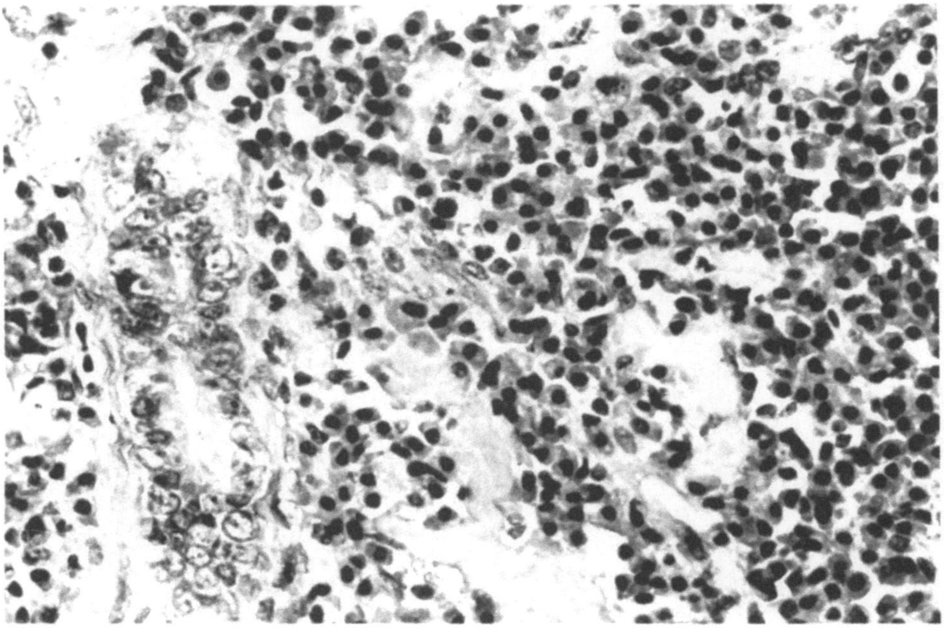

Fig. 20. Purely plasmacellular infiltration surrounding tumor tissue. Bullous dilatation of nuclei in tumor epithelia, distinct nucleoli. HE X 460

only a small insignificant rise in labeling to 16.2% at the earliest phase (5 weeks after surgery).

Separate evaluation was carried out for adenocystic glandular proliferation, anastomosis polyps, dysplastic glands, and carcinomas:

a) *Adenocystic glandular proliferation.* The labeling index was assessed in those areas where the reaction was strongest; it was found to be 10.6%–20.1%, with a mean index of 14.6%. The highest indices were found in advanced nodular proliferation of glands.

b) *Anastomosis polyps.* Focal high labeling reached ^{3}H-indices between 12.3% and 31.5%; the mean value always found in peripheral parts, i.e., near the surface of polyps (Fig. 24).

c) *Dysplastic areas in glands.* The indices reached 18.1% but there were also certain dysplastic complexes with only 6.4% (Fig. 25).

d) The greatest variations, in terms of proliferation kinetics, were observed in *carcinomatous tissue.* In one and the same tumor we were able to identify labeling indices as low as 2% and as high as 21% and more. In areas of extreme proliferative activity, the so-called proliferative zones of a carcinoma, the mean index was 13.2%. These zones were often located near the surface or in peripheral parts of the tumor, at the so-called invasion front (Fig. 26).

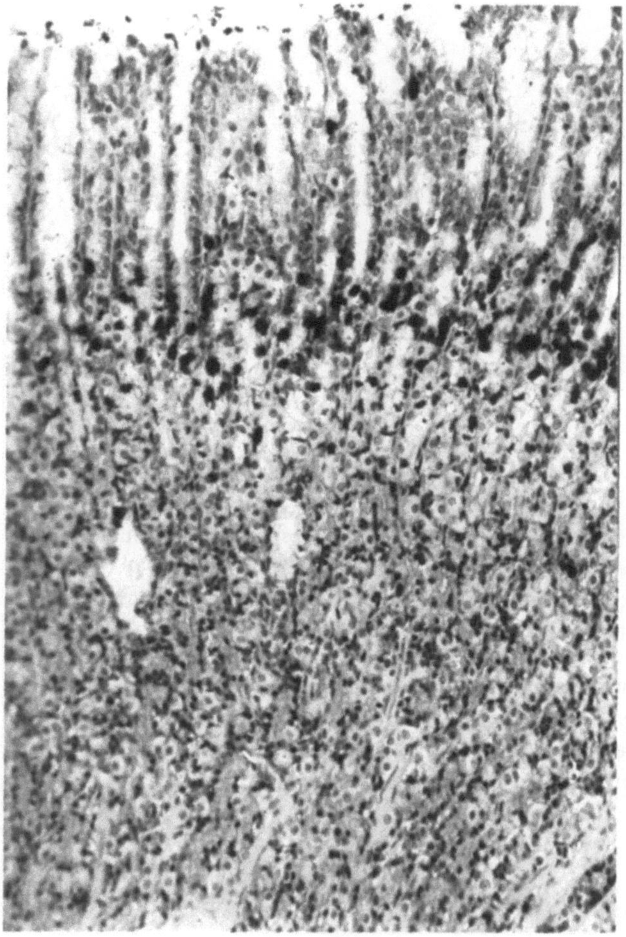

Fig. 21. Corpus mucosa distant from anastomosis. Labeled nuclei are chiefly localized in the gland neck region. Autoradiogram, HE × 180

4. Chronological Aspects of Carcinogenesis Under Different Experimental Conditions

All experimental groups showed regular increase in body weight, unimpaired by the carcinogen (MNNG) or by ALG administration. The mean circumference of the gastroenteroanastomosis was 16 mm in all groups. The reducing incision at the lesser curvature (gastro-gastric anastomosis) had a mean length of 9 mm, corresponding to the shortest connection between the forestomach and the gastroenteroanastomosis. The longest distance between both sites (i.e., between anterior and posterior wall of the corpus) measured 14 mm (a mean value for all resected animals).

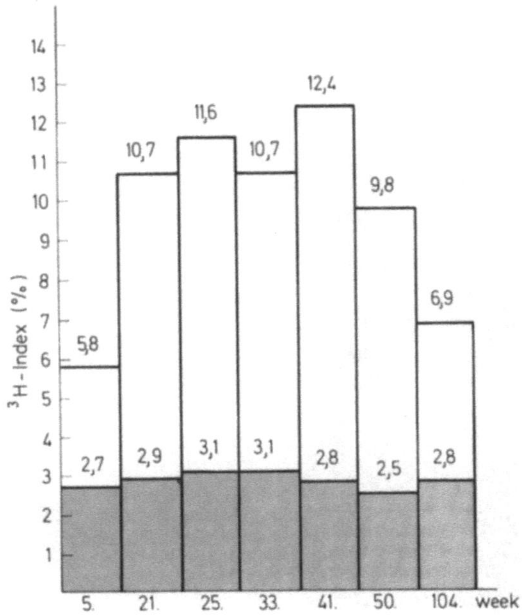

Fig. 22. ^{3}H-index of gastric mucosa in anastomosis (white) as compared to corpus mucosa distant from anastomosis (striped) during postoperative follow-up

Anastomosed parts of the wall were usually overlapped by a hepatic lobule. Tight connections were regularly seen between serosal wall segments and liver. Some adhering strands were also found between the anastomosis and jejunal loops or the pancreas. On the whole, adherences were not very conspicuous and restricted to the area of the anastomosis proper.

a) Follow-up Until the 21st Week of the Assay

During the first 5 weeks after resection, when animals were left untreated, examination of anastomosed mucosal tissue revealed mainly granulocytic infiltration through all layers of the gastric wall in addition to some small focal hemorraghe. Desquamation of sutured mucosal parts was observed in the gastroenteroanastomosis as well as in the reducing suture at the lesser curvature. Subsequently, the development of highly vascular granulation tissue pervaded all layers. In the adjacent submucosa we observed frequent development of marked edema. The surgically joined mucosal tissues either formed a sharply delineated border, or folded up against each other. The development of an anstomotic bulge was evident in all cases and at least histologically visible. This bulge was mostly composed of corpus mucosa; in some isolated cases it consisted of both varieties, and only very rarely did the bulge contain duodenal mucosa alone.

Regeneration of gastric and duodenal glands started early, but irregularly and without polarized orientation. The process involved cystic deformation: some large solitary cysts were found pushing forward the whole anastomotic area. It was a regular sequel to resection that mucosal tissue complexes were dislocated into deeper layers of the wall. These "dystopic" parts of mucosa were frequently the points of origin for cysts

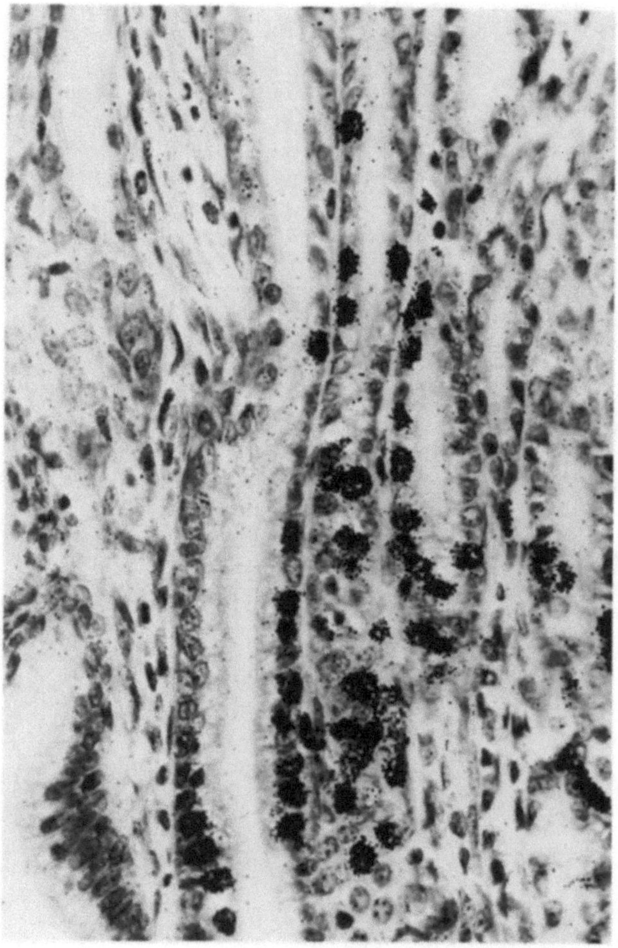

Fig. 23. Corpus mucosa near the anastomosis: irregular distribution of labeled nuclei over all mucosal layers. Autoradiogram, HE X 460

and glandular regeneration. Initial cellular infiltration, of mainly a granulocytic nature, was eventually replaced by lymphocytes, plasmocytes, and macrophages. Mastocytes and neutrophilic, as well as eosinophilic, granulocytes were also a regular finding. These infiltrations were particularly dense around residual sutures found in all strata of the wall. Additionally, we found marked fibroblast activity, accumulation of foreign-body giant cells, and high mitotic activity of neighboring glandular epithelia.

With the beginning of the 6th week after surgery (week 1 of the assay) the resected animals were distributed in the scheduled groups. Animals sacrificed for exact follow-up assessment during weeks 1, 5, 9, 13, 17, and 21, showed no relevant macroscopic differences. Mucosal conditions were unaltered in the groups that received no carcinogen; only one animal of group I developed, in week 8, a polypoid mucosal lesion at the posterior gastric wall near the gastroenteroanastomosis. Carcinogen-exposed animals also

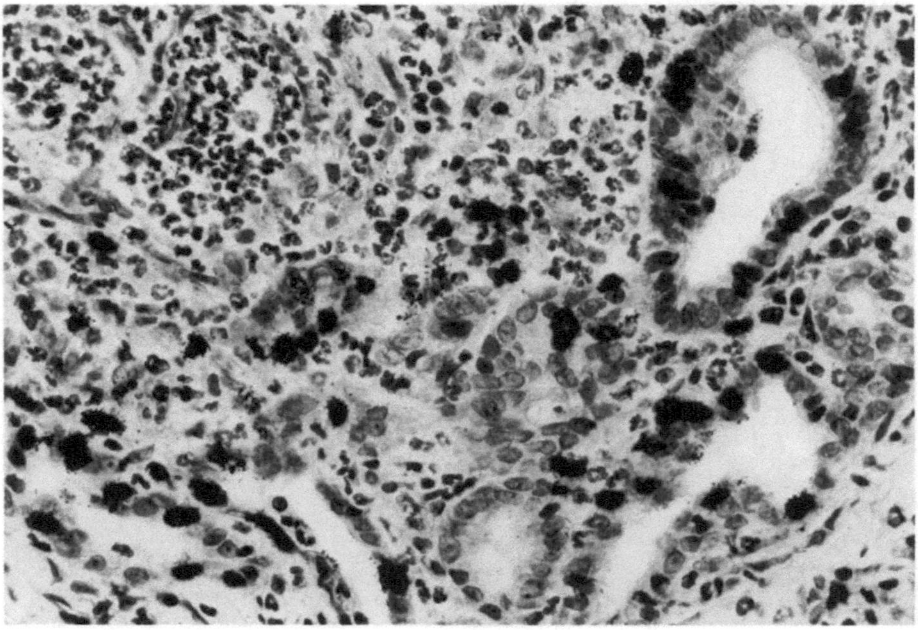

Fig. 24. Labeled nuclei within dysplastic gland tubules of a polyp. Autoradiogram, HE × 460

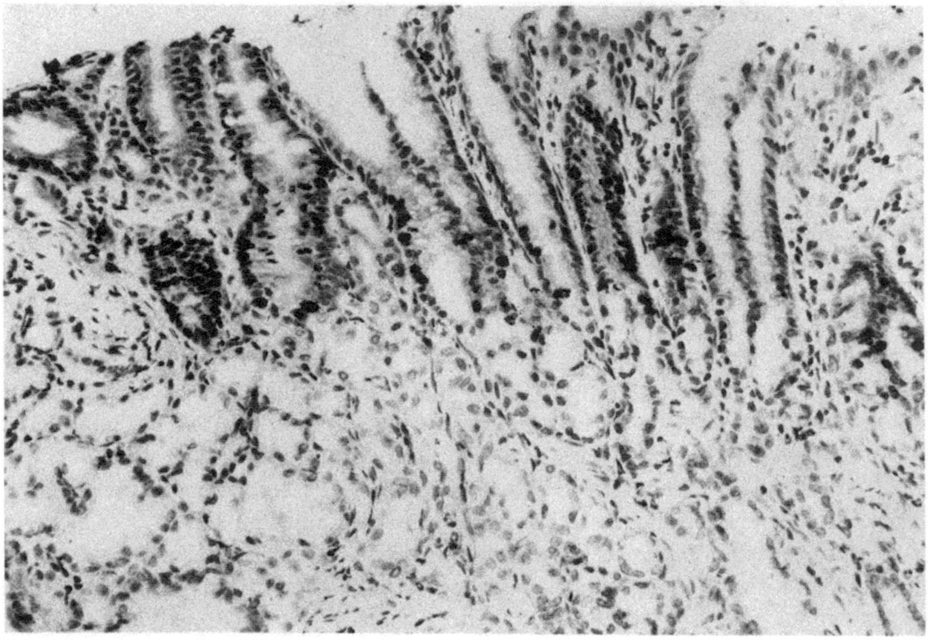

Fig. 25. Some dysplastic gland tubules with strong labeling in corpus mucosa near the anastomosis. Autoradiogram, HE × 225

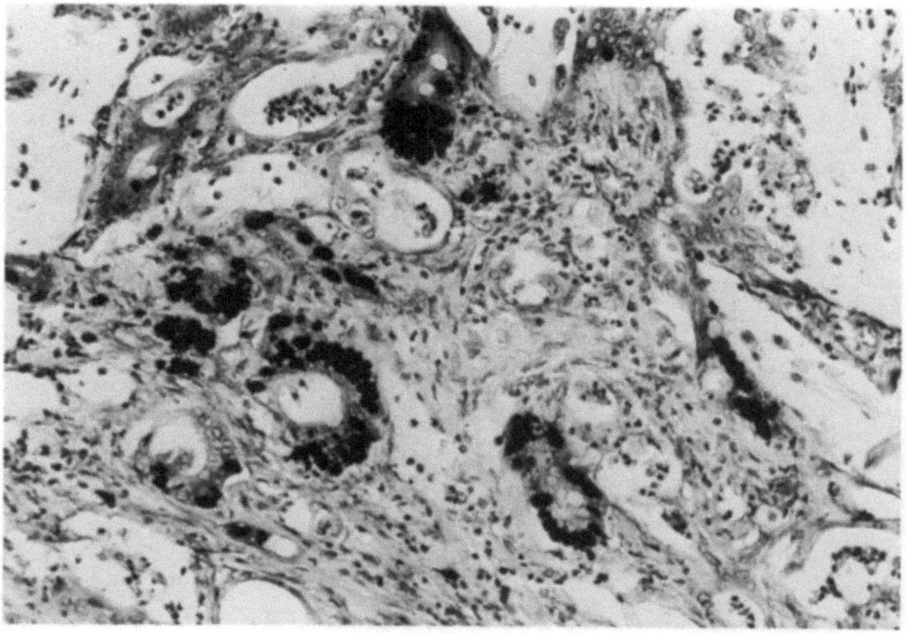

Fig. 26. Numerous labeled nuclei in peripheral portions of the carcinoma (the so-called invasion front). Autoradiogram, HE X 184

failed to show any remarkable peculiarities in this period. There was one polypoid mucosal lesion at the posterior wall in two animals in week 13, and in the anterior wall of two animals in week 17, always in anastomosed mucosal tissue. In some animals the mucosa showed focal or diffuse redness.

Microscopic examination confirmed our macroscopic findings in that it failed to identify marked differences between the groups of the assay. Findings classified macroscopically as polypoid anastomotic foci, could be assessed histologically as an anastomotic bulge with focal enhancement.

As early as 6 weeks after surgery we observed mucosal atrophies in anastomosed regions, manifested in a reduction of parietal and chief cells around the gastroenteroanastomosis and near the reducing suture at the lesser curvature. The atrophism of specific glandular epithelia increased with the course of the assay, but was principally confined to the anastomosed and perianastomotic portions of the mucosa.

Parallel to the increasing atrophy were the regular findings of foveolar hyperplasia, proliferation of undifferentiated gland neck epithelia, and also of an increasing number of mucoid gland neck cells in some gland tubules (Fig. 27). The mucosal areas were involved to varying degrees, and the anastomosis proper showed often complete foveolar hyperplasia.

Dysplasia of glandular epithelia was found, more or less severe, as early as 6 weeks after surgery, its frequency increasing in all groups until week 21 of the assay. Dysplasias occurred exclusively near or in the gastroenteroanastomosis, near or in the

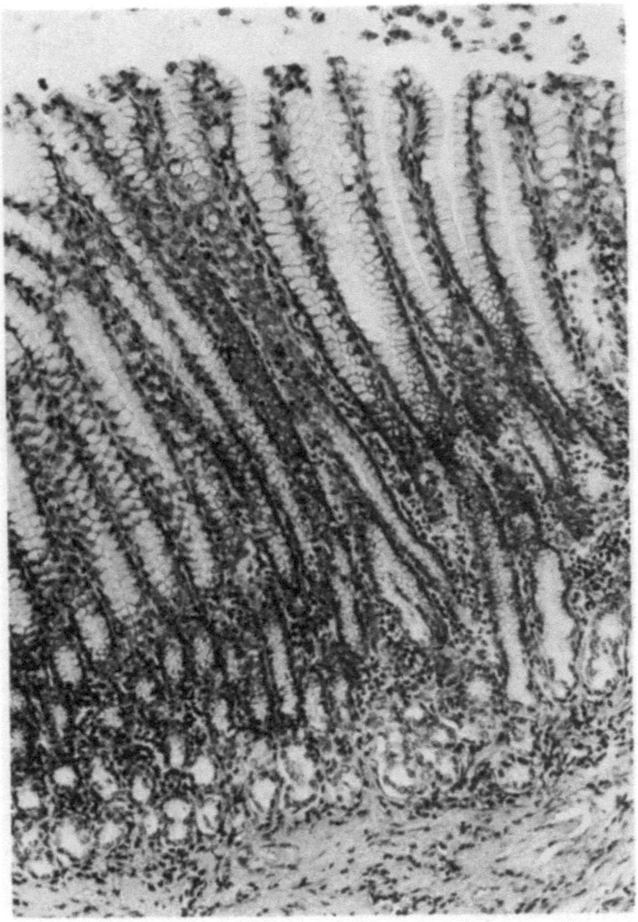

Fig. 27. Severe foveolar hyperplasia of corpus mucosa near the anastomosis, proliferation of undifferentiated and mucoid gland neck cells. Atrophism of specific gastric glands. HE × 114

reducing suture at the lesser curvature, and among advanced adenocystic gland proliferations.

Metaplastic bone formation was first observed near the anastomosis in two animals in week 17 of the assay. Corpus mucosa distant from the anastomosis failed to show any histologic changes that would differ, at the time, from findings in non-resected controls. Uniform tubular corpus glands revealed neither structural nor cellular atypism. Cellular infiltrations of mucosal stroma were as seldom found as in controls.

b) Week 25

Carcinogen exposure ended in the 25th week of the assay in group II. Fifteen animals were sacrificed in each of the groups I and II. Macroscopic and microscopic findings are tabulated in Tables 2 and 3. Evidence of glandular atrophy was found in the anastomosed mucosal tissue in both groups. Glandular dysplasia was also common at this stage, but only in anastomotic areas, whereas mucosal structures distant from the anastomoses were always regular. Chronic granulating or fibrosing inflammation was also found only in anastomosed mucosa.

Group I (OP): Besides the macroscopic and microscopic findings tabulated, we found one fibrosis of the splenic capsule and, in another animal, a serosal cyst of 2 mm diameter above the splenic capsule. Two animals had developed an encapsulated abscess

Table 2. Macroscopic findings at consecutive stages of the assay

Group	Macroscopy	Intervals of the assay (weeks)				
		25	33	41	50	104
I (OP)	a	0/15	–	–	3/10	0/3
	b	3/15	–	–	2/10	0/3
	c	0/15	–	–	0/10	1/3
	d	0/15	–	–	0/10	2/3
II (OP + early MNNG)	a	4/15	8/15	3/10	3/10	1/6
	b	2/15	3/15	2/10	4/10	1/6
	c	0/15	0/15	1/10	0/10	2/6
	d	0/15	0/15	1/10	2/10	2/6
III (OP + late MNNG)	c	–	–	–	–	2/15
	b	–	–	–	–	0/15
	c	–	–	–	–	0/15
	d	–	–	–	–	13/15

Macroscopic findings:
a = Anastomotic bulge
b = Polypoid mucosal lesion
c = Anastomosis polyp
d = Tumor

near the old scars in the abdominal wall. Further, two small abscesses were found in perigastric fatty tissue. Metaplastic bone formation was seen in the gastroenteroanastomotic area in two cases. The mucosa distant from the anastomosis showed minor cysts in two cases, developed mainly in basal gastric glands, but no other remarkable or abnormal findings were observed in the corpus mucosa.

Group II (OP + early MNNG): Mucosal redness was observed as a moderate local manifestation in five animals, more diffuse in three others. One case had an abscess of 3 mm diameter near the lesser curvature. Fibrosis of the splenic capsule was found in two

Table 3. Histologic findings in groups I, II and III of the assay at consecutive stages

Groups	Histologic findings	Intervals of the assay (weeks) 25	33	41	50	104
I (OP)	a	14/15	–	–	10/10	0/3
	b	1/15	–	–	0/10	0/3
	c	2/15	–	–	1/10	1/3
	d	10/15	–	–	5/10	0/3
	e	0/15	–	–	0/10	0/3
	f	0/15	–	–	0/10	0/3
	g	0/15	–	–	0/10	2/3
II (OP + early MNNG)	a	14/15	10/15	8/10	8/10	3/6
	b	0/15	0/15	1/10	1/10	0/6
	c	1/15	0/10	1/10	0/10	1/6
	d	10/15	9/15	8/10	6/10	2/6
	e	0/15	0/15	1/10	0/10	1/6
	f	0/15	0/15	0/10	0/10	0/6
	g	0/15	0/15	0/10	2/10	1/6
III (OP + late MNNG)	a	–	–	–	–	1/15
	b	–	–	–	–	0/15
	c	–	–	–	–	0/15
	d	–	–	–	–	1/15
	e	–	–	–	–	2/15
	f	–	–	–	–	2/15
	g	–	–	–	–	10/15

Histologic findings: a = Anastomotic bulge
b = Anastomosis polyp without dysplasia
c = Anastomosis polyp with dysplasia
d = Adenocystic gland proliferation, intramural
e = Adenocystic gland proliferation, nodular
f = Early carcinoma
g = Advanced carcinoma

cases; two small serosal cysts above the spleen in another. One case developed an incisional hernia at the abdominal wall; another animal showed focal baldness. There was one case of calcification within isolated tubular glands in cystic dilatation near the anastomosis. In corpus mucosa distant from the anastomosis, cysts developed mainly in basal gastric glands in four cases.

c) Week 33

At the end of the 33rd week 15 animals were sacrificed in group II; macroscopic and microscopic findings are listed in Tables 2 and 3. In the area of anastomosed mucosa, the animals showed atrophism of specific gastric glands, glandular dysplasia, and chronic scarring, but no visible alterations as compared to week 25.

Groups II (OP + early MNNG): Besides the tabulated findings we observed the following lesions in the 15 animals of this group: Focal mucosal redness was seen in the gastric stump or in the anastomosis in nine cases, diffuse redness in four others. Two microabscesses developed in the abdominal incision, one near the lower edge of the liver. One animal had suppurating lymphadenitis in a superficial lymph node on the left side, another showed focal fibrosis of the splenic capsule. Distant corpus mucosa showed focal cystic deformation of basal gastric glands in three cases, without any other significant findings.

d) Week 41

In the 41st week of group II (and IV) 10 animals were killed. Macroscopic and microscopic findings are tabulated in Tables 2 and 3. A marked atrophy of specific gastric glands was found in anastomosed mucosal tissue, developing disproportionately and in coincidence with foveolar hyperplasia. The same areas showed also glandular dysplasia to varying degrees of severity.

Group II (OP + early MNNG): Apart from the relevant findings listed we found moderate redness in four animals, stronger focal redness of the mucosa in three and diffuse redness in two animals. An abscess of 3 mm diameter was found in the fatty tissue of the greater omentum of one animal. Inflammatory changes were observed everywhere in anastomosed mucosal tissue, particularly around residual sutures and adenocystic gland proliferations. Dilated glandular cysts of bizarre shape were often filled with granulocytes and cellular detritus. No cystic deformation of gland tubules was found in distant corpus mucosa which had an indifferent appearance, except for some focal inflammatory infiltration.

e) Week 50

In each of the groups I and II 10 animals were killed. Macroscopic and microscopic findings are listed in Tables 2 and 3: Disproportionate atrophism of specific gastric glands in coincidence with distinct foveolar hyperplasia were common findings in anastomosed mucosal tissue in all groups. Glandular dysplasia of all grades was equally found in almost all animals. There were also chronic inflammatory changes (smouldering lesions) to be found in anastomosed mucosal tissue, particularly around residual sutures.

Group I (OP): Besides the relevant findings listed we found local moderate redness of the mucosa in three animals, and severe redness in two, but not polyps or tumors. Cystic deformation of basal gastric glands in distant mucosa was seen in three animals but there were no other mucosal findings of interest.

Group II (OP + early MNNG): Three of the 10 animals killed from this group showed a broad mucosal bulge near or around the gastroenteroanastomosis. Polypoid mucosal lesions were seen in four animals and advanced tumors in the anastomosed mucosa of two cases. One tumor was a polypous mass, 10 mm wide and 6 mm high, of transmural

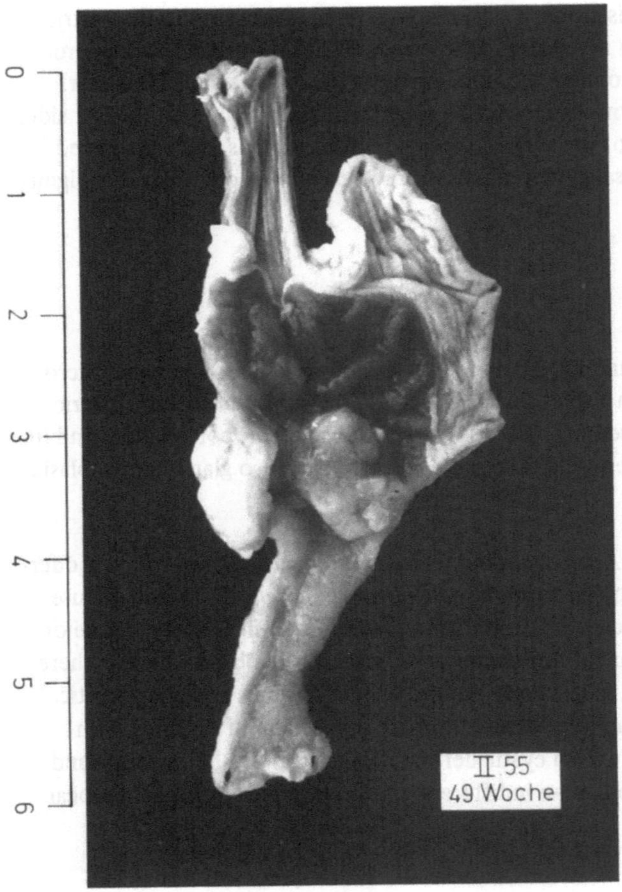

Fig. 28. Circular growth of a transmural carcinoma in the gastroenteroanastomosis. Strong stenosis of gastroenterostomy

growth and circular spread within the gastroenteroanastomosis, stenosing the gastric lumen (Fig. 28). The second tumor was a polypous mass of 13 X 13 X 15 mm growing through the wall at the angle between the gastroenteroanastomosis and the reducing suture (Fig. 29, 30). One lymph node near the lesser curvature and three lymph nodes in mesenteric fatty tissue had increased in size and hardness. One animal showed a small serosal cyst with coarse walls at the outside of the gastroenteroanastomosis. A small focal calcification was found in the right testis of another case; there was one fibrosis of the splenic capsule. Both the above mentioned tumors were identified histologically as advanced adenocarcinoma: one was of polypous mucus-producing type encircling the gastroenteroanastomosis and had invaded adjacent liver tissue in some places. The other carcinoma belonged to the polypous non-mucus-producing type; arising from the reducing suture near the lesser curvature it had nearly reached the serosa, with considerable formation of metaplastic bone tissue. Lymph nodes near this tumor were not invaded by cancerous tissue, but showed massed plasmacellular

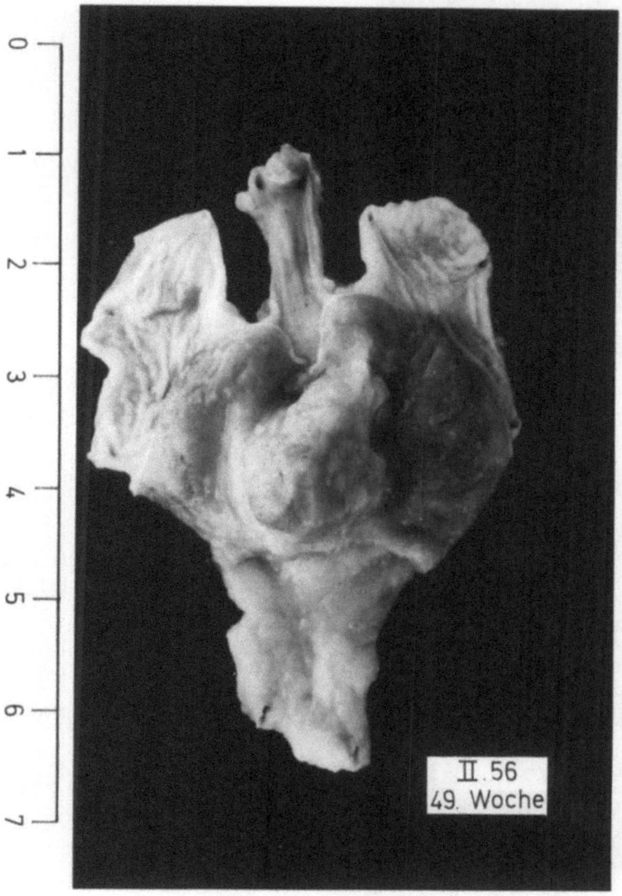

Fig. 29. Large polypous carcinoma at the angle between reducing suture of lesser curvature, and gastroenteroanastomosis

reactions. Distant mucosal tissue showed cystic structures in the glandular epithelia of five cases. Cystic tubules were mainly seen in basal gastric corpus glands.

f) Week 104

Two years after Billroth I resection, 15 animals of group III were killed together with the remaining animals from groups I (three), and II (six). Macroscopic and microscopic findings are tabulated in Tables 2 and 3.

Group I (OP): Of three animals surviving to this stage of the assay, one showed a mucosal polyp of 6 $\times$ 5 $\times$ 5 mm at the junction between lesser curvature and gastroentero-anastomosis, two further polypoid lesions in beadlike arrangement at the anterior wall, and a third polypoid lesion in the dorsal wall of the anastomosis. Both the other ani-

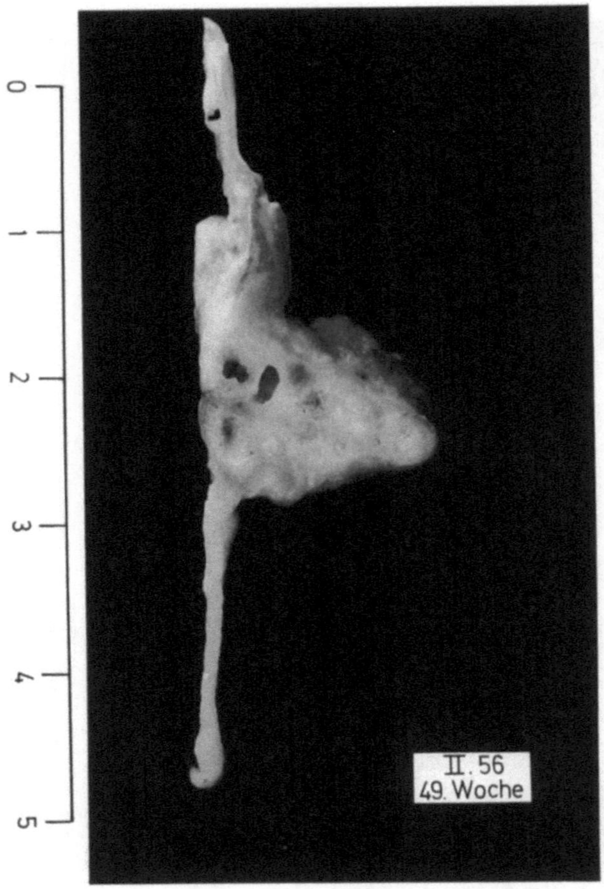

Fig. 30. Longitudinal section of the tumor shown in Figure 29. The carcinoma has pervaded the serosa in one site, although its initial growth was oriented towards the lumen

mals revealed advanced tumors which, macroscopically, arose from anastomosed mucosal tissue. They appeared as whitish polypous mass in focal decay and partly of cystic appearance at their cut surfaces. One of them encircled and stenosed the gastroenteroanastomosis. The tumors showed no clear delineation against adjacent organs (liver, pancreas, fatty tissue of the greater omentum). The largest tumor diameter was 30 mm. Histologically, the mucosal lesion appraised as a polyp was found to be an adenomatous polyp with focal glandular dysplasia of increasing severity and with some isolated bone metaplasia. The macroscopic appearance of both tumors had been that of a mucus-producing adenocarcinoma invading liver, pancreas, and greater omentum, but the histologic pattern was different: Well-differentiated glandular structures were found together with poorly differentiated and anaplastic components. Distant corpus mucosa in these two tumor-bearing animals revealed some light cystic deformation of basal gland tubules and some light focal mucosal hyperplasia.

Group II (OP + early MNNG): Six animals had survived to the 104th week and could be evaluated. Macroscopic lesions were as follows: A mucosal bulge at the anterior wall of the gastroenteroanastomosis in one case; three polypoid mucosal lesions in another; intraanastomotic polyps in two animals; two other animals developed tumors in the angle between the reducing suture and the gastroenteroanstomosis. The sizes of these tumors were 4 X 6 X 7 mm and 14 X 15 X 19 mm. An epidermal ulcus of 1 cm diameter was found above the left shoulder of one animal; another manifested severe kachexia of unknown causation. Histology identified the larger of the tumors as a well-differentiated adenocarcinoma arising from the reducing suture and with predominantly serosal orientation. The other, smaller tumor was an adenocystic gland proliferation with focal glandular dysplasia and some focal bone metaplasia. Distant corpus mucosa showed cystic deformation of mainly basal gastric glands in three cases. Some atypical proliferation of undifferentiated gland neck cells was seen in certain portions of distant corpus mucosa.

Group III (OP + late MNNG): Fifteen animals could be evaluated. Two of them showed a plump circular bulge in the anastomosed mucosa. The remaining 13 animals showed tumors either of polypous lumen-oriented growth, or as nodular masses in primarily serosa-oriented grwoth extending to adjacent organs. All these tumors arose from gastroentero- or gastro-gastric anastomoses.

Tumor sizes varied between 4 X 4 X 4 mm and 90 X 85 X 50 mm. The cut tumor surface had a coarse whitish or a cystic appearance. The cysts were often filled with viscous mucus. Macroscopic infiltration of the liver was seen in three animals. Besides its anastomotic bulge, one animal developed a whitish coarse tumorous mass in the right thoracic muscles, encased in a strong capsule. Another animal developed a subcutaneous tumor of 1 cm diameter some 4 cm behind its left ear. There was a strong fibrosis of the splenic capsule in one case and extended decubital ulcers at both hind legs of another.

In the two cases that developed an anastomotic bulge, histology revealed a thickly protruding mucosal structure in one animal; in the other there was a small carcinoma arising from the gastroenteroanastomosis within an area of adenocystic proliferation. This same animal had also developed a grossly visible mass in the left thoracic muscle, which was identified as a fibromyoma with strong fibrous components. Metaplastic bone formation was observed in five cases.

In two of the 13 macroscopic tumors, histologic examination revealed nodular adenocystic gland proliferations combined with severe focal glandular dysplasia. The remaining 11 tumors were found to be adenocarcinomas of varying differentiation. One carcinoma showed abundant production of mucus (medullary carcinoma) and another was of predominantly signet ring cell type.

Ten of the carcinomas were at an advanced stage of development, with invasion of the liver in two cases, and of liver and pancreas in a third case. One carcinoma was beginning to invade the scarred tissue of the anastomosis. All carcinomas were localized within areas of adenocystic gland proliferation and developed in serosal orientation.

Corpus mucosa distant from the anastomoses showed cystic deformation, sometimes considerable, of corpus glands in 10 cases. Changes were limited to basal glands only in lighter cases. Tumor-bearing animals showed focal, partly atypical, proliferation of undifferentiated gland neck epithelia in distant corpus mucosa.

A combined overview of histologic findings in the individual groups at different stages of the assay, is given in Tables 2 and 3.

IV. Discussion

1. Macroscopic and Microscopic Findings

The experimental model chosen for chemical carcinogenesis in the resected stomach of rats is based on the assay published by *Dahm* and *Werner* in 1973. These authors had found carcinomas in 37.8% of all Billroth-I- or Billroth-II-resected animals after 17–31 weeks from the start of daily carcinogen application. In contrast, carcinoma development was found neither in carcinogen-exposed, unoperated controls, nor in resected but unexposed animals. The carcinogenic agent chosen by *Dahm* and *Werner* was the same as ours, namely N-methyl-N'-nitro-N-nitrosoguanidine. Since the fundamental studies of *Sugimura* and *Fujimura* (1967), this agent has become one of the reliable means for inducing carcinogenesis in the glandular stomach of the rat.

Schlag et al. (1977a) investigated the influence of duodeno-gastric reflux on epithelial tissues in gastroenteroanastomosis. Their studies were made in rats with antecolic gastroenterostomy but no enteroanastomosis, and in another group with Y-anastomosis (Roux' method). Partial resection of the glandular stomach was not performed. The remaining experimental conditions corresponded to those reported by *Dahm* and *Werner* (1973). In the assay of *Schlag* et al. (1977a) no carcinomas could be observed within 35 weeks of follow-up.

Another team (*Rumpf* et al., 1978) studied the influence of vagotomy and Billroth-II resection on chemical carcinogenesis in the rat glandular stomach. Under two different administration schedules (100 mg MNNG/l and 30 MNNG/l), both being carried out over the whole 68 weeks of the assay, the authors found carcinomas in 83% of animals given high doses, and in 50% of those receiving low doses. Thus, the carcinoma yield in both groups was significantly higher than in nonoperated or nonvagotomized animals exposed to the carcinogen.

These findings may only be compared with our results to a limited extent: Due to the differeing questions, experimental conditions had to be quite different, particularly the dosage schedules, methods of carcinogen application, and the duration of the assay itself. The periods observed by the other teams (*Dahm* and *Werner,* 1973; *Schlag* et al., 1977a; *Rumpf* et al., 1978) were much shorter than the postoperative follow-up in our assay (Table 1). Divergent results in other publications may be due to different criteria being employed by the individual workers for carcinoma diagnosis in the rat glandular stomach (*Stewart,* 1971; *Bralow,* 1972; *St. John* et al., 1977). It is particularly difficult in the very early stages of development to distinguish carcinoma from submucosal adenomatous proliferation or diverticula. The only reliable criteria for carcinomatous transformation would be the severity of structural or cellular atypia, and the invasive growth pattern (*Wiebecke* and *Gokel,* 1975).

In our assay we intended not only to induce carcinogenesis but also to identify the exact morphologic stages through which gastric or anastomotic mucosa go to become carcinoma. So far, no reliable criteria have been established for histologic assessment of mucosal changes in the resected stomach with respect to the special conditions of the gastric stump. Teams who had previously studied experimental carcinogenesis in the resected stomach (*Dahm* and *Werner,* 1973; *Schlag* et al., 1977a; *Rumpf* et al., 1978) had adapted their histologic investigation to that classification published by *Saito* et al. (1970) and *Bralow* (1972) which systematized the chronology of mucosal changes developing during carcinogenesis in the non-resected rat stomach. The classification was based on findings compiled after the fundamental work of *Druckrey* et al. (1967) and *Sugimura* and *Fujimara* (1967) had provided models for the induction of adenocarcinomas in the rat stomach at a high incidence rate.

A great number of histologic data have been reported by other authors (*Schauer* et al., 1974; *Fujita* et al., 1974; *Justrabo* et al., 1975; *Uchida* et al., 1976; *Kobori* et al., 1976) who agreed that the majority of mucosal changes, including carcinoma, were observed in the areas of antrum and pylorus near the lesser curvature and were formed on the basis of preceding erosion and ulceration.

We started from a different situation in our study because the antrum was largely removed in Billroth I surgery whereby anatomical conditions were altered. Another fact that was outlined by *Wiebecke* and *Gokel* (1975) played an important role in our studies: *Saito* et al. (1970) defined proliferative reactions at the edge of fresh erosions as "regenerative hyperplasia," and thus interpreted the foregoing lesion as an unspecific stimulus for regeneration of adjacent glands. It appears possible, however, that an erosion is merely the site of the severest toxic damage to cells, whereas hyperplasia at its edge might manifest cell response to a lesser stimulus from the carcinogen (*Wiebecke* and *Gokel,* 1975). In order to prevent severe damage to the stump mucosa by the carcinogen, (i.e., to avoid blurring possible differences in the susceptibility of anastomotic or plain corpus mucosa) we chose a very low dosage for our carcinogen (50 mg/l for 1 month, and 100 mg/l for 5 months). The carcinogen was administered in normal tap water. The low dosage had the advantage of not provoking any ulcers, not even in anastomosed tissue. There were only some single polyps or carcinomas that showed superficial erosion. The following mucosal changes were observed with great regularity:

a) Atrophy of Specific Gastric Glands

This disproportionate pattern is caused by reduction or complete disappearance of chief and parietal cells. The atrophy of specific epithelia increased continuously after surgery and was found regularly after the 25th postoperative week. We observed a slow spreading of atrophy to areas of corpus mucosa that were distant from the anastomosis. Closely anastomosis-related mucosal changes of similar description were also reported by some other authors (*Dahm* and *Werner*, 1973; *Rumpf* et al., 1978).

The fact that specific glandular epithelia of the human stomach are impaired or lost in consequence of surgical resection, has been known since *Konjetzny* (1938) published his first extensive and systematic description of morphologic changes in gastroenteroanastomosis. Mucosal atrophy or chronic atrophic gastritis have been frequently cited, since that time, whenever etiology and pathogenesis of gastric carcinoma in resected or non-resected stomachs are discussed (*Krentz*, 1964; *Morgenstern* et al., 1973; *Siurala*, 1974; *Domellöf* et al., 1977).

b) Hyperplasia of Foveolar Epithelia

Parallel to the reduction of specific glands, all animals in our assay developed hyperplasia of foveolar epithelia in or near the sites of gastroentero- or gastro-gastric anastomoses. Hyperplasia was often accompanied by an increase of mucoid cells in gland necks in the lower part of the mucosa. The typical layers of the mucosa had disappeared. In intermediate mucosal tissue, mucoid gland neck cells were separated from the actual foveolar epithelium by a layer of undifferentiated cells (Fig. 27). Similar lesions have been described by other authors (*Rumpf* et al., 1978). In our material, this morphologic picture was observed with a striking regularity; the proliferation of mucoid epithelia seems to be directly connected with the reduction of specific glandular epithelia.

Proliferations of surface epithelia and of mucoid gland neck cells were equally reported in human findings (*Littler* and *Gleibermann*, 1972).

c) Dysplasia of Glandular Epithelia

This was another regular finding in all groups, increasing from the 25th week and almost general after the 52nd week (Figs. 2, 3, 7). Over a long period these dysplasias were found only in the areas of anastomotic mucosa. Corpus mucosa distant from the anastomosis showed some dysplastic foci as late as 104 weeks after surgery. The same delay was observed in non-resected an untreated animals of the same age. Similar dysplastic changes were also seen in adenocystic gland proliferations.

The histologic picture was always that of irregular gland tubules with marked cellular atypia, but without infiltration. Dysplastic alteration of the mucosa in the resected rat stomach was also described by *Rumpf* et al. (1978). Moreover, lesions of this description have been observed in connection with carcinogenesis in nonoperated rat stomachs (*Uchida* et al., 1976) and in experimental carcinogenesis of ileum and colon induced by DMH (*Nomura* et al., 1978). Any evidence of dysplastic mucosal changes in non-resected human stomachs would be of greatest interest with regard to the definition of precancerous stages as a prerequisite of early diagnosis (*Grundmann, Grundmann* and *Schlake,* 1978; *Oehlert* et al., 1975).

d) Anastomosis Ring or Bulge

The above described changes were observed in both gastroentero- and gastro-gastric anastomoses. In the former they were predominantly found in the so-called anastomosis ring or bulge (Fig. 1) which was a regular finding in all groups of the assay. Plain and even adaptation of gastric and duodenal mucosa was a rare exception. The ring-like bulge consisted mostly of corpus mucosa, in some difficult cases causing a mucosal prolapse into the duodenal lumen. When focally limited, the formation looked like a polypoid lesion of the mucosa (Fig. 4).

Comparable experimental findings have not been published until now, and there were no systematic macroscopic or microscopic follow-up studies of the resected rat stomach. The other papers about this topic (*Dahm* and *Werner,* 1973; *Schlag* et al., 1977a; *Rumpf* et al., 1978) did not include similar lesions. In man, the formation of anastomotic folds or ridges is well known (*Konjetzny,* 1938). In a detailed description of the morphology of gastroenteroanastomosis, *Becker* (1969) had emphasized the fact that the adaptation of both types of mucosa was never a straight and even one, but that both tissues were frequently found overlapping in zig-zag fashion. Mucosal prolapse is also known as one of the frequent complications after gastroenteroanastomosis in man (*Becker,* 1969; *Littler* and *Gleibermann,* 1972; *Griffel* et al., 1974).

Some of the factors responsible for the formation of this bulge may be related to the surgical technique. The beaded polypoid foci recognized by the endoscopist in anastomosed tissues, have been preformed by suture tightening in the bulging edges of the connected mucosas. On the other hand, the "troubled" tissue in the anastomosis must have a part in the formation of the ridge-like folds. The cause of this trouble is seen in the so-called border fighting between two types of epithelium (*Becker,* 1969).

Such a struggle was observed whereever epithelia of different kinds meet at a physiological borderline, and such borders must be of general importance in the origin of certain epithelial tumors (*Hamperl,* 1974). The stomach resection effected in our experimental model (removal of antrum and pylorus) results in an unphysiological bordering of two originally distant epithelia and, in consequence, in an increased "struggle". "Tissue trouble" can be identified in all layers of the anstomosed mucosa where it is manifested in numerous chronic inflammatory and smouldering processes and is accompanied by continuous proliferative and regenerative activity. The anastomotic site constantly shows these processes throughout the whole assay. Obviously the complete and true "healing" of the anastomosed tissues is prevented or delayed by the specific activities that are permanently required of the gastric and intestinal mucosas.

e) Anastomotic Polyps

A natural result of these tissue troubles and continuous regenerative or proliferative activities was seen in anastomotic polyps which always arose in the anastomosis between the reducing suture at the lesser curvature and the gastroenteroanastomosis (Figs. 5, 6). We counted a total of 18 anastomotic polyps of which seven showed small foci of dysplasia (Fig. 7). Five were without cellular atypia.

Polypous tumors in the gastroenteroanastomotic site were also described by *Schlag* et al. (1977a); histologically, these had obviously shown the same adenocystic nature as the polyps found in our material. No polyps of this kind were found in the stomach of unoperated rats, nor did we observe any polypous changes of the mucosa in the non-resected, untreated controls of our assay. Even in non-resected rats under carcinogen exposure such changes are very rare.

Polyps are equally rare in human non-resected stomachs (*Grafe* et al., 1960; *Tomasulo,* 1971). On the other hand, *Domellöf* et al. (1977) found polyps in more than 10% of human resected stomachs; these were predominantly identified as sessile or "regenerative" polyps, or as inflammatory polyps with focal granulomatous structures. Two of these polyps were called adenomatous by the authors. The adenomatous polyp is often interpreted as a premalignant lesion (*Ming* and *Goldmann,* 1965; *Nakamura,* 1970; *Tomasulo,* 1971). Findings of (a) dysplastic glandular epithelia between isolated polyps, (b) subsequently arising polypous adenocarcinomas, and (c) local coincidence of polyp and carcinoma, suggest that anastomotic polyps can be regarded as precursors of the polypous carcinoma.

Apart from these glandular proliferations which are primarily lumen-oriented, and of polypous nature, our special interest was focused on the serosa-oriented glandular proliferations.

f) Serosa-Oriented Adenocystic Proliferation of Glands

Development of these proliferations (Figs. 8, 10) started after the 13th week, either from anastomosed mucosa or from "dystopic" mucosal tissue that had been displaced by surgery. Proliferation proceeded first intramurally (Fig. 8); in later phases it became evident in nodular tumorous masses protruding towards the serosa and showing numerous cysts of different sizes under histologic examination. These adenomatous foci were composed of diverse epithelia: there were undifferentiated cuboid or cylindric cells, secretory cells of goblet type, and unspecific mucoid gland cells in varying proportions. Advanced cases showed foci of glandular dysplasia; chief or parietal cells were never found in this conditions.

Adenomatous glandular proliferation has been interpreted in many different ways; the results published vary accordingly. Some authors fail to mention such adenomatous, partly tumorous glandular proliferation at all, but they report an extremely high incidence of carcinoma in proportion to the period under observation (*Dahm* and *Werner,* 1973). On the other hand, an approximately similar set-up with experimental gastroenterostomy revealed no carcinomas, but adenomatous proliferation of glandular epithelia of partly polypous, partly serosa-oriented nature (*Schlag* et al., 1977a). Both work groups had covered a period of 35 weeks follow-up. In a similar period, *Rumpf* et al. (1978) did not find any carcinoma in their material.

Origin and spread of the glandular proliferation demonstrated that in a resected stomach the more evidence of glandular structures in the lower strata of the wall, even in subserosal tissue, must not be interpreted as proof for malignant tendencies as such. We shall have to look for the actual cause of this remarkable and partly excessive proliferation. Our results suggest that the surgical approach in itself is a considerable stimulus to mucosal proliferation in the artificially connected organs. In connection with the loss of glandular polarity provoked at the anastomotic site, and the loss of correct stratification in the gastric wall (Fig. 8), the natural proliferative potential of the mucosa is in itself responsible for the arising and spreading of adenocystic proliferation. Obviously, epithelial proliferation follows certain given structures, such as the strands of granulomatous tissue (muscular or connective) and residual suture material (Fig. 9). In some advanced cases the proliferations may reach the subserosal area, but will never penetrate the serosa proper. Whenever the serosa is actually penetrated we shall find a predominance of atypical epithelium, that is, a carcinoma.

Very recently some morphologic equivalents to these tumor-like adenomatous gland proliferations were also observed in man. One case was reported as "gastritis cystica polyposa" (prolapse of gastric mucosa within a gastroenteroanastomosis with cystic and invasive epithelial hyperplasia) by *Littler* and *Gleibermann* (1972). The authors found a polypous tumor in an old gastroenterostomy scar; it consisted of hyperplastic mucosa of gastric type with considerable proliferation of surface epithelia and mucoid gland neck cells. The muscularis mucosae was pervaded by specific gastric glands which protruded into the submucosa. Mucus-containing cysts predominated in the submucosa, some of them having already expelled their mucus into the stroma. Some gland tubules invaded the muscularis propria. The morphology of the individual epithelial cells, however, appeared benign.

Another case, mentioned by *Griffel* et al. (1974) as polypous cystic gastritis in an old gastroenterostomy, presented four polypoid tumors in a 26-year-old scar. Histology showed glands of gastric type, some of them in cystic dilatation penetrating the muscularis mucosae and spreading through the submucosa. Cytologically, the appearance of these epithelial cells was quite benign.

In our assay, the development of adenocarcinomas in some of the animals had evidently arisen from the region of such adenocystic proliferation of glands (Fig. 11). Some of these tumors had penetrated the serosa and invaded the adjacent organs (Figs. 14, 15, 16). However, these carcinomatous lesions were evident only after prolonged assay duration. A similar picture was reported of a human case by *Quizilbash* (1975), who observed the coincidence of carcinoma with a cystic gastritis 35 years after partial stomach resection. His interpretation suggests that cystic gastritis might be another link in the chain of factors leading towards carcinoma development.

Cystic hyperplasia of "ectopic" gland tubules in the resected stomach, stretching into deeper regions and sometimes connected with glands of the surface mucosa, have also been mentioned by *Morgenstern* et al. (1973) and *Chakravorty* and *Schatzki* (1975), who saw their origin in the reaction of gastric tissue to the surgical intervention. It appears possible, however, that even lesser stimuli will provoke a rush of proliferation in the mucosa of the rat glandular stomach (*St. John* et al., 1977). These authors fed aspirin to rats over 6 months, and then left them untreated for 6–18 months. In 90% of the animals they found evidence of previous, but healed ulceration. In the area of scarred ulcers they noted an additional glandular growth that penetrated the muscularis propria in some cases and even stretched into subserosal connective tissue in a few others. Epithelia were partly mucus-producing, but without atypia or increased mitotic activity. The surrounding tissue showed frequency of mast cells, plasma cells, and lymphocytes.

These findings suggest the possibility of gastric glands penetrating from the area of aspirin-induced, but now healed, ulcers via the muscularis mucosae into subserosal lipoid tissue. The absence of manifest nuclear atypia and of increased mitotic activity seems to speak against a malignant nature of these changes, which failed to reveal chronological progression. The intrusion of gland tubules into the deeper strata of the gastric walls in a non-resected stomach, seems to be a natural response to repeated traumatic lesions of the mucosa, and to destruction of the muscularis mucosa in combination with repeated regeneratory impulses. As early as 1949, *Lushbaugh* described comparable adenomatous and invasive lesions in the stomach and bowel of monkeys. Consequently, the actual stomach resection represents only the most severe of possible traumatic lesions or destructive damages to the gastric wall.

Pathological pictures of permanence, showing gland tubules spreading throughout the deeper layers of human gastric wall, even without previous surgery, have been described in various forms under the name of gastritis cystica polyposa (*Scotti*, 1973), or gastritis cystica (*Nikolai* and *Müller*, 1965). Inflammatory obstruction or obliteration of excretory gland ducts are being discussed as causes of these diseases.

Cystic gland structures in the mucosal and submucosal layers of the gastric wall are also defined as diffuse heterotopic cystic malformations (*Scott* and *Payne*, 1947; *Obermann* et al., 1963; *Tchertkoff* and *Wagner*, 1966). Carcinomas were found developing in the vicinity of these heterotopic structures (*Ignatius* et al., 1970; *Pillay* and *Petrelli*, 1976).

Iwanaga et al. (1975) reported 12 known cases of diffuse submucosal gastric cysts predominantly combined with a superficially spreading carcinoma. Interpreting these submucosal cysts as the sequelae of gastritis, the authors suggested that they might provoke repeated superficial erosion with subsequent development of multiple surface carcinomas.

Similar cystic gland structures, stretching towards deeper strata of the wall in other segments of the gastrointestinal tract, are present in the colon as in colitis cystica profunda (*Epstein* et al., 1966; *Wayte* and *Helwig*, 1967), and in the ileum as in enteritis cystica polyposa (*Baillie* and *Abell*, 1970).

Occasionally, cystic gland tubules are also found in submucosal tissue of the stalk of adenomatous polyps (*Muto* et al., 1973); a lesion called pseudocarcinomatous invasion. Apparently, the intrusion of gland tubules into deeper layers of the wall may represent an unspecific response to repeated traumatic lesions of the mucosa. These findings emphasize the need for scrupulous accuracy when potentially malignant changes are discussed and interpreted. Any diagnosis of "carcinoma" must be verified and checked against the possibility that adenomatous proliferation of glands may be found in deeper strata of the wall as a result of the naturally strong proliferative potential of the gastric mucosa responding to previous traumatic lesions.

g) Carcinoma

Carcinoma was the severest complication found in the mucosal tissue of anastomoses in our animal material. In strict accordance with the above-mentioned reservations, we were able to identify 14 carcinomas among the 19 tumors diagnosed macroscopically. The remaining five tumors were defined as nodular adenocystic gland proliferations. Two other carcinomas had not been recognized macroscopically and so the total of carcinomas in the mucosal tissue of the anastomotic region was 16. Macroscopically, the tumors developed partly from the reducing suture at the lesser curvature, partly from the gastroenteroanastomosis. As polypous lesions, their growth was lumen-oriented (Fig. 10). When they appeared as nodular tumors, growth was primarily serosa-oriented (Fig. 11). Some tumors presented as growing in both directions. Carcinomas were found in 14.0% of the 114 animals sacrificed during the entire postoperative follow-up.

Of the animals killed in the 104th week, 14 showed a carcinoma in the anastomotic region (i.e., 58.3%). Of the 16 anastomosis carcinomas, two had developed in a polyp and were infiltrating the sclerosed tissue of the stalk. Seven carcinomas showed varied degrees of dedifferentiation down to anaplastic components. One tumor was a medullary (Fig. 12), another a signet ring cell carcinoma (Fig. 13). Four carcinomas were found to be adenocarcinomas, two of them with increased secretory activity. One carcinoma showed polypous lumen-oriented as well as nodular serosa-oriented growth. On the whole, five carcinomas had infiltrated the liver, liver and pancreas, or liver, pancreas, and lipid tissue. Lymph node metastases were not observed.

Carcinomas as seen in our material showed some differences to those described in the literature. Whereas the single instance of a signet ring cell carcinoma (Fig. 13) is indeed a rare finding (*Dahm* and *Werner*, 1973; *Rumpf* et al., 1978), the other carcinomas often show moderate to low-grade differentiation down to anaplastic growth with marked nuclear and cellular polymorphism (Fig. 17). Carcinomas contain numerous foci of increased mitotic activity and, sometimes, atypical mitoses, a finding that contradicts the general opinion of cellular atypia and mitosis being rather infrequent in carcinomas of this description (*Saito* et al., 1970; *Dahm* and *Werner*, 1973).

Infiltration of liver, pancreas, and adjacent lipid tissue, as shown in six cases of our material (Figs. 14, 15, 16), has not been reported previously in experimental anastomosis carcinomas. This divergence of morphologic appearance must be due to the differences of experimental design and set-up. In man, the postoperative latency of carcinoma development in a resected stomach is an average 20 years. The fact that these carcinomas obviously need a long time prompted us to plan follow-up over as long a period as possible, i.e., up to 104 weeks. Consequently, the morphology of carcinoma observed in our assay shows a striking resemblance to the carcinomatous changes in man.

Obviously, metaplastic bone formation within the anastomosed tissues occurs more frequently in experimental animals than in man, as was also reported by other authors (*Dahm* and *Werner*, 1973; *Werner* et al., 1976). Some carcinomas in our material also showed extensive formation of bone tissue; moreover we were able to identify bone metaplasia in "normal" (i.e., non-carcinomatous) gastroenteroanastomoses. The findings were distributed irregularly over all the experimental groups; they were first noted in the 17th postoperative week.

Reports on bone metaplasia in human gastric carcinomas are scarce (*D'Altorio*, 1973; *Yasuma* et al., 1973). *Eid* and *Rohde* (1978) reported a case of tumor-like ossifying changes in the vicinity of a mesocolic slit (after two-thirds resection), which strangled or encircled the anastomosis from the outside.

No convincing similarity to human intestinal metaplasia could be found in our animals, although some foci of duodenal mucosa were occasionally observed in anastomotic regions. Such findings are interpreted, however, not as truly metaplastic changes, but rather as a sign of uneven or mismatched adaptation of gastric and duodenal mucosa in the anastomotic junction itself.

Accumulation of lymphocytes and plasma cells, as well as mastocytes and eosinophilic granulocytes, was observed in anastomosed tissue throughout the duration of the assay. This is possibly an immune response provoked within the anastomosis by the entrance of exogenic antigens via defenseless areas of the mucosa. Anastomosed mucosal tissue after Billroth I surgery is highly predisposed to cancerogenesis. The evidence of histologic changes in none other than anastomotic portions of the mucosa may be seen as proof that cancer development occurs preferably in the anastomosed mucosa.

In our experimental groups, carcinoma development followed two different pathways (Figs. 31, 32). The circular growth of polypous anastomosis carcinoma was a typical feature of gastroenteroanastomosis. The morphologic precursors of this type are seen in the adenomatous anastomotic polyp, in the polyp with dysplastic glandular lesions, and in the carcinoma within a polyp (Fig. 31). The other type of carcinoma development was defined as primarily serosa-oriented growth, with precursors appearing as intramural (later nodular) adenocystic proliferation of glands directed towards the serosa (Fig. 32).

Corpus mucosa at a distance from the anastomosis proper, showed only insignificant morphologic changes, consisting mainly of cysts formed predominantly in the basal gastric glands. These cysts multiplied in the course of postoperative follow-up. Similar cystic structures are a well-known feature in animal experiments (*Morgenstern* et al., 1973); they may be seen in analogy to the glandular cysts in human gastric mucosa that were described only recently (*Gohbrand* and *Krentz*, 1977; *Elster* et al., 1977). A reversible formation of cysts is interpreted as an early symptom of functional disorders in the gastric mucosa.

Fig. 31. The steps of carcinomatous development in or near a gastroenteroanastomosis.
a Anastomotic bulge with some surgically displaced glands in deeper strata,
b Adenotamous anastomotic polyp,
c Adenomatous anastomotic polyp with glandular dysplasia,
d Carcinoma within an adenomatous anastomotic polyp,
e Transmural growth of polypous adenocarcinoma in gastroenteroanastomosis

Fig. 32. The steps of carcinoma development in or near a gastro-gastric anastomosis
a Reducing suture at the lesser curvature = gastro-gastric anastomosis
b Intramural spread of adenocystic gland proliferation,
c Initial serosa-oriented growth of nodular adenocystic gland proliferation with focal dysplasia of gland tubules,
d Transmural growth of adenocarcinoma within gastro-gastric anastomosis

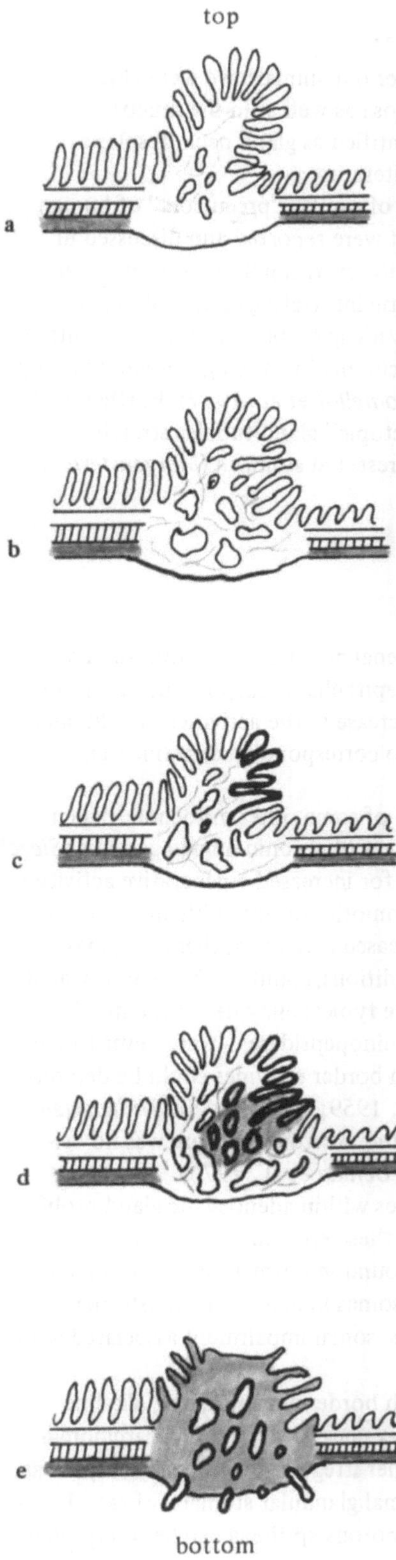

Fig. 31. Legend see page 48

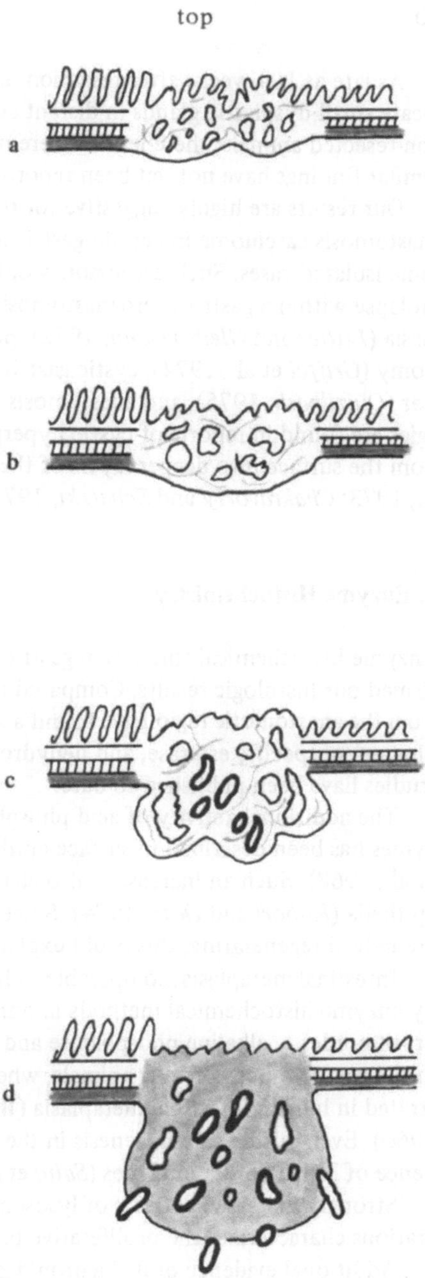

Fig. 32. Legend see page 48

As late as 104 weeks after resection, i.e., in rather old animals, we were able to locate small dysplastic glands in distant corpus mucosa as well as in the mucosa of non-resected animals; these lesions were mainly identified as gland neck dysplasia. Similar findings have not yet been reported in the literature.

Our results are highly suggestive for recognition of similar "precursors" of human anastomosis carcinoma in certain gastric lesions that were reported and discussed in some isolated cases. Such precursors would be gastritis cystica polyposa or mucosal prolapse within a gastroenteroanastomosis with cystic infiltrating epithelial hyperplasia (*Littler* and *Gleibermann,* 1972), polypous cystic gastritis in an old gastroenterostomy (*Griffel* et al., 1974), cystic gastritis plus carcinoma in an old gastroenterostomy scar (*Quizilbash,* 1975), and anastomosis polyps (*Domellöf* et al., 1977). Further analogies are found in reports of cystic hyperplastic "ectopic" gland tubules stretching from the surface into deeper layers of the wall in a resected stomach (*Morgenstern* et al., 1973; *Chakravorty* and *Schatzki,* 1975).

2. Enzyme Histochemistry

Enzyme histochemical findings in gastric and duodenal mucosa of anastomoses confirmed our histologic results. Compared to surface epithelia of corpus mucosa distant from the anastomotic region, we found a striking increase in the activities of acid phosphatase, unspecific esterase, and dehydrogenase. No corresponding experimental studies have been published to date.

The additional activity of acid phosphatase and of some other mitochondrial enzymes has been described in surface epithelial changes of chronic human gastritis (*Siegel* et al., 1968). Such an increase is also characteristic for increased regenerative activity of epithelia (*Kobori* and *Oota,* 1974). Since the anastomotic surface epithelia in our assay are indeed regenerating, this could explain the increased activity of these enzymes.

Intestinal metaplasia, comparable to human conditions, could not be demonstrated by enzyme histochemical methods in our assay. The typical enzymes of the duodenal brush border – alkaline phosphatase and leucine aminopeptidase – were never found in the gastric mucosa of our animals, whereas brush border enzymes could be demonstrated in human intestinal metaplasia (*Wattenberg,* 1959; *Planteydt* and *Willighagen,* 1960). Even during carcinogenesis in the non-resected rat stomach there was no evidence of brush border enzymes (*Saito* et al., 1970; *Uchida* et al., 1976).

Strongly increased activity of lysosomal enzymes within adenocystic gland proliferations characterizes the proliferative potential of these epithelia.

Additional evidence of β-glucuronidase, never found in normal gastric or duodenal rat mucosa, may highlight the possible role of lysosomes in malignant transformation, as discussed in the Chediak-Higashi syndrome (a lysosomal impairment associated with lymphomas, *Dent* et al., 1966).

In adenocystic gland proliferation, typical brush border enzymes, e.g., alkaline phosphatase and leucine aminopeptidase, were always negative. In actual carcinomatous tissues, acid phosphatase activity could be rather irregularly demonstrated; it was completely negative in surface epithelia of the normal glandular stomach of rats. Irregular or changing activity of acid phosphatase in tumorous epithelia can be interpreted as an indicator of varying degrees of differentiation in these epithelial tissues. Acid phosphatase was also demonstrated in human gastric carcinoma (*Planteydt* and *Willighagen,* 1965; *Lev* et al., 1969). In contrast to these findings, unspecific esterase manifested a steady and strong activity in the cancerous epithelia of our experimental anastomosis carcinomas.

The behavior of β-glucuronidase was similar to that of acid phosphatase and unspecific esterase, although its granular reaction in tumorous epithelia was generally weaker. This enzyme has not been demonstrated in normal gastric mucosa of experimental animals. In human gastrointestinal tumors, β-glucuronidase activity is stronger than in the corresponding normal tissues (*Fishman* and *Bigelow,* 1950). This may characterize β-glucuronidase, together with unspecific esterase, as belonging to the small group of enzymes whose activity is increased in tumorous epithelia, in contrast to the reduced activity of the majority of enzymes (*Fishman* et al., 1959). Usually, increased activity of β-glucuronidase signals active cell proliferation or growth of tissues (*Levy* et al., 1948).

The above mentioned brush border enzymes (leucine aminopeptidase and alkaline phosphatase) are principally never to be found in the tumorous epithelia of our animals, in agreement with other experimental findings in non-resected rat stomachs (*Saito* et al., 1970; *Uchida* et al., 1976). In man, however, these enzymes have at least been demonstrated in some gastric carcinomas (*Planteydt* and *Willighagen,* 1965; *Kobori* and *Oota,* 1974).

Special interest focused on β-glucuronidase which was not found in normal gastric mucosa. This enzyme was positive not only in neoplastic areas, but also in all epithelia showing increased proliferative activity outside the normal mucosal complex. The role of β-glucuronidase as an enzyme of cellular growth in general has been confirmed by other studies (*Kondstaal* et al., 1975; *Brown*, 1978).

Our enzyme histochemical studies demonstrated that localization and activities of these enzymes were changed not only in preneoplastic or neoplastic cells, but also in cellular complexes that were still regarded as benign. Therefore, the solution to the problem of if and when malignant transformation occurs in a cell should not be expected from enzyme histochemical methods.

3. Histoautoradiographic Findings

The mucosal changes provoked by Billroth I resection were of particular interest with regard to the interactions between cell differentiation and cell proliferation. Proliferative activity in anastomotic mucosa, and in corpus mucosa distant from the anastomosis, was examined by determining the ^{3}H-index after 1 h radioactive exposure. Proliferative activity and the localization of proliferative zones were also estimated in glandular dysplasia, in anastomosis polyps, in adenocystic glandular proliferation, and in carcinomas. The animals from different groups could be evaluated together at different stages of the assay since the mean average values in the individual groups showed no significant differences in labeling indices which might be caused by altered proliferative activity under low carcinogen exposure.

The ^{3}H-labeling index was three to four times higher in the gastric component of anastomosed mucosa, rising from 5.8% in the 5th week of the assay, to 10.7% in week 21. The labeling index at a high level until the 41st week (week 25: 11.6%; week 33: 10.7%; week 41: 12.4%) (Fig. 22). A slight decrease occurred in week 50 (9.8%); after 2 years (week 104) the index had decreased to 6.9% which was still significantly higher than the index in corpus mucosa distant from the anastomosis. The duodenal compartment of anastomotic mucosa showed a minor increase in labeling indices from their physiologically high values (*Messier* and *Leblond,* 1960). This steady rise of the labeling index in anastomotic areas of the mucosa and the decomposition of proliferative zones in the gland neck region, illustrated by the completely irregular labeling pattern (Fig. 23), are impressive signs of the permanent "trouble" or "disorder" in anastomosed mucosa, and also highly suggestive for the predilection of anastomosed tissue as the site of carcinoma origin.

Although similar results have not been published until now, we found some interesting suggestions in experimental studies of mucosal deficiencies in the stomach. For instance, the administration of aspirin resulted in two different patterns of deficiency (*Yeomans* et al., 1973): Superficial damage which did not touch the ^{3}H-labeled cells of the proliferative zone healed within 24 h. Deeper erosions which had penetrated the proliferative zone revealed increased labeling indices in the neighboring mucosa. Cell turnover was at its peak some 16–18 h after aspirin administration; for complete recovery these deep erosions needed up to 10 days. The authors explained the retarded recovery as a result of the focal destruction of the proliferative zone (*Yeomans* et al., 1973; *Eastwood,* 1977).

The destruction of the proliferative zone, combined with an unchecked displacement or transposition of proliferative cells into various layers of the gastric wall, are very characteristic features in Billroth I resections along with severe structural mismatching of mucosal tissues. Thus, the surgical intervention must cause severe disturbances in the balance or interaction between proliferation and differentiation. Disorders of differentiation were demonstrated in the reduction of highly specific chief and parietal cells in favor of proliferating, unspecific, and mucus-producing cells in anastomosed portions of the mucosa (Fig. 27).

Faulty regeneration of cells, beginning with poorly differentiated cells in the gland neck region, may be a late sequel to this imbalance. Moreover, these poorly differentiated cells are no longer strictly localized in the gland neck region, but are scattered throughout the mucosa as a result of trauma and structural loss (Fig. 23). The considerably increased labeling index and the displacement of the proliferative zone in anastomotic areas can be viewed as causes of malignant transformation; a hypothesis that corresponds well to the fact that "there is a general correlation in all living tissues between the amount of cell regeneration, and the frequency of malignant epithelial tumors" (*Oehlert,* 1969).

However, in the normal gastrointestinal tract with its strong regenerative activity the situation is a different one. Tumors are very rare in the small intestine although it has the highest rate of cell turnover, physiologically. In contrast, the rising labeling index in anastomosed mucosa – coinciding with loss of structural regularity – is highly unphysiological, and it is maintained by chronic irregular stimulation over a very long period. Areas of highest mitotic activity have been shown in previous studies to be predisposed for carcinoma development (*Liavag,* 1968).

It has already been mentioned that we observed morphological changes in conjunction with a particular pattern of proliferation kinetics and a considerable displacement of the proliferative zone, in anastomosed mucosal tissue with severe functional and anatomical impairment. Glandular components identified as "dysplasia" showed a labeling index of up to 18.1%, but equally dysplastic glandular complexes with an index as low as 6.4% also existed (Fig. 25). The particular significance of glandular dysplasia lies in its role as a possible precursor of adenocarcinoma in the non-resected human stomach (*Grundmann,* 1975; *Grundmann* and *Schlake,* 1978; *Oehlert* et al., 1975). Strong variations of labeling indices within glandular dysplasias, as observed in our material, were also found in dimethylhydrazine-induced carcinogenesis in the rat colon (*Nomura* et al., 1978).

Other patho-anatomical changes in the anastomotic area were identified as adenocystic gland proliferations. Their labeling indices, evaluated from tissues showing the highest labeling rates, oscillated between 10.6% and 20.1% (mean index = 14.6%). The highest rates were found in zones of advanced nodular gland proliferation where the strong labeling was interpreted as an expression of the enormous proliferative potential of mucosal epithelia in the stomach. Within anastomotic polyps, the labeling foci attained rates between 12.3% and 31.5% (mean index = 19.6%). These focal peaks of labeling, characterizing proliferative zones, were always found near the periphery, i.e., on the surface of polyp mucosa.

So far, no similar results have yet been published from animal experiments. Findings in human adenomatous polyps, however, show an extension of the proliferative zone and a shifting of peak activity towards superficial layers of the mucosa (*Wiebecke* et al., 1969). Labeling indices in mucosal layers near the surface were markedly higher than those in deeper strata. We may infer that the situation in our experimental anastomotic polyps must be similar to that of adenomatous polyps in man.

The causative factor in the development of anastomotic polyps as well as adenocystic gland proliferations is principally seen in the surgical traumatization of the mucosa. This trauma provokes a focal periodic increase of proliferative activity, producing mainly undifferentiated proliferative gland neck cells and mucoid epithelial cells. Branching neoplastic gland tubules support the structure of the rising polyp or the nodular gland proliferation. The actual proliferative zone is limited to the peripheral portions of both structures, proliferative activity being mainly directed towards the center. In the center itself we find only sporadic mitoses of single cells. Anastomotic polyps and serosa-oriented adenomatous gland proliferations provide a particularly good example of imbalance between differentiation and proliferation – in favor of the latter.

Carcinomas manifested the greatest deviations in terms of proliferation kinetics that were found in our assay (Fig. 26). Labeling rates varied between 2% and over 21% in one tumor. In proliferative tumor zones, the mean labeling index was found to be 13.2%. These zones were always found near the surface or in peripheral parts, i.e., at the so-called invasive front of the tumor (Fig. 26).

Labeling rates in human carcinoma of the unresected stomach were published with differing values: *Klein* et al. (1972) found an index of 32%–33% in poorly differentiated carcinoma, other authors reported values between 23.1% (*Kohli* et al., 1975), 21% (*Castrup,* 1977), or even 8% (*Brückner* and *Kempf,* 1977). Strong variation of labeling indices in one and the same carcinoma – as in our material – have also been demonstrated in experimental colon carcinoma (*Boxler,* 1972).

We also evaluated labeling indices of corpus mucosa distant from the anastomosis in order to see whether the influence of resection would also affect the proliferative activity or the localization of the proliferative zone in these portions. As a mean value of all data collected from these regions in our material, we found a labeling index of 2.84% which was even lower than that of non-resected animals. No shifting of the proliferative zone from the gland necks to other regions was observed in mucosal tissue distant from the anastomosis.

Comparing our results with those of other authors gained from human non-resected stomachs, we found that the labeling indices of the gland neck region of corpus mucosa varied greatly between animal species and in the comparison of animals to humans. In rats, labelling rates have been ascertained at 5.6% (*Wegener* et al., 1971), over 3% (*Rajewsky*, 1966), 3.2% (*Lipkin*, 1965), and 5.3% (*Seelig* et al., 1978). The values for mice are 4% (*Lipkin*, 1965), for hamsters 2.2% (ibid.), and for dogs between 3.5% and 4.7% (*Willems* et al., 1970, 1971a, b). Normal human corpus mucosa shows labeling indices of 9.3% (*Tanaka*, 1968), 10% (*Castrup*, 1977), 12.8% (*Steenbeck* and *Wolff*, 1971), and 10.9% ± 0.7% (*Hansen* et al., 1977).

In addition to morphologic findings, our histoautoradiographic results have documented long-term alterations of proliferative activity and a considerable shifting of proliferative zones. This may explain the predisposition of anastomosed mucosal tissue, following Billroth I resection, for carcinoma development.

4. Chronology of Carcinogenesis Under Different Experimental Conditions

During our assay, the body weight of animals from all groups showed a uniform, steady development neglecting the influence of carcinogen application. Weight development correlated with carcinogen dosage which was scheduled to exclude differences in body weight between exposed and non-exposed animals. Thus, changes in body weight cannot be taken as an early parameter of beginning malignancy, since tumor development obviously precedes any marked alterations of weight in our animals.

The gastroenteroanastomosis had a mean circumference of 16 mm, as elicited from all animals of the assay. During the measurement of circumferences we found no case of stenosis caused by the surgical procedure. The size of the gastric remnant after resection was determined by the length of the reducing suture at the lesser curvature (mean value = 9 mm), and the largest distance between the forestomach and the gastroenteroanastomosis (mean = 14 mm). According to these data, each Billroth-I resection removed som 50% of the glandular stomach in the rats of our assay.

A comparative analysis of the groups during follow-up until week 21, and in later cross-sections at weeks 25, 33, 41, 50, and 104 (Tables 2 and 3) yielded only one significant difference with regard to carcinoma development and the exact date of its beginning. In week 25 when we killed 15 animals in each of the groups I and II, no carcinomas were found. The 15 animals sacrificed from Group II in week 33 and the 10 rats killed from group II in week 41 showed no carcinomas either.

After the assay had been carried over nearly 1 year, the carcinogen-exposed group II showed two carcinomas among 10 animals sacrificed at week 50. As late as 2 years after the start of the assay we were able to detect a number of carcinomas in all experimental groups. In carcinogen-exposed groups we found a carcinoma in one of six animals from group II. The group that had been exposed at a later stage of the assay (week 52, OP + late MNNG, group III) showed carcinomas in anastomosed mucosa in 10 of 15 animals.

It should be emphasized that, in addition to the carcinomas developed in carcinogen-exposed groups, we also found carcinomas in the resected but nonexposed groups. At the end of 2 years we found two carcinomas in three animals of group I (and three in seven nonexposed animals of group IV), all of them in the resected stomach. So far, such carcinomas in the gastric stump of nonexposed animals have not been reported by any other authors. This is probably due to the fact that no other assays have been carried out over so long a period, i.e., 2 years following surgery. We found an interesting publication in this context: *Ackermann* (1967) performed a fundus resection in 59 rats in order to examine its long-term effect on carcinoma development. His study was based on the fact that carcinomas frequently develop in patients with hypochlorhydria or achlorhydria. His idea was to eliminate the acid-forming portion of the stomach by resecting the fundus. Adenocarcinomas were induced in the glandular stomach of two of these 59 rats, one of them in the group receiving methylcholanthrene after the resection. The other carcinoma arose in an animal from the group receiving only 0.02 *M* HCl as drinking water after resection. *Ackermann*'s own interpretation of the results was that the 0.02 *M* HCl, which had been given in order to compensate for the deficient acid in the stomach, must have acted as a chronic irritant or even as a carcinogen on the sensitized achlorhydric stomach. Resection as a possible cause was not discussed.

Our findings – carcinomas developing 2 years after surgery even in nonexposed animals – are in accordance with the results of *Schlag* et al. (1977a). During 35 weeks follow-up after surgery these authors had observed adenomatous glandular proliferations, but no carcinomas. The most significant result seems to be that they found no difference between carcinogen-exposed and nonexposed animals as concerns the progress of morphologic changes.

Accordingly, our observations of carcinomas after 2 years follow-up in all groups suggest some relevant conclusions. Although the number of animals in our groups is too small for a statistical evaluation of the carcinoma yield, the results may serve to determine one common factor: the Billroth-I resection. Thus it must be that resection proper, given a sufficient interval after surgery, provokes the development of a carcinoma in the rat stomach. We have to bear in mind that spontaneous adenocarcinoma is a very rare finding in the glandular stomach of rats, both wild and domestic (*McCoy*, 1909; *Bullock* and *Curtis*, 1930; *Ratcliffe*, 1940; *Crain*, 1958; *Lindt*, 1968; *Wiebecke* and *Gokel*, 1975), and that our "spontaneous," i.e., nonexperimental carcinomas, have all been observed within anastomosed mucosal tissue.

The long post-operative interval required for carcinoma development in our nonexposed groups is highly suggestive of the situation in human gastric carcinogenesis. Usually, the average interval between gastric resection and evidence of carcinoma in the gastric remnant is about 20 years (*Peitsch* and *Burkhardt*, 1976; *Wolf* et al., 1977; *Domellöf* et al., 1977).

Carcinoma development in animals after Billroth-I resection has considerable bearing on the discussion of carcinogenesis in the human resected stomach. Obviously,

Billroth-I resection alone is apt to create an environment that favors the development of carcinomatous changes during a long postoperative period. The occurrence of carcinomas in our nonexposed group I (and IV) focused our interest on the resection and its sequela. The most important of these are (1) troubled tissue, (2) atrophy of specific gastric glands, and (3) gastroduodenal reflux.

1. "Troubled tissue" in the area of anastomosed mucosal tissues could be demonstrated through the whole assay. The surgical procedure implies severe local traumatization of the mucosa necessarily inducing structural changes, formation of scars on the resection level, and permanent irritation of traumatic mucosa by inadequate stimuli. Consequently, the anastomosed tissues will heal slowly and imperfectly or not at all. The "troubling" of tissues within anastomosed mucosa is impressively illustrated by our autoradiographic findings.

2. Atrophy of specific gastric glands in the anastomosis area was an early finding in all our groups, as reported in the discussion of anatomical changes in the anastomosed mucosal tissues (Fig. 3).

3. Beside anatomical restructuration and imbalance of the interaction between differentiation and proliferation (Fig. 27), the *gastroduodenal reflux* must be seen as an important pathogenetic factor for prolonged mucosal irritation (*Duplessis,* 1962; *Lawson,* 1964; *Rothmund,* 1977; *Schumpelick* et al., 1977). After human gastroduodenostomy, this reflux plays an important role insofar as the coordination of gastric closure and duodenal systole is severely impaired by the surgical intervention (*Schumpelick* et al., 1977). Naturally, the anastomosed mucosal tissues are most heavily affected by the reflux phenomena (*Gjeruldsen* et al., 1968; *Morgenstern* et al., 1973). Normally, the duodenal fluid contains, among other substances, bile acids and lysolecithin which are well-known detergents capable of breaking the mucosal barrier and affecting the lipid component of cell membranes (*Davenport,* 1967b; *Ivey* et al., 1970). Other compounds breaking the mucosal barrier are alcohol and salicylates. Alcoholic "damage" and salicylic damage to the mucosal barrier in the canine stomach were found to induce increased rediffusion of H^+ ions (*Davenport,* 1965, 1967a, b).

The influence of bile acids was shown to induce reproducible damage to the gastric mucosa (*Schumpelick,* 1975). In addition to bile acids, the intragastral concentration of lysolecithin is an important factor (*Johnson* and *McDermott,* 1974; *Clemencon,* 1976). The cytotoxic potential of lysolecithin may provoke the destruction of cell membranes in mucosal epithelia, and may break down the difference between intravascular, interstitial, and intragastral concentration of hydrogen ions (*Davenport,* 1968). Evidence for the in vitro transformation of bile acids – via physiological desoxycholic acid and other intermediates – to methyl cholanthren, a well-known carcinogen, was collected in some other studies (*Dannenberg,* 1958).

In contrast to the nonexposed group I (and IV, partly) of our assay manifesting carcinoma development after 2 years, group II which was exposed to carcinogen during the first 24 weeks of the assay, yielded the first two carcinomas after nearly 1 year. Thus, the effect of the rather low carcinogenic dose relates only to the date, but not to the number or to the morphology of subsequently developing carcinomas.

It is interesting to compare the groups II and III, i.e., early and late exposure to the carcinogen. Despite the different onsets of exposure, both groups received the same total dosage and both were maintained at a similar interval between carcinogen cessation and sacrifice, i.e., about 25 weeks. In group II, two animals had developed carcinomas at week 50, whereas 10 carcinomas were found in the 15 animals of group III at week 104. Evidently it is the extended postoperative interval which alters the result of an otherwise identical schedule of carcinogen exposure. Corresponding findings have not been presented from other experimental studies. The comparison serves to emphasize the decisive roles of the resection and of the postoperative period in the development of anastomosis carcinoma.

5. Conclusion

The five questions posed in the introduction, may now be answered as follows:

1. Experimental carcinoma in the Billroth-I resected stomach may develop via two histologic precursors with corresponding prestages, characterized by different grades of glandular dysplasia. One pathway of carcinogenesis proceeds via adenomatous polyps to fully developed polypous adenocarcinoma (Fig. 31); the other via adenocystic gland proliferations to primarily serosa-oriented (endophytic) anastomosis carcinoma (Fig. 32).

2. The enzyme histochemical methods used in our study, are not completely adequate for the safe identification of prestages of gastric stump carcinoma: The changes in localization and activity of enzymes, as seen in or near the anastomosis, are not only observed in preneoplastic and neoplastic cells, but also within benign glandular regeneration.

3. The problem of chronic atrophic gastritis and its possible pathogenetic influence on the development of gastric stump carcinoma cannot be definitely solved by the results of our material. Gastritic manifestations, even without dysplasia or carcinomatous transformation, were constantly associated with all anastomosed areas of the mucosa.

4. Prolonged alterations, i.e., predominant increase of proliferative activity and an extensive displacement of the proliferative zone, are found in anastomosed mucosal tissue as a result of severe imbalance between differentiation and proliferation. This must be interpreted as an important pathogenetic factor in the development of anastomosis carcinoma.

5. The accumulated evidence that carcinomas consistently take their origin from the anastomotic site and that they also occur in nonexposed animals suggests that Billroth-I gastric resection must itself be an important risk factor for the development of anastomosis carcinoma.

V. General Implications and Deductions

Experimental induction of carcinomas by N-methyl-N'-nitro-N-nitrosoguanidine is possible not only in the normal galndular stomach of the rat (*Sugimura* et al., 1969; *Saito* et al., 1970; *Bralow,* 1972; *Uchida* et al., 1976), but also in the resected stomach (*Dahm* and *Werner,* 1973; *Schlag* et al., 1977a; *Rumpf* et al., 1978). It was, however, not known that carcinomas can be induced in the resected rat stomach by Billroth-I surgery alone (i.e., without carcinogen application).

The present extensive studies show for the first time that the mere trauma of Billroth-I surgery can suffice to promote carcinoma in anastomosed mucosal tissue. This holds good in gastroenteroanastomosis, as well as in gastro-gastric junctions (i.e., in the reducing suture at the lesser curvature). Obviously the nature of the basic disease originally causing the necessity of gastric resection is of little relevance to gastric carcinogenesis since the rats operated in our assay had no previous history of stomach disease.

In those animals only subjected to Billroth-I surgery without other treatment, resulting tissue troubles and gastroduodenal reflux were identified as the only possible causes for carcinoma development. Consequently, these are the factors which might offer an approach for eliminating the "damaging" effects of gastric surgery, at least partially.

Tissue troubles and their sequelae caused by surgical intervention can be reduced by an adequate surgical technique when performing the anastomosis (*Schönleben* et al., 1979). This requires, in particular, the use of completely resorbable suture material (polyglycolic acid) in order to keep foreign body irritation and reaction as limited as possible (such as suture abscesses and granulomas); the displacement of mucosal tissue into deeper layers of the wall by way of permanent suture sheathing must be carefully avoided. A further postulate, careful adaptation of the corresponding wall layers on the gastral as well as on the duodenal level avoids, or at least reduces, tissue troubles. The lumina of both organs must be most carefully matched in size and circumference to prevent one-sided folding, shrinking, or stretching when the sutures are closed.

Gastroduodenal reflux can also be avoided or limited by modified surgical techniques. Some true clinical alternatives are seen in Billroth-I with isoperistaltic interposition of a defunctionalized jejunal loop, or in retrocolic Billroth-II surgery with gastroenterostomy performed after Roux' Y-method (*Bünte,* 1976). Experimental investigation of these techniques has shown that the significant increase of intragastral bile acid and lysolecithin concentration (after direct Billroth-I gastroduodenostomy) can be effectively limited according to the length of the interposed jejunal loop (*Schumpelick* et al., 1977).

The postoperative interval of 104 weeks was demonstrated to be long enough to imitate human conditions, which means that in experimental animals, as well as in man, the risk of developing gastric stump carcinoma increases with the postoperative duration. This interval between surgery and development of anastomosis carcinoma may be shortened (under experimental conditions) by certain factors. Carcinogen application has a direct effect by accelerating the malignant transformation of gastric mucosal epithelia. Another direct pathway is modulation of the immune surveillance. Both may provide some explanation for the great variation in postoperative intervals of human patients. Morphologic studies have elicited another aspect. The criteria of "early gastric carcinoma," established for carcinomas in the non-resected human stomach, are not applicable to carcinoma arising in an anastomosis because the definition is strictly correlated with the intact anatomical architecture of the gastric wall. Consequently, the identification or definition of early gastric carcinoma in anastomosed mucosal tissue, in analogy to the non-resected stomach, appears neither possible nor meaningful. On the other hand, it is of the highest importance that the carcinoma in the resected stomach be detected as early as possible, i.e., in a stage of minimal extension. We have to remember that in an anastomosed mucosa in general structural disarray, carcinomas may arise even in those small mucosal complexes that have been surgically dislodged and transported to the deeper strata of the wall. This might explain why certain anastomosis carcinomas are never detected by endoscopy or, if at all, then only at a very advanced stage. Allowing for the necessary caution when experimental findings are transferred to clinical problems, we might venture the following interpretation:

Our results have demonstrated that Billroth-I surgery is in itself a provocation for cancerogenic predisposition, i.e., Billroth-I resection must be viewed as a risk for carcinoma development in the gastric stump. Practical interferences would suggest regular check-ups in the follow-up of all resected patients. Examination should include combined gastroscopy and biopsy, the latter being made along anastomosed mucosal areas in conjunction with a prescribed schedule and in close cooperation with the endoscopist.

VI. Summary

The histogenesis of carcinomas in the resected stomach was studied with light microscopic, enzyme histochemical, and autoradiographic methods in the following experimental assay: In a total of 400 Wistar rats, 356 animals were subjected to gastric resection with subsequent gastroduodenostomy Billroth-I. Animals surviving the 5th week after surgery were divided into four groups. Group I was left without further treatment. Group II was given the carcinogen N-methyl-N'-nitro-N-nitrosoguanidine (MNNG) in its drinking water for 6 months, starting the 6th week after surgery. Group III was treated with MNNG following the same schedule as group II, but the exposure started as late as 1 year after surgery. Group IV was subjected to an additional treatment with antilymphocyte globulin with or without carcinogen exposure. The results will be published separately. In each of the groups I and II (and IV), 10–15 animals were sacrificed at fixed intervals until week 50 of the assay. Fifteen animals of group III, and all surviving animals of the other groups, were sacrificed in the 104th week, i.e., 2 years postoperatively. In group I (OP), carcinomas were only at the latest stage, week 104. In group II (OP + early MNNG) carcinomas were already found in week 50. Of the 15 animals from group III (OP + late MNNG) sacrificed during week 104, 10 had developed a carcinoma.

Carcinoma development in the Billroth-I resected stomach can be shown to follow two pathways via precursors and prestages that may be identified and differentiated by their degree of glandular dysplasia. One pathway is via adenomatous anastomotic polyps to fully developed polypous anastomosis carcinoma; the other via adenocystic gland proliferation to the serosa-oriented, endophytic anastomosis carcinoma.

The prestages of these carcinomas in the resected stomach are not adequately identified by the histochemical methods used in our assay; the observed changes in enzyme localization and activity occurred not only in preneoplastic or neoplastic tissues, but also in benign glandular regeneration. Chronic atrophic gastritis was commonly found, and constantly associated with, all anastomosed mucosal tissues, even those without dysplasia or carcinomatous transformation.

Prolonged alterations in terms of enhanced proliferation and massive shifting or displacing of proliferative zones were found in anastomosed mucosa as a result of severe imbalance in the interactions between differentiation and proliferation. These alterations must be seen as an important pathogenetic factor in the development of anstomosis carcinoma in the Billroth-I resected stomach.

The finding that carcinomas arise in anastomosed mucosal tissues, in carcinogen-exposed, and in nonexposed animals highlights the risk involved in Billroth-I surgery and the necessity to minimize or prevent conditions predisposing for malignant transformation. Improved and modified techniques and careful follow-up should help to decrease the risk.

References

Ackermann, N.B.: Fundic resection in rats and its long term effect on development of gastric cancer. Gastroenterology *53,* 280–287 (1967)

D'Altorio, R.A.: Calcification in a gastric mucinous adenocarcinoma. Dig. Dis. *18,* 419–422 (1973)

Baillie, E.E., Abell, M.R.: Enteritis cystica polyposa. Am. J. Clin. Pathol. *54,* 643–649 (1970)

Baroni, C.D., Scelsi, R., Peronace, M.L., Uccini, S.: Heterologous antilymphocyte serum hastens the growth of 7,12 Dimethylbenzanthracene induced tumors in mice. Br. J. Cancer *28,* 221–226 (1973)

Becker, V.: Pathologische Anatomie des resezierten Magens. In: Magenoperation und Magenoperierter. Bartelheimer, H., Maurer, H.J., Schreiber, H.W., Müller-Wieland, K. (eds.), pp. 135–167. Berlin: de Gruyter 1969

Boller, R.: Der operierte Magen. Wien: Urban und Schwarzenberg 1947

Boxler, K.: Autoradiographische Bestimmung des Generationszeitzyklus von 1,2-Dimethylhydrazin-induzierten Adenokarzinomen des Rattenkolon. Inaugural-Dissertation zur Erlangung der Doktorwürde in der gesamten Medizin. Aus dem Pathologischen Institut der Universität München, 1972

Bralow, S.P.: Experimental gastric carcinogenesis. Digestion *5,* 290–310 (1972)

Brown, C.A.: The cytochemical demonstration of β-glucoronidase in colon neoplasms of rats exposed to azoxymethane. J. Histochem. Cytochem. *26,* 22–27 (1978)

Brückner, R., Kempf, P.: Zur Früherfassung des Ulkuskarzinoms des Magens (In vitro-Untersuchungen mit H^3-Thymidin). Aktuelle Gastrologie *6 (2),* 163–167 (1977)

Bünte, H.: Persönliche Mitteilung (1976)

Bullock, F.D., Curtis, M.R.: Spontaneous tumors of the rat. Cancer Res. *16,* 1–115 (1930)

Burstone, M.S.: Histochemical comparison of naphtol AS-phosphates for the demonstration of phosphatases. J. Natl. Cancer Inst. *20,* 601–615 (1958)

Burstone, M.S.: Enzyme histochemistry and its application in the study of neoplasms. New York, London: Academic Press 1968

Burstone, M.S., Keyes, P.H.: Studies on calcification. I. The effect of inhibition of enzyme activity on developing bone and dentin. Am. J. Pathol. *33,* 1229–1235 (1957)

Castrup, H.J.: Proliferationskinetische Studien bei chronischer Gastritis und Magenkarzinom. Aktuelle Gastrologie *6 (2),* 151–158 (1977)

Cerilli, G.J., Treat, R.C.: The effect of antilymphocyte serum on the adult mouse. Transplantation *8,* 774–782 (1969)
Chakravorty, R.C., Schatzki, P.F.: Gastric cystic polyposis. Am. J. Dig. Dis. *20,* 981–989 (1975)
Clemençon, G., Baumgartner, R., Leuthold, E., Miller, G., Neiger, A.: Das Karzinom des operierten Magens. Dtsch. Med. Wochenschr. *101,* 1015–1020 (1976)
Crain, R.C.: Spontaneous tumors in the Rochester Strain of Wistar rat. Am. J. Pathol. *34 (1),* 311–335 (1958)
Dahm, K., Werner, B.: Experimentelles Anastomosencarcinom. Ein Beitrag zur Pathogenese des Magenstumpfcarcinoms. Langebecks Arch. Chir. *333,* 211–236 (1973)
Dannenberg, H.: Über die endogene Krebsentstehung. Dtsch. Med. Wochenschr. *83,* 1726–1731 (1958)
Davenport, H.W.: Damage to the gastric mucosa: effects of salicylates and stimulation. Gastroenterology *49/2,* 189–196 (1965)
Davenport, H.W.: Ethanol damage to canine oxyntic glandular mucosa. Proc. Soc. Exp. Biol. *126,* 657–662 (1967a)
Davenport, H.W.: Salicylate damage to the gastric mucosal barrier. N. Engl. J. Med. *276,* 1307–1312 (1967b)
Davenport, H.W.: Destruction of the gastric mucosal barrier by detergents and urea. Gastroenterology *54,* 175–181 (1968)
Davis, B.J., Ornstein, L.: High resolution enzyme localization with a new diazo reagent, "hexazonium paraosaniline". J. Histochem. Cytochem. *7,* 297–298 (1959)
Dent, P.B., Fish, L.A., White, J.G., Good, R.A.: Chediak-Higashi syndrome. Observations on the nature of the associated malignancy. Lab. Invest. *15,* 1634–1642 (1966)
Domelöff, L., Eriksson, S., Helander, H.F., Janunger, K.-G.: Lipid islands in the gastric mucosa after resection for benign ulcer disease. Gastroenterology *72,* 14–18 (1977)
Druckrey, H., Preussmann, R., Ivankovic, S., Schmähl, D., unter Mitarbeit von Afkham, J., Blum, G., Mennel, H.D., Müller, M., Petropoulos, P., Schneider, H.: Organotrope carcinogene Wirkungen bei 65 verschiedenen N-Nitrose-Verbindungen an BD-Ratten. Z. Krebsforsch. *69,* 103–201 (1967)
Du Plessis, D.J.: Gastric mucosal changes after operations on the stomach. South Afr. Med. J. *34,* 101–108 (1962)
Eastwood, G.L.: Progress in Gastroenterology. Gastrointestinal Epithelial Renewal. Gastroenterology *72,* 962–975 (1977)
Eder, M.: Neuere morphologische Aspekte der Magen-Darm-Tumoren. In: Fortschritte der Krebsforschung. Schmidt, C.G., Walter, O. (eds.), pp. 119–127. Stuttgart, New York: Schattauer 1969
Eid, M., Rohde, E.: Fibroplasia osteoplastica post oerationem – eine seltene Komplikation bei Magenresektionen nach Billroth II. Zentralbl. Chir. *103,* 182–184 (1978)
Elster, K., Eidt, H., Ottenjann, R., Rösch, W., Seifert, E.: Drüsenkörperzysten, eine polypoide Läsion der Magenschleimhaut. Dtsch. Med. Wochenschr. *102,* 183–187 (1977)
Epstein, S.E., Ascari, W.Q., Ablow, R.C., Seaman, W.B., Lattes, R.: Colitis Cystica Profunda. Am. J. Clin. Pathol. *45,* 186–201 (1966)
Fishman, W.H., Baker, J.R., Borges, R.F.: Localization of β-glucuronidas in some human tumors. Cancer *12,* 240–245 (1959)
Fishman, W.H., Bigelow, R.: A comparative study of the morphology and glucuronidase activity in 44 gastrointestinal neoplasm.s J. Natl. Cancer Inst. *10,* 1115–1122 (1950)
Fujita, M., Taguchi, T., Takami, M., Usugane, M., Takahashi, A., Shiba, S.: Carcinoma and related lesions in dog stomach induced by oral administration of N-methyl-N'-nitro-N-nitrosoguanidine. Gann *65,* 207–214 (1974)
Gjeruldsen, S.T., Myren, J., Fretheim, B.: Alterations of gastric mucosa following a graded partial gastrectomy for duodenal ulcer. Scand. J. Gastroenterol. *3,* 465–470 (1968)
Gohrband, G., Krentz, K.: Drüsenkörperzysten der Magenschleimhaut. – Ein neuer gastroenterologischer Begriff. Leber Magen Darm *7,* 58–61 (1977)

Grafe, W., Thorbjarnarson, B., Pearce, J.M., Beal, J.M.: Benign neoplasms of stomach. Am. J. Surg. *100*, 561–569 (1960)

Griffel, B., Engleberg, M., Reiss, R.: Multiple polypoid cystic gastritis in old gastroenteric stoma. Arch. Pathol. *97*, 316–318 (1974)

Grundmann, E.: Histologic types and possible initial stages in early gastric carcinoma. Histologische Typen und mögliche Vorstadien des Magen-Frühkarzinoms. Beitr. Pathol. *154*, 256–280 (1975)

Grundmann, E., Schlake, W.: Sonderformen des Magen-Frühkarzinoms und ihre möglichen Vorformen. Vortrag anläßlich des X. International Magen-Symposions in Berlin, 10.–12. Mai 1978

Gschnitzer, F.: Magenstumpfkarzinom. 144. Tagung der Vereinigung Niederrheinisch-Westfälischer Chirurgen in Essen, 6.–8. Oktober 1977

Hamperl, H.: Praecancerose und Carcinoma in situ. In: Handbuch der Allgemeinen Pathologie. Grundmann, E. (ed.), Vol. VI/5, pp. 350–415. Berlin, Heidelberg, New York: Springer 1974

Hansen, O.H., Johansen, A.A., Larsen, J.K., Pedersen, T., Svendsen, L.B.: Relationship between gastric acid secretion, histo-pathology, and cell proliferation kinetics in human gastric mucosa. Gastroenterology *73*, 453–456 (1977)

Hayashi, M., Nakajima, Y., Fishman, W.H.: The cytologic demonstration of β-glucuronidase employing naphtol AS-B glucuronide and hexazonium pararosanilin; a preliminary report. J. Histochem. Cytochem. *12*, 293–297 (1964)

Henning, N.: Über die Grenzen der Diagnostik des Magenkarzinoms. Münch. Med. Wochenschr. *108*, 293–300 (1966)

Howell, S.B., Dean, J.H., Esber, E.C., Law, L.W.: Cell interactions in adoptive immune rejection of a syngeneic tumor. Int. J. Cancer *14*, 662–674 (1974)

Hunt, T.E.: Mitotic activity in the gastric mucosa of the rat after fasting and refeeding. Anat. Rec. *127*, 539–550 (1957)

Ignatius, J.A., Armstrong, C.D., Eversole, S.L.: Multiple diffuse cystic disease of the stomach in association with carcinoma. Gastroenterology *59*, 610–614 (1970)

Ito, S., Winchester, R.J.: The fine structure of the gastric mucosa in the rat. J. Cell Biol. *16*, 541–577 (1963)

Ivey, K.J., Den Besten, L., Clifton, J.A.: Effect of bile salts on ionic movement across the human gastric mucosa. Gastroenterology *59*, 683–690 (1970)

Iwanaga, T., Koyama, H., Takahashi, Y., Taniguchi, H., Wada, A.: Diffuse submucosal cysts and carcinoma of the stomach. Cancer *36*, 606–614 (1975)

Jacobsen, N.O., Jorgensen, F.: Further enzyme histochemical observations on the segmentaction of the proximal tubules in the kidney of the male rat. Histochemistry *34*, 11–32 (1973)

Johnson, A.G., McDermott, J.S.: Lysolecithin: a factor in the pathogenesis of gastric ulceration? Gut *15*,710–713 (1974)

Justrabo, E., Martin, M.S., Michiels, R., Martin, F., Bastien, H., Knopf, J.F., Cabanne, F.: Experimental gastro-intestinal neoplasma and hepatic cysts in rats induced by N-methyl-N'-nitro-N-nitrosoguanidine. Pathol. Eur. *10*, 61–71 (1975)

Klein, H.O., Lennartz, K.J., Gross, R., Eder, M., Fischer, R.: In-vivo- und In-vitro-Untersuchungen zur Zellkinetik und Synchronisation menschlicher Tumorzellen. Dtsch. Med. Wochenschr. *97*, 1273–1282 (1972)

Kobayashi, S., Prolla, J.C., Kirsner, J.B.: Late gastric carcinoma developing after surgery for benign conditions. Am. J. Dig. Dis. *15*, 905–912 (1970)

Kobori, O., Gedigk, P., Totovic, V.: Early changes of glandular stomach in Wistar rats ingesting N-methyl-N'-nitro-N-nitrosoguanidine (MNNG): With special reference to light microscopic, electron microscopic and enzyme histochemical study of the regenerating epithelium induced by MNNG. Z. Krebsforsch. *87*, 127–138 (1976)

Kobori, O., Oota, K.: Mucous substance and enzyme histochemistry of nonneoplastic and neoplastic gastric epithelium in man. Acta Pathol. Jpn. *24*, 119–130 (1974)

Kohli, Y., Hashimoto, Y., Takeda, S., Kawai, K.: Cell kinetics of gastric carcinoma and other gastric lesions in rats by N-methyl-N'-nitro-N-nitrosoguanidine with or without Tween 60. Gann *66,* 133–140 (1975)

Kondstaal, J., Makkink, B., Overdiep, S.H.: Enzyme histochemical patterns in human tumors. 1. Hydrolytic enzymes in carcinomas of the colon and the breast. Eur. J. Cancer *11,* 105–110 (1975)

Konjetzny, G.E.: Der Magenkrebs. Stuttgart: Enke 1938

Krentz, K.: Gastroskopische und saugbioptische Befunde am operierten Magen. Dtsch. Med. Wochenschr. *89/II,* 664–671 (1964)

Kuru, M.: Pathophysiologie und Früherkennung des Magenkrebses. Münch. Med. Wochenschr. *108,* 737–747 (1966)

Lawson, H.H.: Effect of duodenal contents of the gastric mucosa under experimental conditions. Lancet *1964 I,* 469–472

Lev, R., Howard I. S, Jerzy Glass, G.B.: The enzyme histochemistry of gastric carcinoma in man. Cancer *5,* 1086–1093 (1969)

Levy, G.A., Kerr, L.M.H., Campbell, J.G.: β-Glucuronidase and cell proliferation. Biochem. J. *42,* 462–468 (1948)

Liavag, I.: Mitotic activity of gastric mucosa. Acta Pathol. Microbiol. Scand. *72,* 43–63 (1968)

Lindt, S.: Magen. In: Handbuch der speziellen pathologischen Anatomie der Haustiere. Dobberstein, J., Pallaske, G., Stünzi, H. (eds.), Vol. V/1, pp. 409–526. Berlin, Hamburg: Parey 1968

Lipkin, M.: Cell proliferation in the gastrointestinal tract of man. Fed. Proc. *24,* 10–15 (1965)

Littler, E.R., Gleibermann, E.: Gastritis cystica polyposa. Cancer *29,* 205–209 (1972)

Lojda, Z., Gossrau, R., Schiebler, T.H.: Enzymhistochemische Methoden. Berlin, Heidelberg, New York: Springer 1976

Lojda, Z., Havrankova, E., Slaby, J.: Histochemical demonstration of intestinal hetero-β-galactosidase (glucosidase). Histochemistry *42,* 271–286 (1974)

Lojda, Z., Ploeg, M. van der, Duijn, P. van: Phosphates of the naphtol AS series in the quantitative determination of alkaline and acid phosphataseactivities "in situ" studied in polyacrylamide membrane model system and by cytospectrophotometry. Histochemie *11,* 13–23 (1967)

Lushbaugh, C.C.: Infiltrating adenomatous lesions of the stomach, cecum, and rectum of monkeys similar to early human carcinoma in situ. Cancer Res. *9,* 385–394 (1949)

MacDonald, W.C., Trier, J.S., Everett, N.B.: Cell proliferation and migration in the stomach, duodenum, and rectum of man: radioautographic studies. Gastroenterology *46,* 405–417 (1964)

McCluskey, R.T., Bhan, A.K.: Cell-mediated reaction in vivo. In: Mechanisms of tumor immunity. Green, I., Cohen, St., McCluskey, R.T. (eds.), pp. 1–25. New York: Wiley & Sons 1977

McCoy, G.W.: A preliminary report on tumours found in wild rats. J. Med. Res. *16,* 285–296 (1909)

McGinty, F., Delides, G., Harrison, D.: The significance of enzyme histochemical patterns in carcinomas of the large intestine in man. Gut *14,* 502–505 (1973)

Meijer, A.E.F.H.: Semipermeable membranes for improving the histochemical demonstration of enzyme activities in tissues sections. I. Acid Phosphatase. Histochemie *30,* 31–39 (1972)

Meijer, A.E.F.H., Vloedman, A.H.T.: Semipermeable membranes for improving the histochemical demonstration of enzyme activities in tissue sections. II. Nonspecific esterase and β-glucuronidase. Histochemie *34*, 127–134 (1973)

Messier, B., Leblond, C.P.: Cell proliferation and migration as revealed by radioautography after injection of thymidine-H^3 into male rats. and mice. Am. J. Anat. *106,* 247–284 (1960)

Ming, S., Goldman, H.: Gastric Polyps. Cancer *18,* 721–726 (1965)
Morgenstern, L., Tatsuo Yamakawa, Seltzer, D.: Carcinoma of the gastric stump. Am. J. Surg. *125,* 29–38 (1973)
Muto, T., Bussey, H.J.R., Morson, B.C.: Pseudo-carcinomatous invasion in adenomatous polyps of the colon and rectum. J. Clin. Pathol. *26,* 25–31 (1973)
Nachlas, M.M., Monis, B., Rosenblatt, Seligman, A.M.: Improvement in the histochemical localization of leucine aminopeptidase with a new substrate, L-leucyl-4-methoxy-2-naphthylamide. J. Biophys. Biochem. Cytology *7,* 261–264 (1960)
Nakamura, T.: Pathohistologische Einteilung der Magenpolypen mit spezifischer Betrachtung ihrer malignen Entartung. Chirurg *41,* 122–130 (1970)
Nikolai, N., Müller, D.: Das klinische und pathologisch-anatomische Bild der Gastritis cystica. Bruns' Beitr. Klin. Chir. *210,* 367–378 (1965)
Nomura, K., Schlake, W., Grundmann, E.: New aspects of intestinal carcinogenesis by 1,2-dimethyl-hydrazine dichloride (DMH) and the influence of Anti-Lymphocyte globulin (ALG) on its progress. Z. Krebsforsch. *92,* 17–34 (1978)
Oberman, H.A., Lodmell, J.G., Sower, N.D.: Diffuse heterotopic cystic malformation of the stomach. N. Engl. J. Med. *269,* 909–911 (1963)
Oehlert, W.: Regeneration, Hyperplasie und Cancerisierung am Beispiel der epithelialen Wechselgewebe. In: Handbuch der Allgemeinen Pathologie. Bücher, F. (ed.), Vol. 6/II, pp. 244–374. Berlin, Heidelberg, New York: Springer 1969
Oehlert, W.: Cellular proliferation in carcinogenesis. Cell. Tissue Kinet. *6,* 325–335 (1973)
Oehlert, W.: Klinische Pathologie des Magen-Darm-Traktes. Histologische Diagnose und Differentialdiagnose am gastroenterologischen Biopsiematerial. Stuttgart, New York: Schattauer 1978
Oehlert, W., Keller, P., Henke, M., Strauch, M.: Die Dysplasie der Magenschleimhaut. Dtsch. Med. Wochenschr. *100,* 1950–1956 (1975)
Padykula, H.A., Strauss, E.W., Ladman, A.J., Gardner, F.H.: A morphological and histochemical analysis of the human jejunal epithelium in nontropical sprue. Gastroenterology *40,* 735–765 (1961)
Pearse, A.G.E.: Histochemistry, theoretical and applied. Vol. 2. Edinburgh, London: Churchill Livingstone 1972
Peitsch, W., Burkhardt, K.: Zur Pathogenese und Klinik des Magenstumpfcarcinoms. Langenbecks Arch. Chir. *341,* 195–203 (1976)
Pillay, I., Petrelli, M.: Diffuse cystic glandular malformation of the stomach associated with adenocarcinoma. Cancer *38,* 915–920 (1976)
Planteydt, H.T., Willighagen, R.G.J.: Enzyme histochemistry of the human stomach, with special reference to intestinal metaplasia. J. Pathol. Bacteriol. *80,* 317–323 (1960)
Planteydt, H.T., Willighagen, R.G.J.: Enzyme histochemistry of gastric carcinoma. J. Pathol. Bacteriol. *90,* 393–398 (1965)
Qizilbash, A.H.: Gastritis cystica and carcinoma arising in old gastrojejunostomy stomach. Can. Med. Assoc. J. *112,* 1432–1433 (1975)
Rabbat, A.G., Jeejeebhoy, H.F.: Heterologous antilymphocyte serum (ALS) hastens the appearance of methylcholanthrene-induced tumours in mice. Transplantation *9,* 164–166 (1970)
Raekallio, J.: Histochemical studies on vital and postmortem skin wounds. Experimental investigation on medicolegally significant vital reactions in an early phase of wound healing. Ann. Med. Exp. Biol. Fenn. *39,* Suppl. 6, 1–105 (1961)
Raekallio, J.: Histochemical demonstration of enzymatic response to injury in experimental skin wounds. Exp. Mol. Pathol. *4,* 303–310 (1965a)
Raekallio, J.: Die Altersbestimmung mechanisch bedingter Hautwunden mit enzymhistochemischen Methoden. Lübeck: Schmidt-Römhild 1965b
Rajewsky, M.F.: Zellproliferation in normalen und malignen Geweben: H^3-Thymidin-Einbau in vitro unter Standardbedingungen. Biophysik *3,* 65–93 (1966)

Ratcliffe, H.L.: Spontaneous tumors in two colonies of rats of the "Wistar Institute of Anatomoy and Biology." Am. J. Pathol. *16*, 237–254 (1940)

Rösch, W., Elster, K.: Gastrointestinale Präkanzerosen. Baden-Baden, Brüssel, Köln, New York: Witzstrock 1977

Rosenow, J.H., McDonald, J.R.: The histology and histopathology of the gastroenteric stoma with especial reference to gastrojejunitis. Gastroenterology *2*, 161–179 (1944)

Rothmund, M.: Duodenogastrischer Reflux. Z. Gastroenterol. *15*, 192–201 (1977)

Rothmund, M.G., Deisler, A., Kaufmann, A., Höhn, P.: Duodenogastrischer Reflux nach Vagotomie und Pyloroplastik. Langenbecks Arch. Chir. *340*, 167–178 (1976)

Rumpf, P., Schacht, U., Palomba, P., Kremer, K., Schmitz, H., Borchard, F.: Chemisch induzierte Karzinogenese des Rattenmagens nach Vagotomie und Resektion. Z. Gastroenterol. *16*, 85–94 (1978)

Saegesser, F., Jämes, D.: Cancer of the gastric stump after partial gastrectomy (Billroth II principle) for ulcer. Cancer *29*, 1150–1159 (1972)

Saito, T., Inokuchi, K., Takayama, S., Sugimura, T.: Sequential morphological changes in N-methyl-N'-nitro-N-nitrosoguanidine in the glandular stomach of rats. J. Natl. Cancer Inst. *44*, 769–783 (1970)

Schauer, A., Kunze, E., Ober, M.: "Early carcinoma" des Magens im Tierexperiment. Deutscher Krebskongress, München, Februar 1974

Schlag, P., Meister, H., Feyerabend, G., Merkle, P.: Der Einfluß des duodenogastrischen Refluxes auf das Epithel an der gastroenteralen Anastomose. Langenbecks Arch. Chir. *344*, 207–217 (1977)

Schlag, P., Wonka, W., Meyer, H., Feyerabend, G., Merkle, P.: Bakterielle Besiedlung und Nitritbildung im Magen nach Gastroenterostomie. Langenbecks Arch. Chir. *344*, 109–114 (1977a)

Schmidt, A.J.: Cellular biology of vertebrate regeneration and repair. Part 4. Chicago: University of Chicago Press 1968

Schönleben, K., Langhans, P., Schlake, W., Kautz, G., Bünte, H.: Zur Prophylaxe des Magenstumpfkarzinoms. Acta Hepatogastroenterol. (in press) (1979)

Schumpelick, V.: Der Einfluß der Galle auf das Stressulkus der Ratte. Langenbecks Arch. Chir. *338*, 265–274 (1975)

Schumpelick, V., Begemann, F., Grossner, D., Lauchart, Kessler, G.: Gastroduodenostomie und duodenogastraler Reflux. Langenbecks Arch. Chir. *344*, 179–188 (1977)

Scott, H.W., Payne, T.P.B.: Diffuse congenital cystic hyperplasia of stomach clinically simulating carcinoma – Report of a case. Bull. Johns Hopkins Hosp. *81*, 448–455 (1947)

Scotti, T.M.: Simian gastropathy with submucosal glands and cysts. Arch. Pathol. *96*, 403–408 (1973)

Seelig, L.L., Winborn, W.B., Weser, E.: Changes in gastric glandular cell kinetics after small bowel resection in the rat. Gastroenterology *74*, 1–6 (1978)

Shearer, W.T., Fink, M.P.: Immune surveillance system: Its failure and activation. Prog. Hematol. *10*, 247–310 (1977)

Sherman, F.G., Quastler, H.: DNA synthesis in irradiated intestinal epithelium. Exp. Cell. Res. *19*, 343–360 (1960)

Siegel, H.I., Lev, R., Glass, G.B.J.: Enzyme histochemistry of chronic atrophic gastritis. Am. J. Dig. Dis. *13*, 974–986 (1968)

Siurala, M.: Chronische Gastritis und Magenkarzinom. Bioptische Untersuchungen. Zentralbl. Chir. *90*, 1472–1478 (1965)

Siurala, M.: Atrophic gastritis: A possible precancerous condition. Neoplasma *21*, 253 (1974)

Stalsberg, H., Taksdal, S.: Stomach cancer following gastric surgery for benign conditions. Lancet *1971 II*, 1175–1177

Steenbeck, L., Wolff, G.: Histoautoradiographische Untersuchungen der menschlichen Magenschleimhaut bei chronischer Gastritis und Magenkarzinom. Arch. Geschwulstforsch. *38/2*, 132–138 (1971)

Stevens, C.E., Leblond, C.P.: Renewal of the mucous cells in the gastric mucosa of the rat. Anat. Rec. *115*, 231–245 (1953)

Stewart, H.L.: Experimentally induced gastric adenocarcinomas. Lab. Invest. *25*, 672–674 (1971)

St. John, D.J.B., Yeomans, N.D., Bourne, C.A.J., Boer, W.G.R.N.: Aspirin-induced glandular dysplaisa of the stomach. Arch. Pathol. Lab. Med. *101*, 44–48 (1977)

Strickland, R.G., Mackay, I.R.: A reappraisal of the nature and significance of chronic atrophic gastritis. Am. J. Dig. Dis. *18*, 426–440 (1973)

Sugimura, T.S., Fujimura, S.: Tumor production in glandular stomach of rat by N-methyl-N'-nitro-N-nitrosoguanidine. Nature *216*, 943–944 (1967)

Sugimura, T., Fujimura, S., Kogure, K., Baba, T., Saito, T., Nagao, M., Hosoi, H., Shimosato, Y., Yokoshima, T.: Production of adenocarcinomas in glandular stomach of experimental animals by N-methyl-N'-nitro-N-nitrosoguanidine. Gann Monographs *8*, 157–196 (1969)

Tanaka, J.: Autoradiographic studies on the cell proliferation the human gastric mucosa in supravital condition. Acta Pathol. Jpn. *18 (3)*, 307–318 (1968)

Taub, R.N., Deutsch, V.: Antilymphocyte serum. Pharmacol. Ther. A *2*, 89–111 (1977)

Tchertkoff, V., Wagner, M.B.: Diffuse cystic malformation of stomach. N.Y. State J. Med. *66*, 2049–2052 (1966)

Teir, H., Räsänen, T.: A study of mitotic rate in renewal zone of nondiseased portions of gastric mucosa in cases of peptic ulcer and gastric cancer, with observations on differentiation and so-called "Intestinalization" of gastric mucosa. J. Natl. Cancer Inst. *27*, 949–971 (1961)

Thomas, E., Pearse, A.G.E.: The fine localization of dehydrogenases in the nervous system. Histochemie *2*, 266–282 (1961)

Tomasulo, J.: Gastric polyps. Cancer *27*, 1346–1355 (1971)

Trainin, N., Linker-Israeli, M.: Influence of immunorestoration on the formation of urethan-induced lung adenomas. J. Natl. Cancer Inst. *44*, 893–900 (1970)

Trier, J.S.: Morphological alterations induced by methotrexate in mucosa of human proximal intestine: 1. Serial observations by light microscopy. Gastroenterology *42*, 295–305 (1962)

Uchida, Y., Schlake, W., Roessner, A., Rühland, D., Themann, H., Grundmann, E.: Development of tumors in the glandular stomach of rats after oral administration of carcinogens. I. Histological Findings. Z. Krebsforsch. *87*, 199–212 (1976)

Wanke, M.: Magen. In: Spezielle pathologische Anatomie. Doerr, W., Seifert, G., Uehlinger, E. (eds.), Vol. II/1, pp. 117–1044. Berlin, Heidelberg, New York: Springer 1971

Wattenberg, L.W.: Histochemical study of aminopeptidase in metaplasia and carcinoma of the stomach. Arch. Pathol. *67*, 281–286 (1959)

Wayte, D.M., Helwig, E.B.: Colitis cystica profunda. Am. J. Clin. Pathol. *48*, 159–169 (1967)

Wegener, K., Dörmer, M., Krempien, B.: Urämie und Proliferation in der Magenschleimhaut. Autoradiographische Untersuchungen über Teilphasen des Zellzyklus und der Generationszeiten der Magenschleimhautepithelien urämischer Ratten. Virch. Arch. (Cell Pathol.) *8*, 186–195 (1971)

Werner, B., Dahm, K., Breucker, H.: Ossification in cancer of the stomach. Z. Krebsforsch. *86*, 147–154 (1976)

Wiebecke, B., Gokel, J.M.: Experimentelle Cancerogenese des Magen-Darm-Kanals. A. Magen. In: Handbuch der allgemeinen Pathologie. Grundmann, E. (ed.), Vol. VI/7, pp. 693–730. Berlin, Heidelberg, New York: Springer 1975

Wiebecke, B., Löhrs, U., Brandts, A., Eder, M.: Vergleichende tierexperimentelle und bioptische Untersuchungen zur Morphogenese der Dickdarmpolypen. Verh. Dtsch. Ges. Pathol. *53,* 239–243 (1969)
Wiendl, H.-J.: Zur Frühdiagnose des Magenkarzinoms. Gastroskopische, histologisch-zytologische und zytophotometrische Untersuchungen. Stuttgart: Enke 1975
Willems, G., Galand, P., Chretien, J.: Autoradiographic studies on cell population kinetics in dog gastric and rectal mucosa. Lab. Invest. *23,* 635–639 (1970)
Willems, G., Galand, P., Vansteenkiste, Y., Zeitoun, P.: Cell population kinetics of zymogen and parietal cells in the stomach of mice. Z. Zellforsch. *134,* 505–518 (1972)
Willems, G., Vansteenkiste, Y., Smets, P.H.: Effects of ethanol in the cell proliferation kinetics in the fundic mucosa of dogs. Am. J. Dig. Dis. *16,* 1057–1063 (1971b)
Willems, G., Vansteenkiste, Y., Verbeustel, S.: Autoradiographic study of cell renewal in fundic mucosa of fasting dogs. Acta Anat. *80,* 23–32 (1971a)
Wolf, O., Pannenborg, G., Voigtsberger, P.: Über das primäre Magenstumpfkarzinom. Zentralbl. Chir. *102,* 1183–1187 (1977)
Yasuma, T., Hashimoto, K., Miyazawa, R.: Bone formation and calcification in gastric cancer. – Case report and review of literature. Acta Pathol. Jpn. *23,* 155–172 (1973)
Yeomans, N.D., St. John, D.J.B., de Boer, W.G.R.M.: Regeneration of gastric mucosa after aspirin-induced injury in the rat. Am. J. Dig. Dis. *18,* 773–780 (1973)

Morphology and Morphogenesis of Experimentally Induced Small Intestinal Tumors

P. HÖHN

I. Introduction

1. Concepts on the Causal Genesis of Human Intestinal Tumors

The action of chemical substances has a significant role in the genesis of human tumors. It is assumed that most human tumors are induced by exogenous chemical noxae (*Schmähl,* 1970; *Heidelberger,* 1975; and others). In the course of intensive efforts to discover the principles of tumor etiology, important insights have resulted in recent years. These are that chemical carcinogens do not only arise as products of our technological civilization, but that they also occur in nature as potent solitary carcinogens and cocarcinogens (e.g., as plant products). For review, see *Hecker* (1972) and *Preussmann* (1975). Not only "complete" carcinogens are significant for the genesis of tumors, but also substances which are first transformed to the actual carcinogenic compound in the organism (*Schmähl,* 1975). The causal significance of exogenous noxae in carcinogenesis is indicated by the fact emphasized by *Bauer* (1963) that malignant tumors occur predilectively at those sites in the body which are in direct or indirect contact with the environment. This applies especially to the intestinal tract.

Extensive geographical, pathological, and socioeconomic studies indicate that alimentary factors must be responsible for the high incidence of intestinal tumors (about 15% of all carcinomas are alleged to be located in the intestinal tract) in Northern Europe and North America, since intestinal tumors are only rarely observed in regions with other conditions of life (Africa, Asia, and South America) (*Wynder* and *Shigematsu,* 1967; *Haenszel* and *Correa,* 1971; *Burkitt,* 1971; *Haenszel* et al., 1973; *Berg* and *Howell,* 1974; *Zaldivar* and *Wetterstrand,* 1976; and others). Epidemiological studies reveal a coincidence between the high proportion of fat in the food as well as meat consumption on the one hand and the occurrence of intestinal tumors on the other (research team led by *Wynder*, 1967, 1974; and others). The proportion of the fat in the food is again strictly correlated with the composition and concentration of cholesterol and bile acid metabolites as well as certain fatty acids in the intestinal lumen (*Wynder* and *Reddy,* 1974; *Reddy,* 1975; *Sperry* et al., 1976). Some of the latter are suspected of possessing a carcinogenic action (*Lacassagne* et al., 1966; *Coombs* et al., 1973; *Hill,* 1974; and others). Since the fat content of the food has a great effect on the composition of the intestinal flora (*Wynder* and *Reddy,* 1973), it is also possible that the terminal carcinogen (or carcinogens) is formed indirectly through bacterial metabolism of the bile acid and cholesterol degradation products (*Hill,* 1975; and others).

2. Genesis of Adenomas and Carcinomas in Human Small Intestine

In contrast to the large intestine, tumors derived from cylindrical epithelial cells arise only rarely in the small intestine although this accounts for almost 90% of the internal surface of the intestinal tract. Carcinoids and other tumors deriving from endocrine cells of the intestinal tract will not be discussed here. A possible cause of this "resistance" of the small intestinal mucosa to carcinogenic influences may include the following factors: a) short duration of contact between the mucosa and the carcinogen(s) which may be contained in the fluid chyme because of its rapid passage, b) lower concentration of the carcinogenic substance(s) in the fluid small intestinal contents than in the large intestinal contents concentrated by reabsorption of water (*Alrich* et al., 1960), and c) low content of microorganisms in the small intestinal lumen (*Hess* et al., 1975). However, there are as yet no definite clues to explain the lower incidence of primary, small intestinal epithelial tumors in man. On the other hand it could be demonstrated in animal experiments that the small intestinal mucosa reacts less "sensitively" to the action of carcinogenic substances than the large intestinal mucosa (*Gennaro* et al., 1973). This different resistance of small and large intestine towards carcinogenic substances is, at least in part, caused by the lower activity of "DNA repair" mechanisms in the colon epithelia compared to the epithelial cells of the small intestinal mucosa (*Kanagalingam* and *Balis,* 1975).

The figures in the literature on the incidence of cancer of the human small intestine show a relatively wide scatter. As a whole, 3%–6% of all benign and malignant intestinal tumors are thought to be localized in the small intestine (cf. *Otto* et al., 1976). About 30% of benign small intestinal tumors are adenomas (*River* et al., 1956; *Grözinger* and *Schüler,* 1970), which affect proximal and distal regions of the small intestine at about the same frequency (*Wood,* 1967), although adenomas tending to malignant transformation with villous components are said to be localized more frequently in the duodenum than in the rest of the small intestine (*Mir-Madjlessi* et al., 1973). Histologically, adenomas of the small intestine show a similar constitution to those of the large intestine. Tubular adenomas and villous adenomas are distinguished as well as mixed forms of these two tumor types, the tubulo-villous adenomas (*Moersch* et al., 1962; *Ebert* and *Zuidema,* 1965; *Keeley* and *Gottlieb,* 1969; *Morson* and *Dawson,* 1974). A malignant transformation of the adenomas is regarded as probable (*Steinberg* and *Shieber,* 1972; *Mir-Madjlessi* et al., 1973; *Silbermann* et al., 1974; cf. literature on the problem of the "polyp-carcinoma sequence": *Kurzon* et al., 1974; *Morson,* 1974; *Muto* et al., 1975; *Otto* et al., 1976).

Carcinomas of the small intestine arise mainly in the duodenum. The second most frequent localization is the jejunum (*Wood,* 1967). According to *Kümmerle* and *Schier* (1973) 10 times as many carcinomas are found in the duodenum than in the rest of the small intestine when the carcinoma frequency in this region of the intestine is correlated with the length of the rest of the small intestine. Histologically, more than 90% of the tumors involve adenocarcinomas with varying degrees of differentiation. A small percentage involves signet ring cell carcinomas and anaplastic carcinomas (*Wood,* 1967) or still rarer tumor forms such as adenoacanthomas and squamous epithelial carcinomas (*Busch* and *Wodak,* 1966).

3. Mode of Action of 1,2-Dimethylhydrazine and Related Substances in Cancerification of the Intestinal Mucosa

Knowledge on carcinogenesis in the intestinal mucosa has become more profound in recent years since some carcinogenic substances have been available with which benign and malignant tumors of the small and large intestine could be induced (review: *Wiebecke,* 1975). The substance which is today preferentially used for experimental induction of intestinal tumors is 1,2-dimethylhydrazine (DMH) synthesized by *Druckrey* et al. (1967). After subcutaneous injection, it gives rise with an almost 100% rate of induction to mostly multiple tumors of the small and large intestine in experimental animals (rat: *Schauer* et al., 1969; mouse: *Wiebecke* et al., 1969; *Evans* et al., 1972; golden hamster: *Osswald* et al., 1969; *Toth*, 1972; and others).

The point of departure of DMH synthesis was the detection of cycasin (methylazoxymethanol-β-D-glucoside), a "natural" carcinogen chemically related to DMH. Cycasin can be extracted from the roots, leaves, and fruits of a tropical-subtropical palm species (Guam: Cycas circinalis; Japan: Cycas revoluta). After feeding to rats, it induces kidney and liver tumors as well as benign and malignant epithelial large intestinal tumors (*Laqueur* et al., 1963; *Laqueur*, 1965; *review: Magee* et al., 1975). The carcinogenic action of cycasin was shown only after intestinal passage and not after parenteral application. In the intestinal tract, cycasin is hydrolyzed by the action of bacterial enzymes (e.g., α-glucosidase) with release of the actual carcinogenic substance, methylazoxymethanol (MAM) (*Matsumoto* and *Strong*, 1963). Because of the lack of bacterial enzymes, cycasin has no carcinogenic action in rats reared germ free (*Laqueur*, 1964; *Laqueur* et al., 1967) whereas MAM induces tumors independent of the route of application (enteral or parenteral), even in germ-free animals (*Laqueur* and *Spatz*, 1968). Cycasin and MAM also possess transplacental carcinogenic (*Spatz* and *Laqueur*, 1967) and mutagenic actions (*Garbridge* et al., 1969). Similar to cycasin, DMH is converted to MAM in the organism, i.e., the degradation of both substances leads to the same activation mechanism. The metabolism of DMH to MAM probably takes place in the liver. The noncarcinogenic MAM-glucuronide then passes with the bile into the duodenum, is transported from here with the intestinal contents into the colon and is thought to be hydrolyzed by the action of bacterial glucuronidase into the

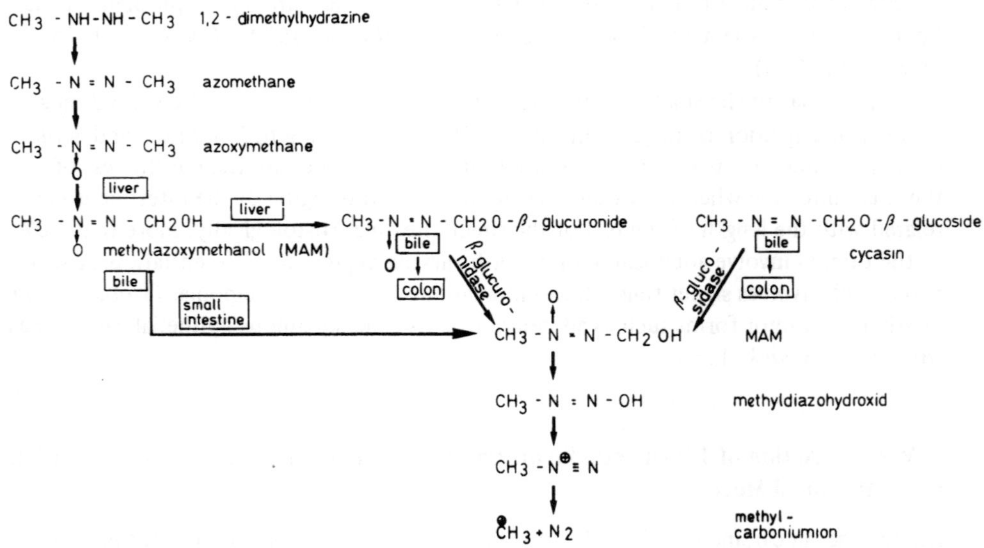

Fig. 1. Biotransformation pathway of 1,2-dimethylhydrazine and cycasin according to *Druckrey* (1970) and *Weisburger* (1971)

carcinogen MAM and glucuronic acid (Fig. 1; Weisburger, 1971; *Burdette,* 1974; and others). On the other hand, when larger DMH amounts are applied, the conjugation capacity of the liver appears to be exceeded and nonconjugated MAM passes with the bile into the duodenum (*Weisburger,* 1972). This assumption is supported by the finding that tumors appear almost exclusively in the rectum and colon after application of a low dose of DMH in rats (*Ward* et al., 1973), whereas in the majority of experimental animals tumors are also detectable in the small intestine (especially the duodenum and upper jejunum) after application of a higher dose (*Wiebecke* et al., 1973). Experimental surgical (*Wittig* et al., 1971) and biochemical investigations (*Fiala,* 1975 and 1977) have shown that the degradation products of DMH (azoxymethane and MAM) are transported only to a slight extent via the biliary tract, but mainly via the blood vessels in the intestinal mucosa (*Pozharisskij* et al., 1976).

In view of the organotropic action of DMH (*Druckrey,* 1970, 1972), the final biotransformation of the DMH metabolites must occur either spontaneously or under the influence of tissue-specific enzyme activities at the site of carcinogenesis (*Fiala,* 1975; *Zedeck* and *Brown,* 1977). The end product of the biotransformation of DMH as terminal carcinogen is the alkylating methyl carbonium ion (*Druckrey* et al., 1965; *Preussmann* et al., 1969) which is thought to cause a methylation of the nucleic acids in the intestinal epithelia (*Matsumoto* et al., 1965; *Hawks* et al., 1972). It is generally known that the highly reactive radicals formed in the endoplasmic reticulum and then transported to the cell nucleus of the target cell may trigger carcinogenesis through their binding to nucleic acids (mutation theory) or through a reaction with intracytoplasmic regulatory proteins (protein deletion theory) (review: *Grundmann,* 1972; *Stier,* 1973).

Studies on the biotransformation of DMH, of which the pathway has by no means been entirely clarified (cf. *Fiala,* 1977), may also contribute to our understanding of carcinogenesis in the human intestinal tract since it is to be assumed that the local (probably intraepithelial) metabolism of carcinogenic substances and the biochemical processes involved in humans and experimental animals show parallels. This applies all the more since the light microscopic morphology of the epithelial intestinal tumors of man and the experimentally induced intestinal tumors of experimental animals is very similar, irrespective of the carcinogenic substance used (*Spjut* and *Spratt,* 1965; *Spjut,* 1972; *Pozharisskij,* 1972; *Ward,* 1974; *Toth* et al., 1976); thus, these tumors can be classified histologically in close compliance with the nomenclature of human pathology (*Wiebecke,* 1975). Experimental studies have further shown that some of the alimentary (e.g., high-fat food), metabolic (e.g., concentration and composition of bile acids in the intestine lumen), and microbiological factors considered to be significant for human intestinal carcinogenesis also promote the genesis of tumors in experimental carcinogenesis (*Ward* et al., 1973; *Narisawa* et al., 1974; *Chomchai* et al., 1974; *Reddy* et al., 1975; *Reddy,* 1975; *Schmähl* et al., 1976; *Wittig* and *Wildner,* 1976; *Broitman* et al., 1977). Taken as a whole, these studies indicate that 1,2-dimethylhydrazine is a substance with which tumor induction and the individual phases of tumor development in the human intestinal tract can be followed in model terms in animal experiments.

II. Animal Material and Methods of Investigation

Animal material: Male rats of a Wistar strain, bred by the Institute for Pathology at the University of Mainz, were used for the studies. The animals were given food (Altromin R 10 mixed food) and water ad libitum.

The intestinal tumors were induced with 1,2-dimethylhydrazine dihydrochloride (DMH; from the company Merck-Schuchardt). Composition of the aseptically prepared injection solution: 1.86 g DMH-dihydrochloride in 100 ml of a neutral 0.01 *M* – methylene-diamine tetracetic acid solution (pH 6.5; ***Druckrey*** et al., 1967). A dose of 21 mg DMH/kg body weight was injected subcutaneously paravertebrally once a week.

Methods of Investigation

Light microscopy: Embedding of the material in paraffin. Staining: hematoxylin-eosin and PAS.

Autoradiography: Tritiated thymidine was applied intravenously (10^{-3} Ci[^{3}H]-thymidine/kg body weight dissolved in 1 ml of distilled water; specific activity: 2.0 Ci/10^{-3} Mol) 1 h before the animals were killed. Segments of normal small intestine and intestinal tumors were fixed for 24 h in neutral buffered 4% formalin and afterwards embedded in paraffin. The deparaffinated irrigated 4 μ thick sections were coated with a photographic layer (Ilford L4, nuclear research emulsion in gel form, dipping method), exposed for 21 days, developed, and stained with hematoxylin-eosin. The [^{3}H]-thymidine labeling index was determined in percent (%) in the section preparations by counting 1000 epithelial cells per normal intestinal segment or per tumor integrated over the entire level of the mucosa or tumor.

Electron microscopy: The tumors were fixed intravitally. A 1% bufferd OsO_4 solution (0.1 *M* Sörensen buffer, pH 7.3) was dropped on to the tumor surface (cf. ***Thoenes*** and ***Langer,*** 1969). Truncated tissue pyramids were excised from the tumor with a razor-blade. Postfixation in a 1% OsO_4 solution (0.1 *M* Sörensen buffer, pH 7.3) for 1–2 h at 4°C; dehydration in an ascending alcohol series and embedding in Epon.

Preparations of thin sections with the ultramicrotome Reichert Om U_2; postcontrasting of the thin sections with lead citrate and uranyl acetate. Preparation of the electron microscopic pictures with the Elmiscope I (Siemens).

Scanning electron microscopy: The normal intestinal segments were cut open in a longitudinal direction and the tumors were pinned on to thin cork slabs immediately after removal from the body and fixed for 4 h in a buffered (0.1 *M* Sörensen buffer, pH 7.2) 6.25% glutaraldehyde solution. After rinsing three times (30 min each time) in 0.1 *M* Sörensen buffer (ph 7.2), the tissue was dehydrated in an ascending acetone series. Frigen 11 and 13 was afterwards substituted for acetone in the preparations, which were dried using the critical point procedure (LWU critical point apparatus). Samples prepared in this way were glued to the preparation stands and introduced into an osmium tetroxide vapor atmosphere. A metal layer about 20 μ thick (gold or carbon-gold) was deposited on the preparations by sublimation. The preparations were evaluated with a scanning electron microscope (REM) "Stereoscan" mark IIA at a voltage of 15–30 k*V*.

Enzyme histochemistry: The light microscopic-histochemical investigations were performed on fresh cryostat sections (thickness of sections: 8 μ). The specificity of all enzyme reactions was controlled by introducing the cryostat sections into incubation solutions without substrate.

Alkaline phosphatase: Fixation (24 h) of the tissue in a 4% formaldehyde solution (*Pearse*, 1968) adjusted to pH 7.2 with a 0.067 *M* phosphate buffer and containing 7.5% sucrose. The tissue was afterwards stored in "Holt's mixture" (*Holt*, 1959).

Incubation solutions: Gössner (1958) and *Burstone* (1958). Control studies with inhibitory substances: preincubation of the sections in 0.01 *M* L-cysteine solution (pH 9.2); simultaneous incubation with 0.01 *M* sodium floride (NaF), 0.005 *M* and 0.05 *M* L-phenylalanine in the incubation solution.

Ultrahistochemistry of the alkaline phosphatase: Preparation of the tissue and incubation solution according to *Hugon* and *Borgers* (1966a, b). Duration of incubation: 5 min at 4°C. Control incubation with inhibitory substances: simultaneous incubation with 0.01 *M* NaF, 0.005 *M* and 0.05 *M* L-phenylalanine.

Acid phosphatase: Fixation and pretreatment of the tissue as in the alkaline phosphatase incubation solution: *Gomori* (1950), *Barka* and *Anderson* (1962). Control investigations with inhibitory substances: preincubation of the sections in 0.01 *M* L-cysteine solution (pH 5.0); simultaneous incubation with 0.01 *M* NaF, 0.05*M* L-phenylalanine and L-tartaric acid in the incubation solution.

Ultrahistochemistry of the acid phosphatase: Preparation of the tissue after *Hugon* and *Borgers* (1966a, b). Incubation solution: *Barka* (1964). Duration of incubation 15–20 min at 37°C. Control incubation with inhibitory substances: simultaneous incubation with 0.01 *M* NaF and 0.05 *M* L-phenylalanine in the incubation solution.

Adenosine triphosphatase (ATPase): Histochemical detection after von *Deimling* (1964). Control investigations with inhibitory substances: simultaneous incubation with 0.005 *M* 2,3-dimercapto-1-propanol (BAL) and 0.33 m*M* strophanthin G (*Ouabain).*

5'-Nucleotidase: Histologic detection according to von *Deimling* (1964). Control investigations: simultaneous incubation with 0.001 *M* nickel chloride ($NiCl_2$; *Pearse,* 1968).

Neutral α-glucosidase: Histologic detection according to *Lojda* (1965).

Leucyl-β-naphthylamidase (LNA): Histologic detection according to *Nachlas* et al. (1957). Control investigations: preincubations with 0.5 *M* β-phenylpropionate (BPP) in 0.01 *M* acetate buffer (pH 6.5) as well as in a 0.001 *M* p-hydroxymercuribenzoate (p-HMB) solution (*Pearse,* 1972).

Glucose-6-phosphatase (G-6-P): Histochemical detection according to *von Deimling* (1964). Control investigations: preincubation with 0.01 *M* L-cysteine in 0.2 *M* Tris buffer (pH 7.2).

Nonspecific esterase: Histochemical detection according to *Nachlas* and *Seligman* (1949) modified after *Barka* and *Anderson* (1962). Control investigations: *Pearse* (1972); preincubation of the sections in 10^{-3} *M* and 10^{-5} *M* diethyl-p-nitro-phenylphosphate (E 600, Mintacol) in 10^{-4} *M* p-chloromercuribenzoate (PCMB) and in 10^{-5} *M* eserine.

Glucose-6-phosphate-(G6PD), glutamate-(GDH), *3-hydroxybutyric acid-*(HBDH), *isocitrate-*(IDH),*lactate-*(LDH), *malate-*(MDH) and *succinate-*(SDH)*dehydrogenases* (according to *Pearse,* 1972).

Monoamine oxidase (MAO): Histochemical detection according to *Glenner* et al. (1957) Control investigations: simultaneous incubation with 10^{-6} *M* p-chloromercuribenzoate.

Histochemistry of Acid Glycoproteins

Light microscopy: Iron binding reaction according to *Hale* (1946) modified after *Graumann* and *Clauss* (1958).

Electron microscopy: Iron binding reaction in the modification of *Sonntag* and *Arnold* (1973).

Disc Electrophoresis: Electrophoretic separation of the LDH and MDH isoenzymes.

Animal material: Groups of six untreated rats were investigated on the 19th, 20th, and 21st fetal day, postnatally on the 1st, 10th, 15th, 20th, and 25th day of life as well as 3–4 months old adult rats. Normal mucosa was excised in the duodenum (1 cm distal to the pylorus) and in the distal ileum (1 cm before the opening of the small intestine into the cecum). The normal small intestinal mucosa and the tumor tissue (0.1 g in each case) were homogenized in cold Ringer solution; centrifugation of the homogenate and dilution with 40% sucrose solution (dilution: 0.1 ml of homogenate in 1.9 ml sucrose solution). This mixture (0.3 ml) is transferred to the electrophoresis tubes which are ready for use.

Preparation of the electrophoretic gels and detection of enzymes: Preparation of gels according to *Dietz* et al. (1967) and *Gabbert* (1973). Duration of electrophoresis: 90 min at a voltage of 300 V and a current strength of 2.5 m*A* per electrophoresis tube. Incubation solution for detection of LDH: *Nachlas* et al. (1958) with phenazine methosulfate in the incubation solution (0.25 mg/10 ml incubation solution). Incubation solution for detection of MDH: *Pearse* (1972) with phenazine methosulfate in the incubation solution (the same concentration as for LDH).

III. Findings

1. Macroscopy of Experimentally Induced Intestinal Tumors

In 250 rats, tumors could be demonstrated in the small and large intestine after an induction period of 90–200 days and a total dose of 200–450 mg DMH/kg body weight. After longer application (after about 150 days) multiple intestinal tumors arise in almost all experimental animals. It is not possible to specify the precise number of tumors since numerous densely packed tumors appear in advanced stages of cancerification, especially in the duodenum, descending colon, and rectum; in some experimental animals, these form a closed confluent tumor formation. For this reason, one can only specify the incidence of tumors in the individual intestinal regions (Fig. 2): tumors in the duodenum and proximal jejunum in 82 rats, lower jejunum in 15, ileum in 9, cecum in 7, ascending colon in 60, middle third of the colon in 62 and in the descending colon and rectum in 85 experimental animals. These figures show that tumors have arisen at the same time in different segments of the intestine in individual rats.

The following types of tumors can be distinguished macroscopically:

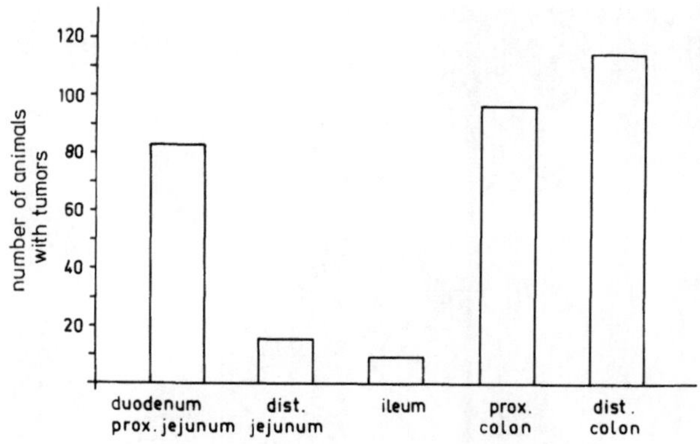

Fig. 2. Tumor development in the intestine of 250 rats after tumor induction with 1,2-dimethylhydrazine

a) Polypous tumors which either have a pedicle or are mounted with a broad base in the mucosa (Fig. 3a and c). Whereas pedunculate polypous tumors are frequently encountered in the colon, this tumor form can be demonstrated only very rarely in the duodenum and the jejunum. Here are mostly found polypous tumors with a broad base which are shown histologically to be predominantly adenomas and well differentiated adenocarcinomas.

b) Superficial, only slightly raised and partly ulcerated tumors (Fig. 3b and c). This is the most frequent kind of tumor in the duodenum and upper jejunum. The flat-growing tumors sometimes show an extent of several centimeters. Histologically, these are often shown to be adenocarcinomas and solid carcinomas.

2. Light Microscopy of Experimentally Induced Small Intestinal Tumors.

Experimentally induced intestinal epithelial tumors (Fig. 4) can be classified in analogy to the human intestinal epithelial tumors (Table 1).

Table 1. Histologic classification of the intestinal tumors induced with 1,2-dimethylhydrazine

Adenomas (Fig. 4)	Carcinomas
Tubular adenoma (adenomatous polyp)	*Adenocarcinoma* with or without production of mucus
Tubulo-villous adenoma (adenomatous-villous polyp)	*Carcinoma solidum:* signet ring cell carcinoma, undifferentiated carcinoma
Villous adenoma (villous polyp)	

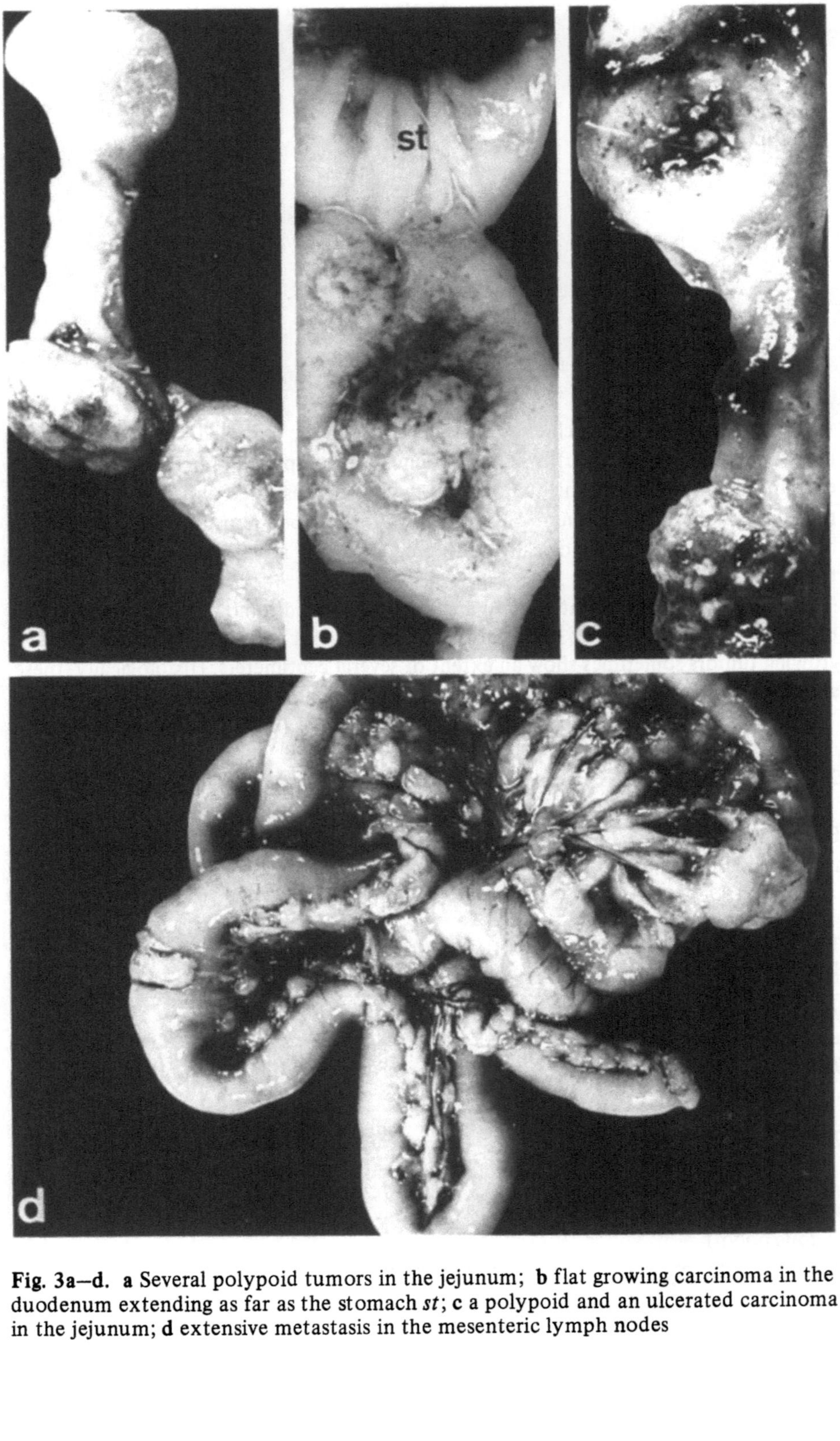

Fig. 3a–d. **a** Several polypoid tumors in the jejunum; **b** flat growing carcinoma in the duodenum extending as far as the stomach *st*; **c** a polypoid and an ulcerated carcinoma in the jejunum; **d** extensive metastasis in the mesenteric lymph nodes

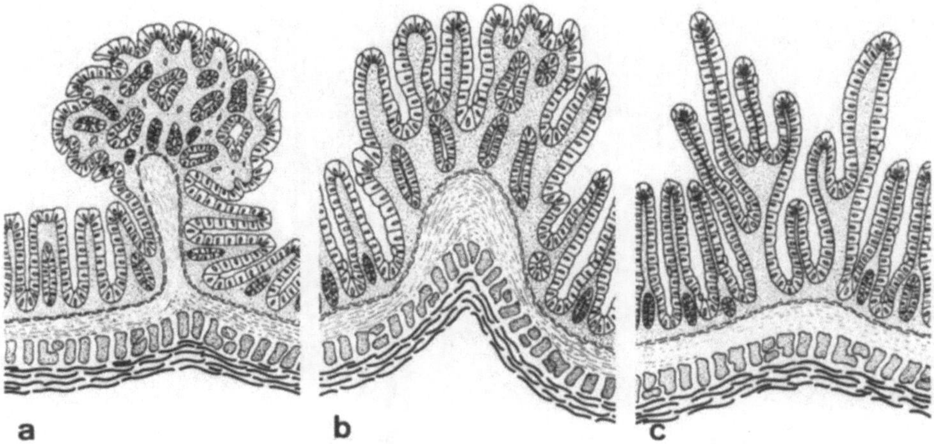

Fig. 4a–c. Schematic representation of various forms of adenoma in the intestinal mucosa: **a** tubular adenoma (adenomatous polyp); **b** tubulo-villous adenoma (adenomatous-villous polyp); **c** villous adenoma (villous polyp)

Adenomas: In the proximal small intestine of the experimental animals predominate broad-based, tubulo-villous adenomas with a quantitative proportion of villous components which varies from tumor to tumor (cf. Fig. 5a). Purely villous adenomas (which also rarely occur in the colon), and the pedunculate tubular adenomas (which are characteristic for the colon) are only rarely found in the small intestine of the present experimental material. Particularly the smaller adenomas show a fungiform or fan-shaped growth. One, therefore, observes in the periphery of these tumors only adenomatous areas near to the surface with a sharp boundary to the basally situated normal mucosa or crypt zone; in the center of the tumors the "adenomatous" change extend as far as the base of the crypt.

The tumor cells show the "rodlike dedifferentiation" familar from human pathology with a mainly monostratified arrangement and polar structure. In accordance with a high proliferative activity of these tumors, abundant mitoses can be demonstrated. In the individual tumors, focally occurring nuclear atypias indicate an incipient carcinomatous transformation. Adenomas with a carcinomatous transformation in the region of the base of the tumor and incipient tumorous infiltration of the muscularis/mucosae and the submucosa are frequently found (Fig. 5b).

Carcinomas: The experimentally induced carcinomas of the small intestine mainly involve adenocarcinomas with varying degrees of maturation. The adenocarcinomas derived from adenomas are frequently well differentiated, mostly show only a slight tendency to infiltration, and only rarely invade the subserous connective tissue. They form elongated, narrow glandular tubes of which the epithelia are predominantly monostratified in arrangement with polar differentiation (Fig. 5c and d). Tumor cells

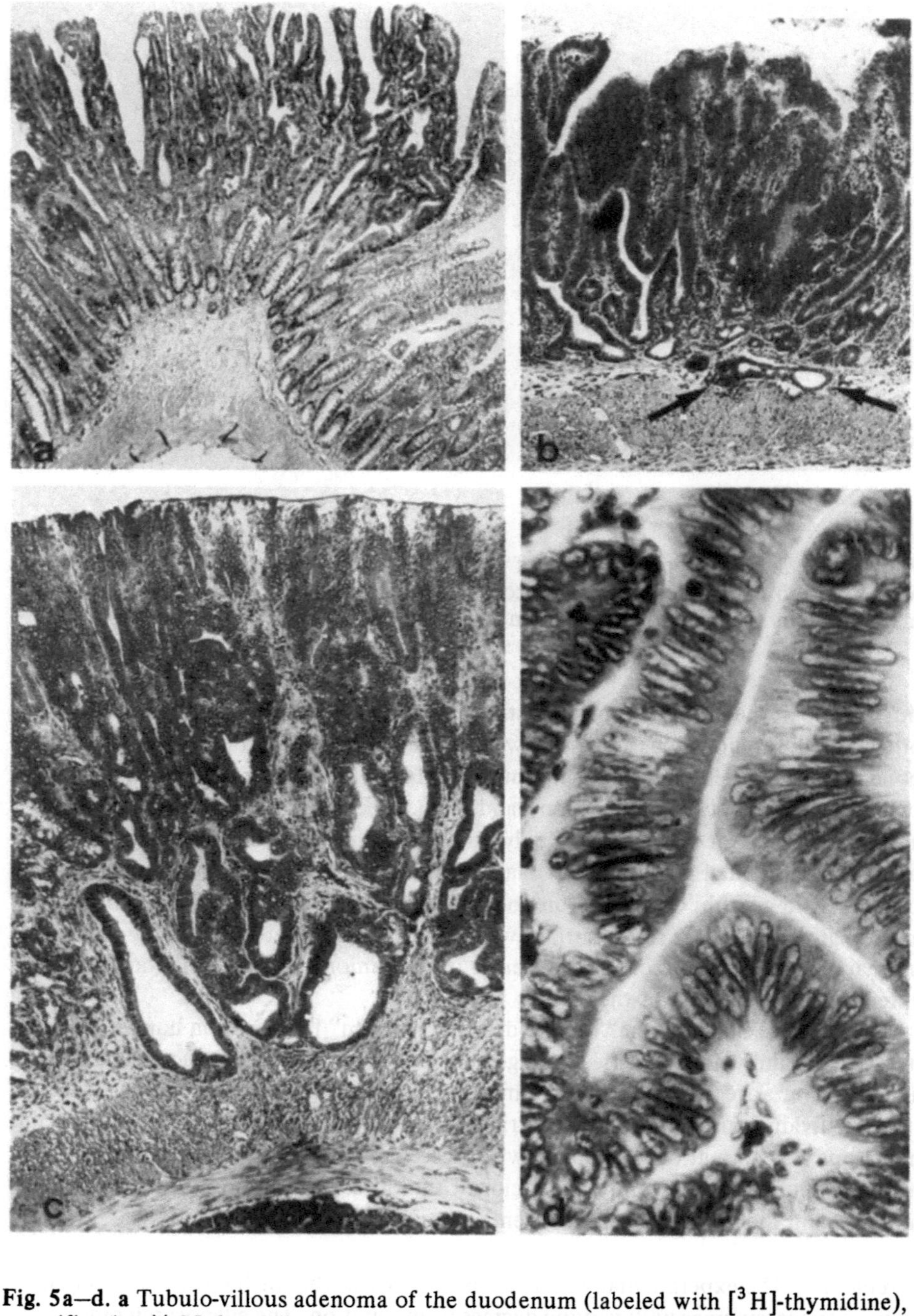

Fig. 5a–d. a Tubulo-villous adenoma of the duodenum (labeled with [^{3}H]-thymidine), magnification × 35; **b** small adenocarcinoma (derived from a tubular adenoma) with tumorous infiltration of the submucosa *(arrows)*, magnification × 23; **c** adenocarcinoma of the duodenum with incipient infiltration of the muscularis propria, magnification × 85; **d** gland with monostratified and multistratified tumor cells, magnification × 560. Staining a–d: hematoxylin-eosin

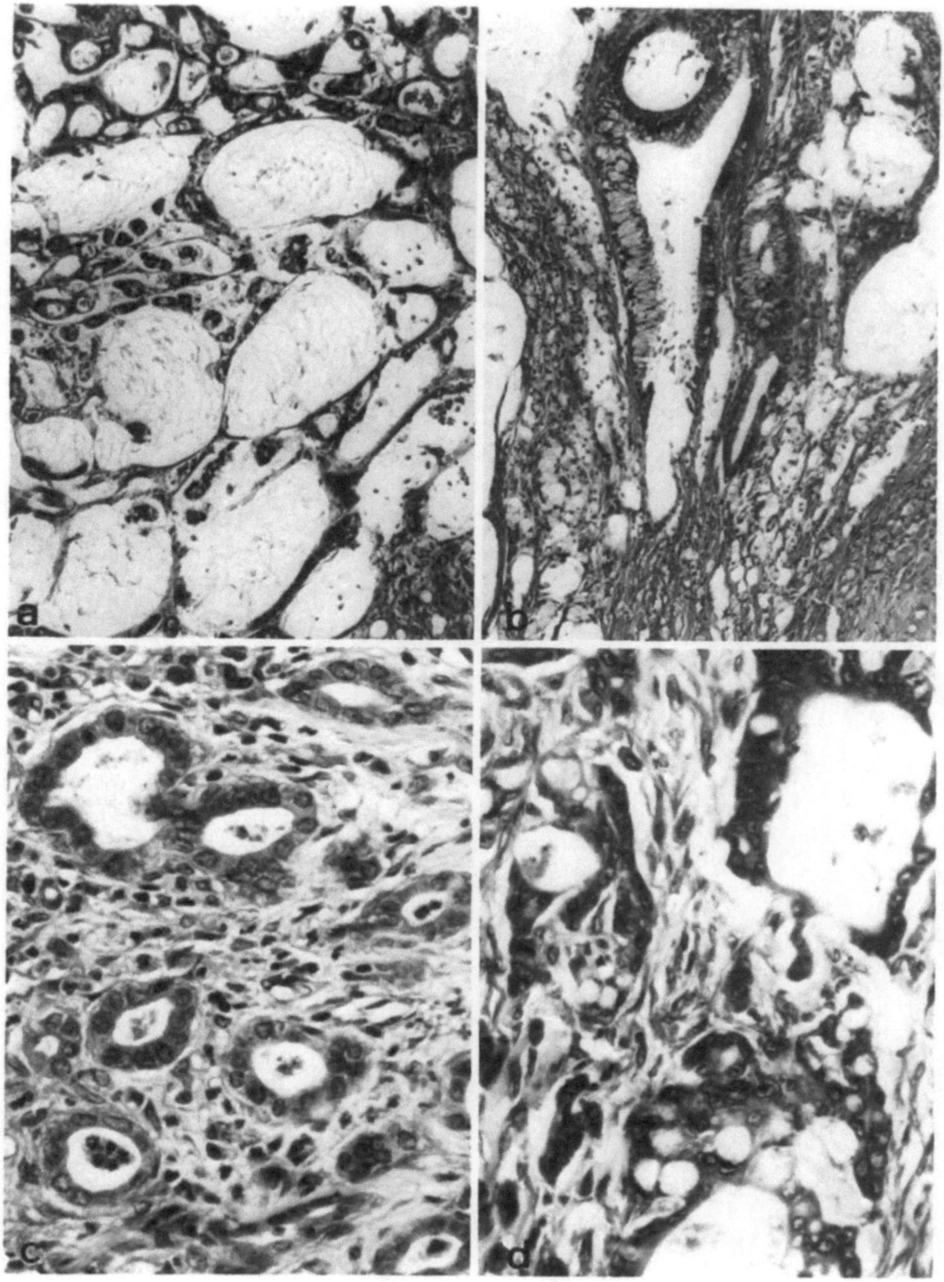

Fig. 6a–d. Adenocarcinomas of the duodenum: **a** and **b** mucus-producing adenocarcinoma with mucus-filled, dilated glands, magnification X 88; **c** adenocarcinoma with pronounced mesenchymal tumor component ("scirrhous adenocarcinoma"), magnification X 350; **d** poorly differentiated adenocarcinoma, magnification X 560. Staining a–d: hematoxylin-eosin

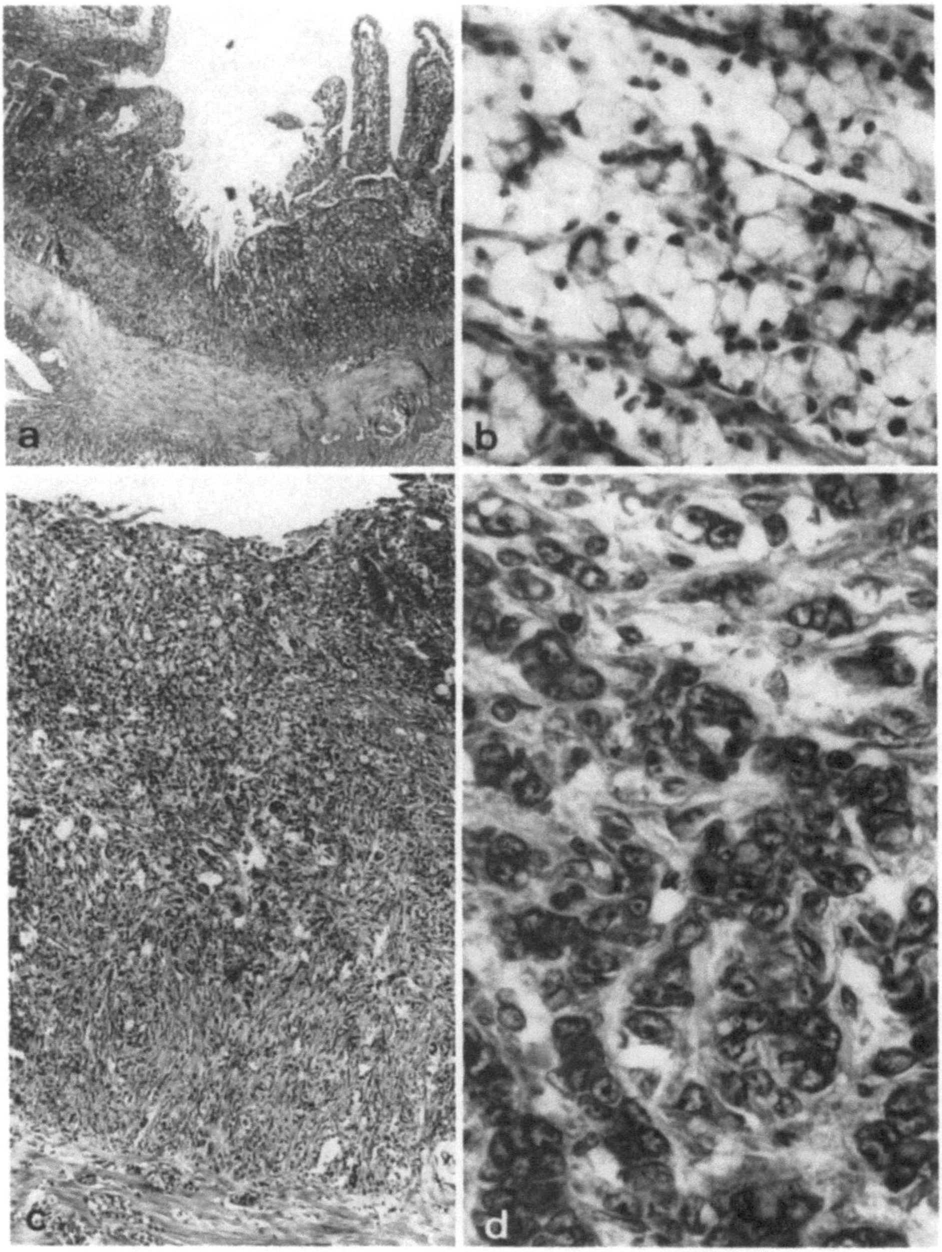

Fig. 7a–d. Solid carcinomas of the duodenum: **a** and **b** superficial ulcerated signet ring cell carcinoma with tumorous infiltration of all layers of the intestinal wall, magnification X 35 (a) and X 350 (b); **c** and **d** scirrhous (anaplastic) carcinoma with tumorous infiltration of all layers of the intestinal wall, magnification X 88 (c) and X 560 (d). Staining a–d: hematoxylin-eosin

of the enterocyte type predominate; one also recognizes isolated epithelia with mucus formation. Adenocarcinomas with mainly mucus-producing epithelial components (gallert carcinomas) are rare in the small intestine (Fig. 6a and b). In tumor areas with production of mucus, the histologic picture is characterized by cystically dilated, mucus-filled glands exhibiting a monostratified epithelial coating. Such tumors show a more aggressive growth than adenocarcinomas without a mucus-producing epithelial component and infiltrate the muscularis propria and the subserosa more frequently than the latter. Besides these, a special form of the adenocarcinoma is occasionally found. These are only rarely observed in the human intestine and are designated "scirrhous adenocarcinomas." The characteristic feature of these tumors is the dense, fibroplastic tissue components with only a few widely separated glands (Fig. 6c).

There are fluid transitions from the well-differentiated adenocarcinomas to adenocarcinomas with a low degree of differentiation which, in turn, in places cannot be sharply demarcated from the solid carcinomas. They develop irregularly formed, in some cases bizarre glands which are often built up from only a few epithelial cells with a multistratified arrangement without discernible polar differentiation (Fig. 6d).

The solid carcinomas as well as the poorly differentiated adenocarcinomas almost exclusively involve endophytic tumors with pronounced infiltrative growth and flat erosions or ulcerations which are also crater-like in some cases. Even in small carcinomas which cannot be seen macroscopically, the tumor cells often intersperse the entire intestinal wall. They spread preferentially in the loose connective tissue of the submucosa and subserosa and invade lymphatic vessels. In solid carcinomas are found mostly mucus-producing tumor cells in which the proportion of pure signet ring cell carcinomas is relatively high (Fig. 7a and b). On the other hand, solid carcinomas without mucus-producing tumor cells are rarer. They occur under the histologic picture of a scirrhous or anaplastic carcinoma and showed just an aggressive behavior as the signet ring cell carcinomas (Fig. 7c and d).

Metastases could be demonstrated in the majority of experimental animals with intestinal tumors. The intestinal carcinomas mostly metastasize in the mesenteric lymph nodes (Fig. 3d), but the other lymph node regions in the abdominal cavity and the retroperitoneal lymph nodes are often also affected. In an advanced stage of cancerization, conglomerate tumors frequently develop between the duodenum, stomach, and hilus of the liver with continuous tumorous infiltration of the liver and the diaphragm as well as transformation of the mesentery and the omentum into a homogenous tumor slab. Lymph node metastases in the pulmonary hilus (12 ×), liver metastases (14 ×) and pulmonary metastases with formation of a pleuritis carcinomatosa (8 ×) are found very much more rarely. The lymph node metastases mostly derive from solid carcinomas while liver and lung metastases are always derived from solid carcinomas.

3. Autoradiographic Findings with Special Consideration of the Morphogenesis of Experimentally Induced Small Intestinal Tumors

In the normal small intestinal mucosa, about 30% of the epithelial cells in the lower two-thirds of the crypts (proliferation compartment) show a [^{3}H]-thymidine labeling

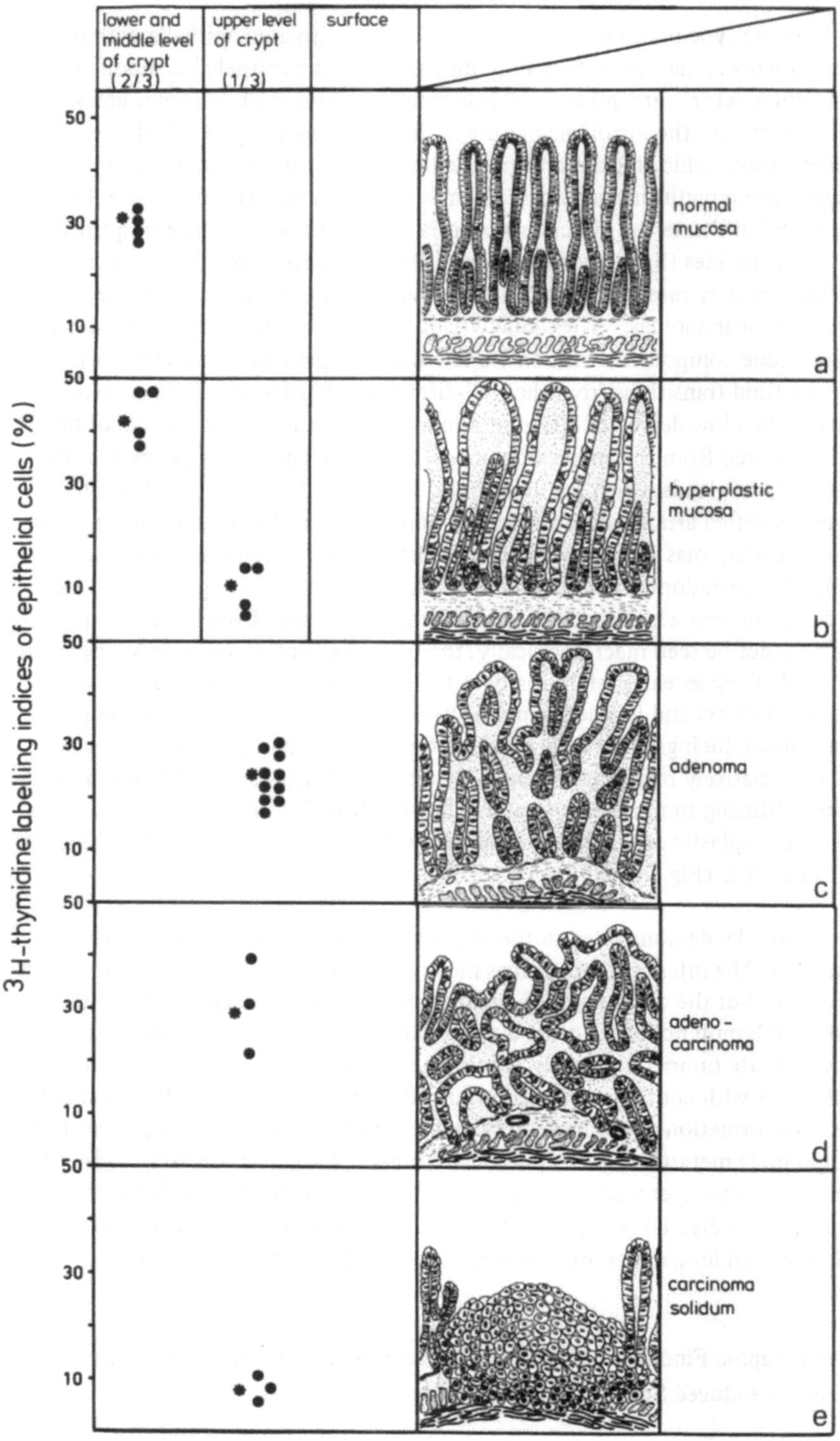

Fig. 8a–e. (Legend see page 85)

whereas epithelial labeling is no longer demonstrable in the upper third of the crypt (differentiation compartment) and in the region of the villi (functional compartment) (Fig. 8a; cf. *Eder,* 1969; *Watson* and *Wright,* 1974). Mucosal hyperplasias develop within mucosal areas of normal appearance, but also in the vicinity of tumors. The epithelial cells of the hyperplastic mucosa do not differ light microscopically from the crypt and villous epithelium of the adjacent mucosa with normal structure. One hour after application of [^{3}H]-thymidine, the labeling maximum in the epithelial cells of the mucosal hyperplasias is shown to be in the same place as in the normal proliferation compartment, although the mean value of the labeling index is over 40%. In contrast to the proliferation conditions in the normal mucosa, in the hyperplastic areas isolated epithelial cells in the upper third of the crypt are also labeled, i.e., the zone of proliferation has advanced to the surface (Fig. 8b, 9a and b). Besides this, one observes within the crypt zones of both hyperplastic and nonhyperplastic mucosal areas, circumscribed abrupt epithelial transformations which are manifested light microscopically by an increase in the cytoplasmic basophilia and a greater stainability of the cell nuclei (Fig. 9c and d). In the further course of cancerization, these proliferating epithelial cells replace the normal epithelial population of the differentiation compartment; the goblet cells become smaller at the same time. In connection with the restricted differentiation capacity of the crypt epithelia caused by the extension of the proliferation zone, the architecture of the mucosal surface is also altered. The small intestinal villi become shorter and broader, sometimes with development of villous bridges and furcations (Fig. 9c).

Adenomas and carcinomas derive from these circumscribed crypt areas with increased epithelial proliferation. The form of their growth is determined by the site of the centers of proliferation. When the proliferation maximum is situated at the surface, exophytic tumors develop (e.g., polyps with villous components – Figs. 5a, 10a and b). On the other hand, when it is more in the area of the middle crypt zones, exophytic-endophytic tumors with the tendency to flat, lawn-like growth developed: Adenomas with a broad base and which are slightly raised developed, and adenocarcinomas protruding only slightly above the level of the mucosa are formed (Figs. 5c, 10c and d). The latter are typical tumor forms of the proximal small intestine. Additionally carcinomas with a high degree of malignancy and without precursors which can be morphologically demonstrated with certainty develop in the duodenum and proximal jejunum; these

---

Fig. 8a–e. [^{3}H]-Thymidine labeling index: **a** of the normal small intestinal mucosa with a labeling maximum of the epithelial cells in the lower two thirds of the crypts, no labeling in the upper one third of the crypts; **b** of the hyperplastic mucosal areas with the labeling maximum in the two lower thirds of the crypts, labeled epithelial cells also in the upper third of the crypts; **c** of adenomas; **d** of adenocarcinomas with labeled tumor cells in all regions of the tumor ([^{3}H]-thymidine labeling index integrated over the entire tumor area); no regional counting of the tumor cells and no differentiation between the various forms of adenoma and adenocarcinoma; **e** of solid carcinomas with a labeling maximum in the peripheric tumor zone ([^{3}H]-labeling index integrated over the entire tumor area); no regional counting of the tumor cells and no differentiation between the various forms of solid carcinoma. Symbols within the scheme: *dots* = individual values of [^{3}H]-thymidine labeling index (per investigated normal intestinal region or tumor); *asterisks* = mean values of the [^{3}H]-thymidine labeling indices

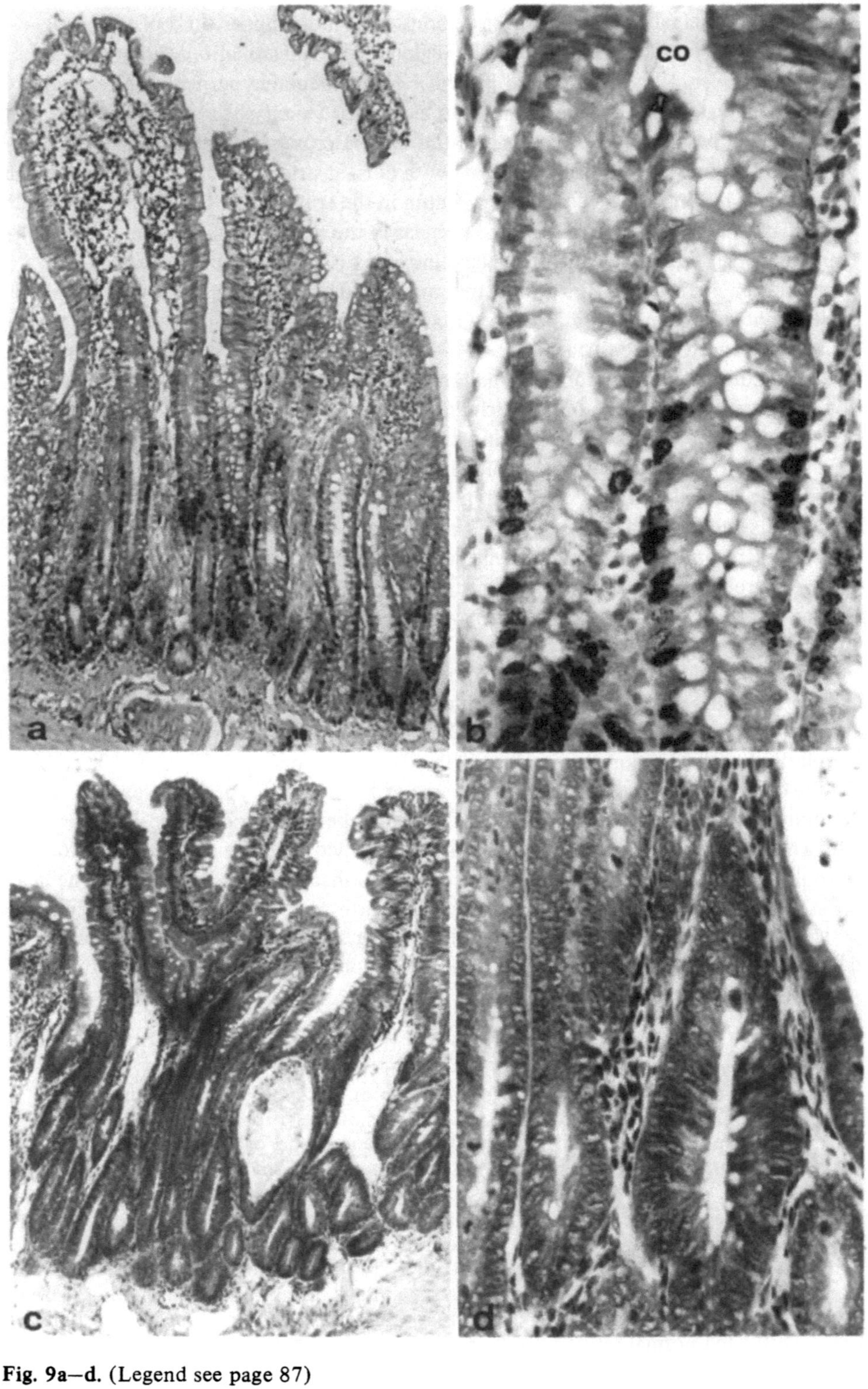

Fig. 9a–d. (Legend see page 87)

rapidly invade the deeper layers of the intestinal wall. Histologically, these carcinomas are poorly differentiated adenocarcinomas and solid carcinomas. As long as these carcinomas have not yet broken through the intestinal wall, the maximum [^{3}H]-thymidine incorporation is mostly localized in a narrow margin at the base of the tumor (Fig. 11). Whereas the mean value of the [^{3}H]-thymidine labeling index in the adenomas and adenocarcinomas is 25%–30% (Fig. 8c and d) and thus is only slightly lower than in the proliferation compartment of the normal small intestinal mucosa, the solid carcinomas show a surprisingly low rate of proliferation. There is a labeling index between 5% and 10% integrated over the entire area of the individual solid carcinomas (Fig. 8e). However, the proliferative behavior of the tumor cells shows appreciable regional differences within the solid carcinomas. Whereas mostly only a few tumor cells are labeled in the center of the carcinomas, a higher proliferative activity is found in the edge zones or offshoots which infiltrate the adjacent tissue. An accentuation of the [^{3}H]-thymidine labeling can also be registered in the vicinity of blood vessels. Such an arrangement of the [^{3}H]-thymidine-labeled tumor cells is manifested especially in the carcinomas which have broken through the muscularis propria and spread in the loose subserous connective tissue (Fig. 11d).

4. Electron Microscopic Findings

a) Ultrastructure of Normal Small Intestinal Mucosa

One can dispense with a broader description of ultrastructural findings at this point, since there is a large number of relevant review studies (*Trier* and *Rubin,* 1965; *Trier,* 1968; *Toner,* 1968; *Toner* et al., 1971; and others). Only the histogenetic findings in

---

Fig. 9a–d. Mucosal hyperplasia in the duodenum: **a** and **b** [^{3}H]-thymidine labeling maximum in the region of the base of the crypts and individual labeled epithelial cells in the apical halves of the crypts (*co* = crypt opening), magnification × 88 (a) and × 350 (b); **c** and **d** focal extension of the zones of proliferation in individual small intestinal crypts and marked reduction of the goblet cells, magnification × 88 (c) and × 350 (d). Staining a–d: hematoxylin-eosin

Fig. 10a–d. **a** and **b** Tubulo-villous adenoma of the duodenum with a maximum of [^{3}H]-thymidine incorporation in the epithelial cells of the apical tumor zones, a second center of proliferation at the base of the tumor, magnification × 88 (a) and × 350 (b); **c** and **d** adenocarcinoma of the duodenum with [^{3}H]-thymidine labeling of the epithelial cells in the entire tumor and labeling maximum in the middle and apical parts of the tumor, magnification × 88 (c) and × 350 (d). Staining a–d: hematoxylin–eosin

Fig. 11a–d. **a** Poorly differentiated adenocarcinoma, **b** and **c** signet ring cell carcinoma of the duodenum: maximum of [^{3}H]-thymidine labeling in the tumor cells at the base of the tumors; **d** tumor cord of a solid carcinoma in the subserous connective tissue of the jejunum: only slight [^{3}H]-thymidine incorporation with a maximum in the periphery of the tumor, magnification × 88 (a and b), × 350 (c) and × 35 (d). Staining a–d: hematoxylin–eosin

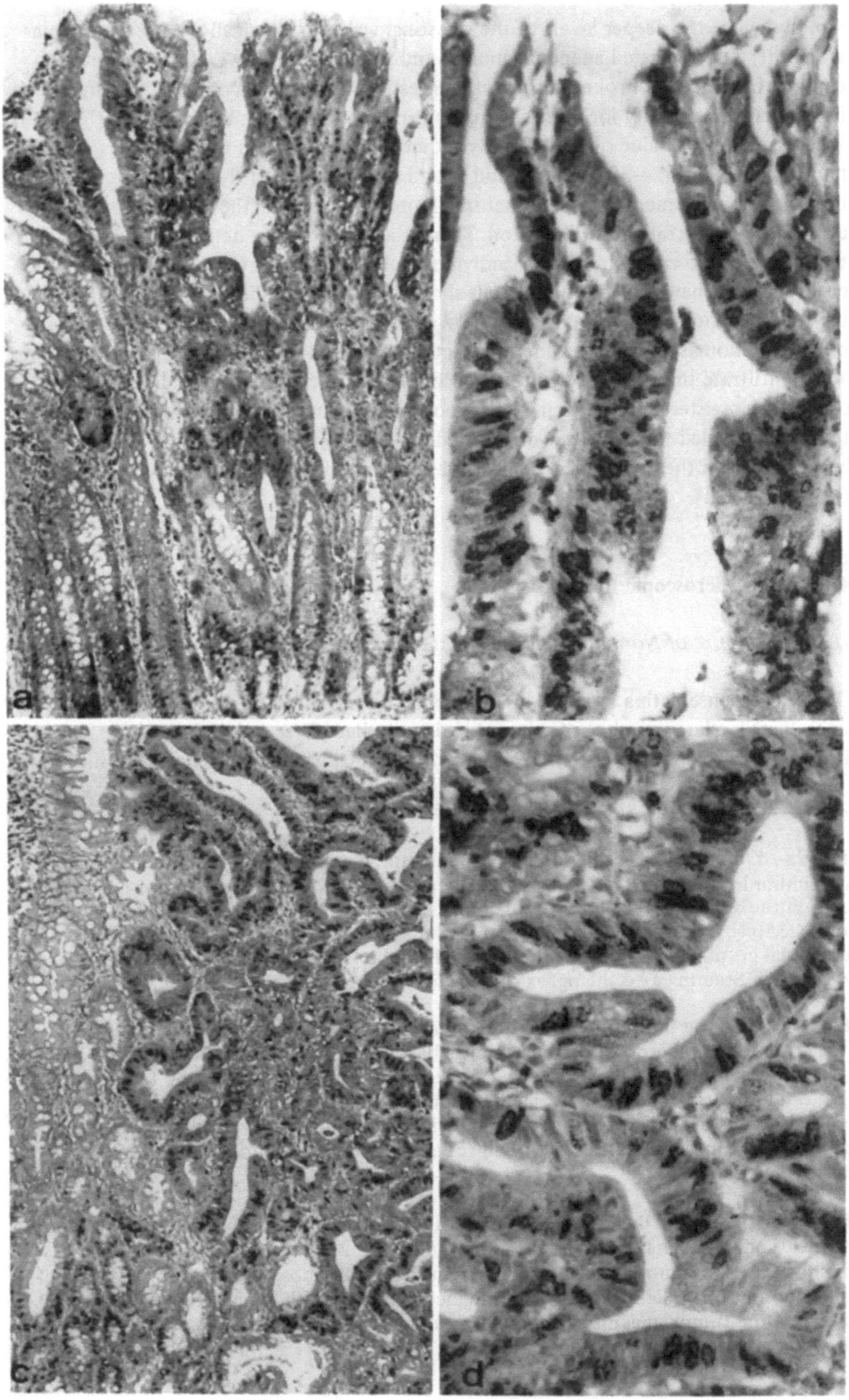

Fig. 10a–d. (Legend see page 87)

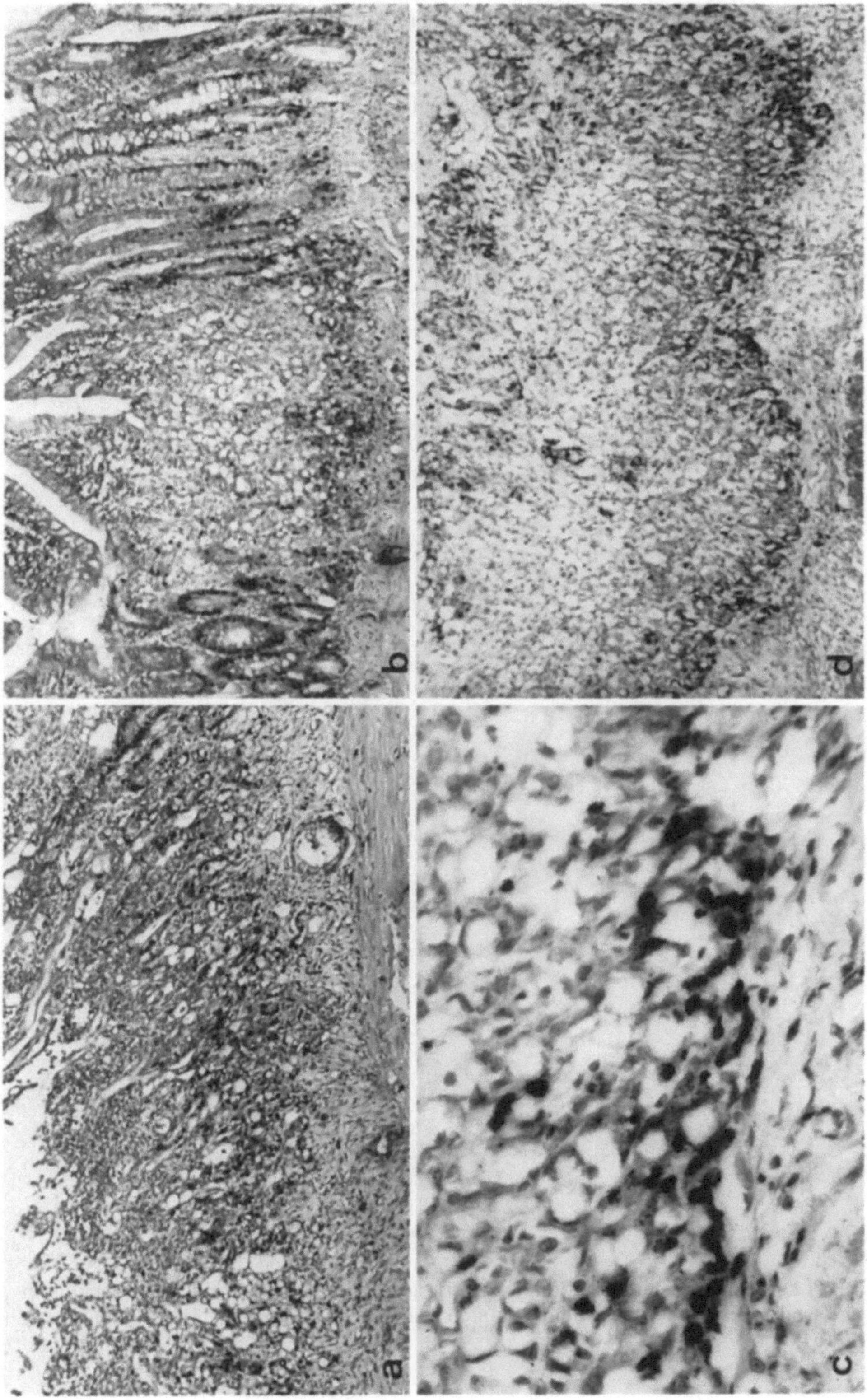

Fig. 11a–d. (Legend see page 87)

the normal small intestinal mucosa which are relevant to the topic will be dealt with in the following treatise.

A total of four epithelial cell groups with different differentiation can be distinguished in the small intestinal mucosa: the cylindrical epithelia of the villi which are capable of resorption (enterocytes, columnar cells), the mucous-producing goblet cells, the Paneth cells and the "endocrine cells of the gastrointestinal tract." Some authors

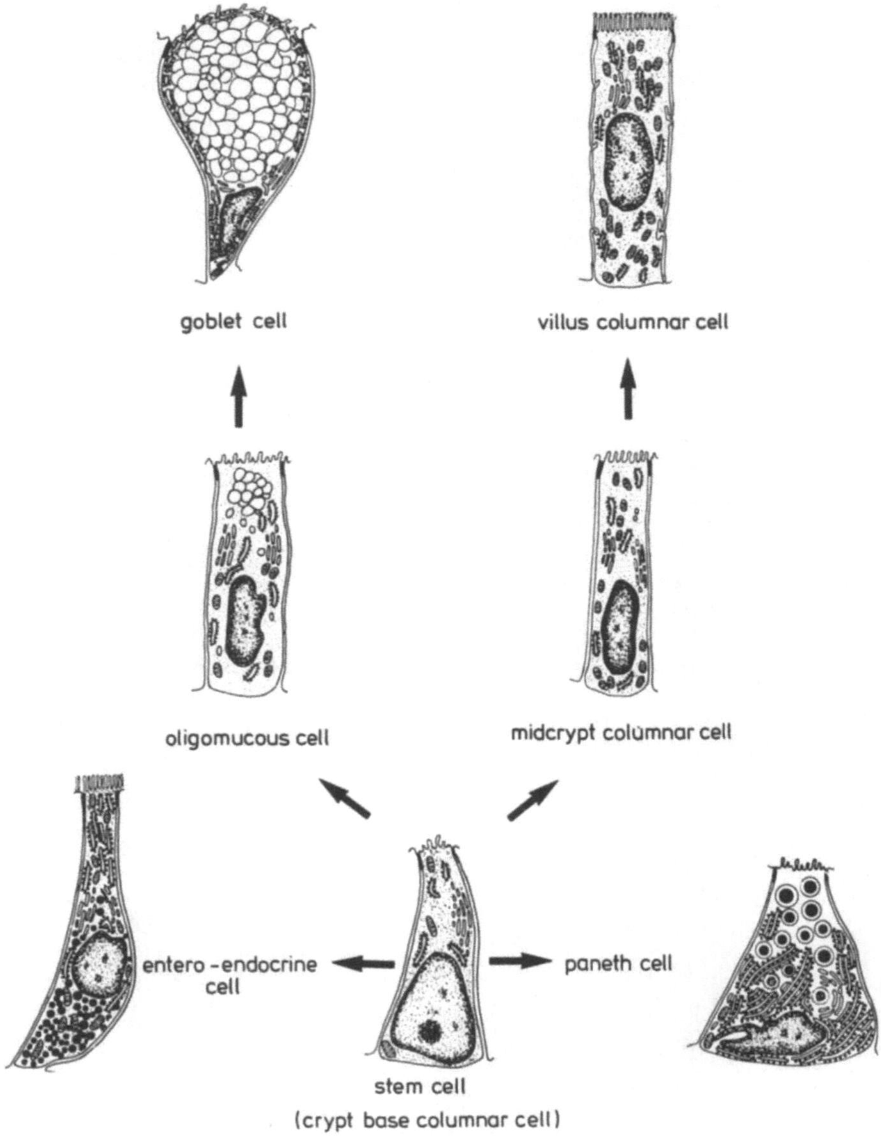

Fig. 12. Schematic representation of the histogenesis of the four kinds of epithelium in the small intestine derived from a common stem cell (according to *Leblond* and *Cheng*, 1976)

assume that a specific stem cell is responsible for the formation of each of these four epithelial groups (*Trasher* and *Greulich,* 1966). More recent electron microscopic and autoradiographic studies have revealed, however, that all epithelial cell groups of the small intestine probably derive from a common stem cell (*Cheng* and *Leblond,* 1974; *Leblond* and *Cheng,* 1976; Fig. 12) as is also postulated for the epithelia of the stomach (*Corpron,* 1966; *Rubin* et al., 1968) and the colon (*Cheng* and *Leblond,* 1971). The stem cell situated at the base of the crypts is termed the "crypt base columnar cell" by *Chang* and *Leblond* and is identical with the "undifferentiated crypt cell" described by *Trier* (1963, 1964). Since Paneth cells and entero-endocrine cells are not an essential cellular constituent of the experimentally induced tumors, the morphogenesis of these cell forms will not be dealt with in more detail here.

The *undifferentiated crypt epithelial cell* possesses a large basally situated cell nucleus which takes up about 25%–30% of the cell volume. The apical cell membrane only develops scanty microvilli with uneven height and irregular arrangement. Only a few cellular organelles are found in the cytoplasm compared with mature enterocytes, but there are abundant free ribosomes. Secretory granules are frequently present in the apical cytoplasm. In the vicinity of undifferentiated crypt epithelia mucus-producing epithelial cells are found which are partly in the process of maturation and in some case already mature; Paneth cells and entero-endocrine cells are also found.

The *cylindrical epithelia of the middle third of the crypts* are longer than the undifferentiated epithelial cells at the base of the crypt. The microvilli become higher and show a regular arrangement. The cell organelles (mitochondria, granular endoplasmic reticulum, and Golgi apparatus) are increased in number; the number of the free ribosomes in the cytoplasm is reduced. These epithelial cells are capable of division just as the nondifferentiated crypt epithelial cells.

Maturation to *enterocytes* (Fig. 13) which are no longer capable of division takes place during further migration to the crypt orifice. The final morphological differentiation is attained by the cylindrical epithelia at the orifice of the crypts or at the base of the small intestinal villi with development of the 1–2 μ high brush border as the most striking structural characteristic. First beginning at that time the brush border enzymes develop their activity (*Padykula,* 1962; *Oehlert,* 1969) and the "surface coat" attains its full development (*Weiser,* 1973). According to the theory of *Cheng* and *Leblond* (1974, 1976), the nondifferentiated crypt epithelial cell is also the stem cell for goblet cells. The development of goblet cells which are no longer capable of division takes place, via an intermediate cell, from the *"oligomucous cell"* which is still capable of division (*Merzel* and *Leblond,* 1969; *Cheng* and *Leblond,* 1974). The apical cell membrane of the oligomucous cell possesses only scanty microvilli. Immediately under the protruding apical cell membrane are found a few densely packed mucus droplets surrounded by a membrane. The cell nucleus is at the base of the epithelium. One discerns a well differentiated Golgi complex supranuclearly with numerous parallel and partly enlarged cisternae. In the vicinity of the Golgi complex are found profiles of the glandular endoplasmic reticulum and mitochondria.

From the oligomucous cells developed the *goblet cells* (Fig. 13) which are localized both in the small intestinal crypts and in the region of the villi. The apical cell membrane of the goblet cells mostly forms only a few irregularly arranged microvilli. The most striking structural characteristics are the numerous densely packed mucus droplets

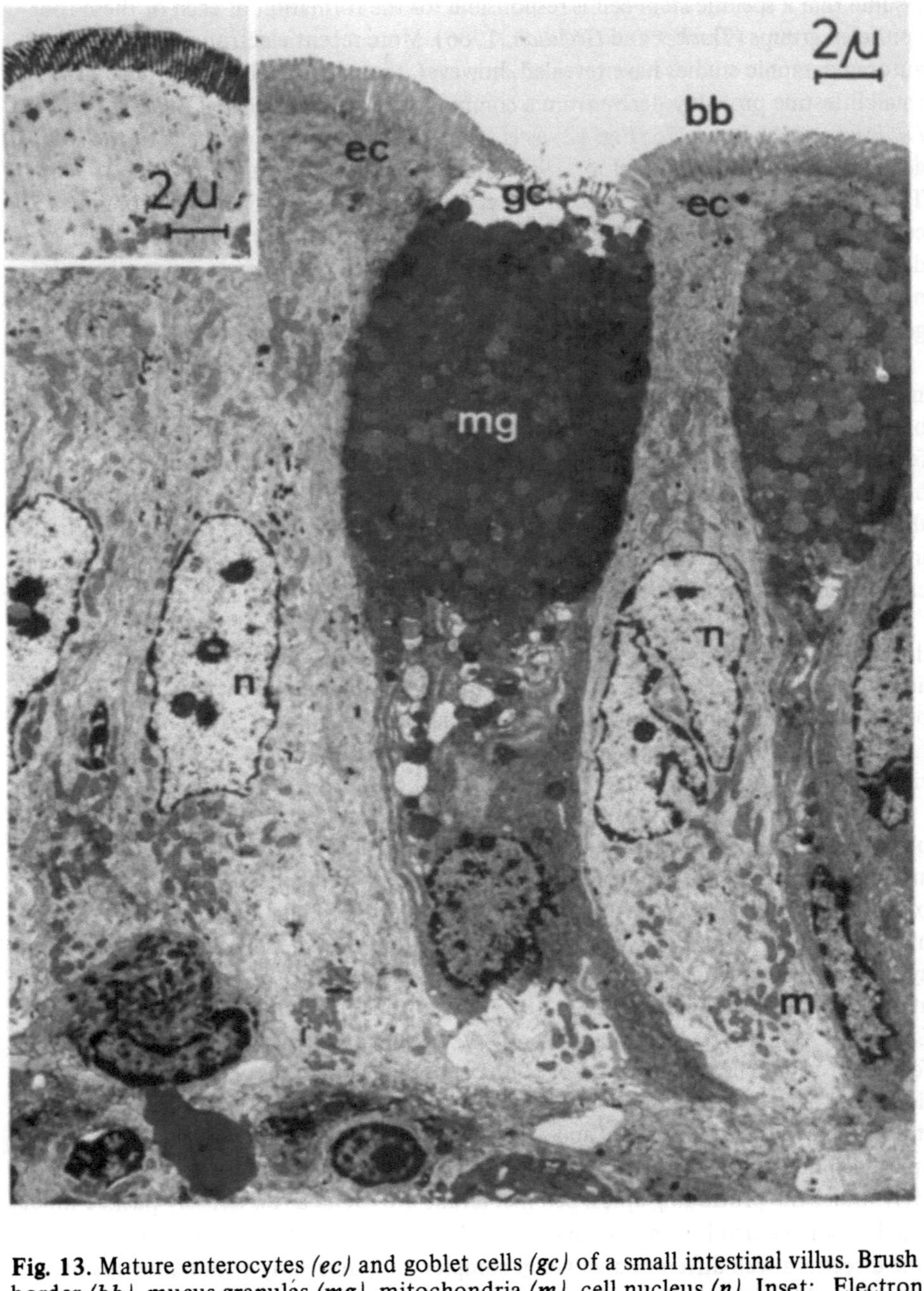

Fig. 13. Mature enterocytes *(ec)* and goblet cells *(gc)* of a small intestinal villus. Brush border *(bb)*, mucus granules *(mg)*, mitochondria *(m)*, cell nucleus *(n)*. Inset: Electron microscopic-histochemical representation of alkaline phosphatase with a distinct positive enzyme reaction in the brush border, magnification X 4500, inset: X 3500

surrounded by a membrane in the supranuclear cytoplasm by which the cell organelles and the cell nucleus are pushed to the base of the epithelium. There is a well-differentiated Golgi complex between mucous granules and cell nucleus and abundant profiles of the granular endoplasmic reticulum and mitochondria.

Scanning electron microscopic findings on the normal small intestinal mucosa

With low magnification, one recognizes the leaf-like villi of the small intestinal mucosa with their even height and regular arrangement (Fig. 14a). At irregular intervals, the villi show ring-like transverse constrictions. With higher magnification one sees the surface of the enterocytes protruding forward in the center and falling away to the lateral cell membrane. Each individual enterocyte adjoins 5–6 adjacent epithelial cells. The surface structures of the enterocytes mostly can not be distinguished clearly since they are covered by a 0.2–0.6 μ high fiber film, the so-called surface coat (*Bennett,* 1963: glycocalyx) (Fig. 14b) which cannot be dissolved away even by the action of proteolytic agents (*Ito,* 1965; *Swift* and *Mukherjee,* 1976). The surface coat consists of sulfated acid glycoproteins which can be demonstrated histochemically with the iron colloid reaction of *Hale* (Fig. 15a). The surface coat is detached only above small areas of villi and one distinguishes the 1–2 μ long and 0.1 μ wide microvilli (Fig. 14b – inset). There are pore openings in the enterocyte association (Fig. 14b) in the depth of which the goblet cell surface (with only a few irregular microvilli) can be distinguished.

b) Ultrastructure of Experimentally Induced Small Intestinal Tumors

α) Adenomas

Adenomas of the small intestine do not exhibit a uniform cytological picture and epithelial cells with varying differentiation are found even within one and the same tumor. However, in the main, tumor cells are involved which are comparable with epithelial cells in the lower and middle third of the crypts of the normal mucosa: adenoma cells of the enterocyte precursor type and mucus-producing cells which sometimes resemble the oligomucous cells.

Tumor cells of the enterocyte type show a marked variance with regard to the number, height, and arrangement of the *microvilli* which are relatively highly developed in a few tumor cells (Fig. 16a) and display an irregular architecture in other tumor cells (Fig. 17a). The glycocalyx over the microvilli is mostly much less developed than in normal enterocytes so that the surface structure can also be well observed under the scanning electron microscope. The scanning electron microscopic image of differentiated tumor cells differs only slightly from that of normal enterocytes (Fig. 16b and c). The *interepithelial adhesion complexes* resemble those of the normal epithelium. Directly at the apex, the tumor cells are linked together by a zonula occludens. The zonula adherens as well as desmosomes varying in number and size adjoin distally. Some epithelial cells possess a smooth lateral cell membrane, whereas others show pronounced interdigitations of the membrane. The adhesion complexes between individual cells are only poorly developed, so that wide intercellular spaces arise into

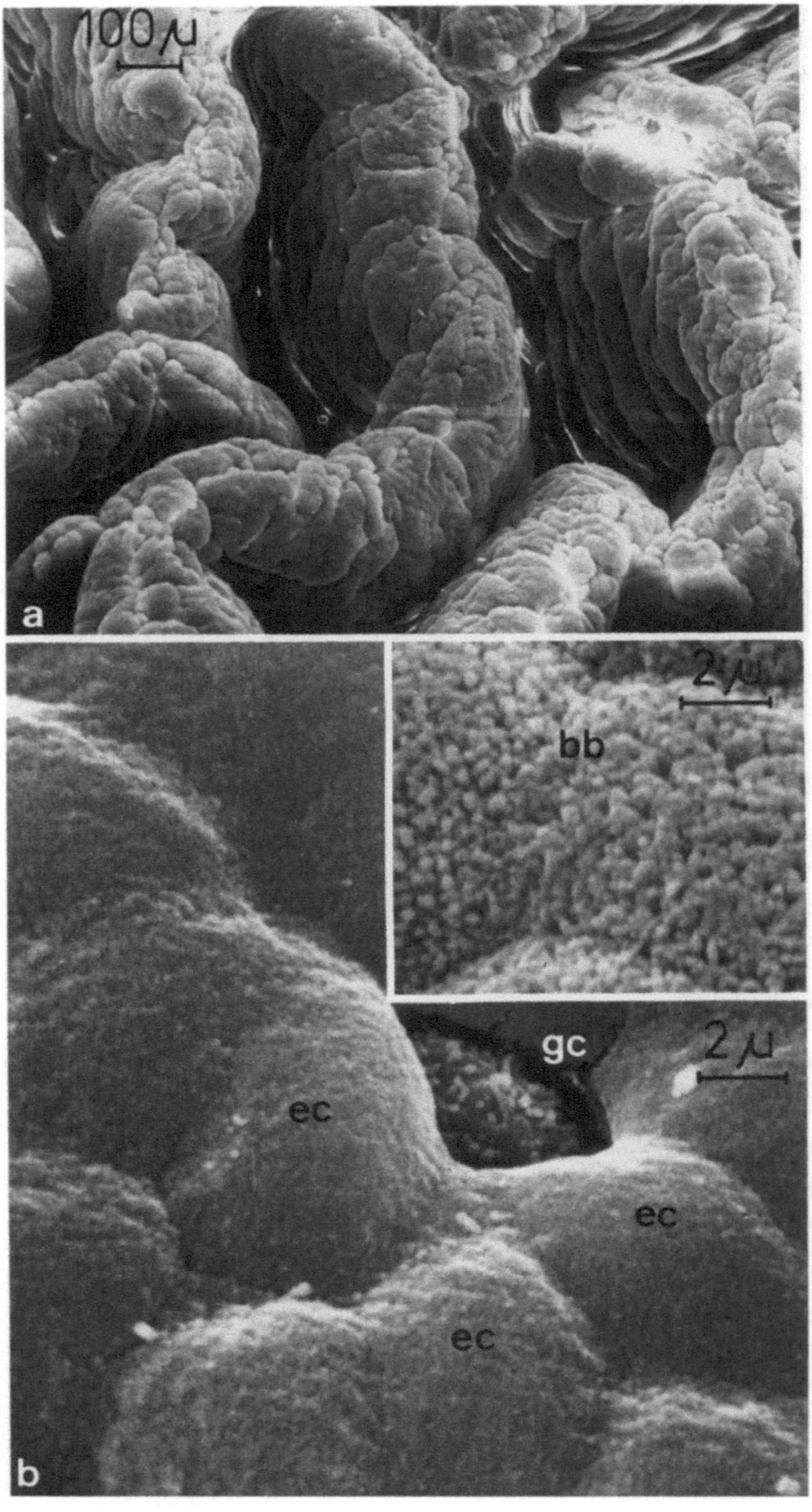

Fig. 14a and b. (Legend see page 95)

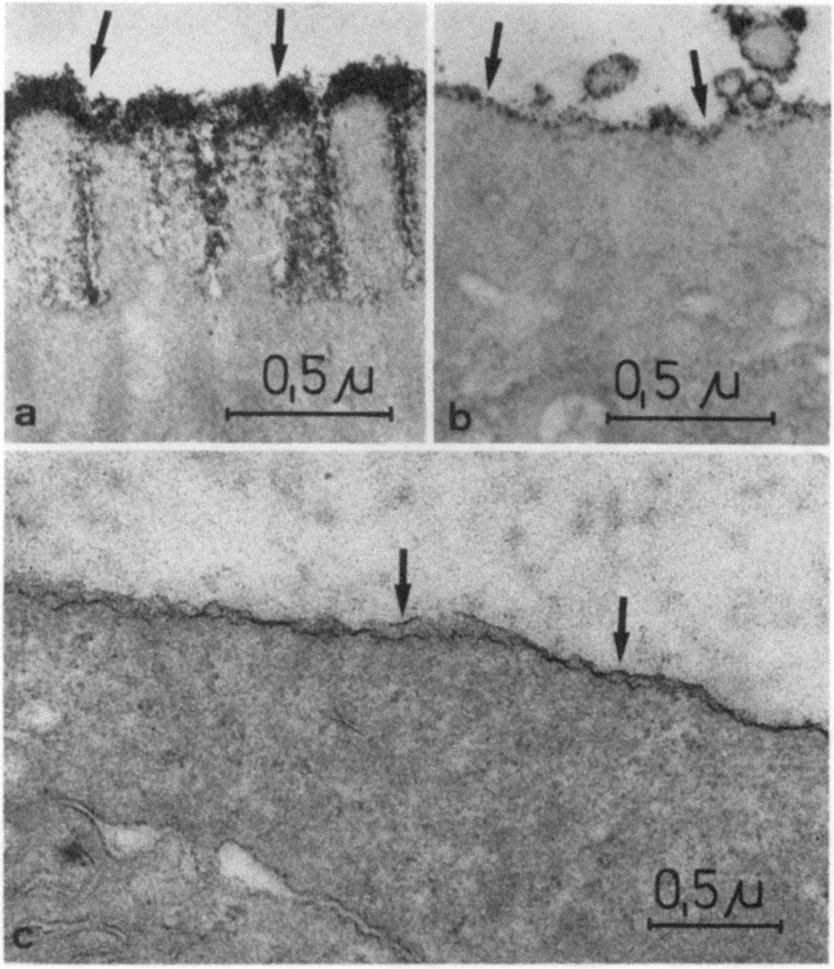

Fig. 15a–c. Ultrahistochemical representation of the glycocalyx *(arrows)* with the iron colloid reaction in a normal enterocyte **a**, in a tumor cell of an adenocarcinoma **b**, and in a tumor cell of a solid carcinoma **c**, magnification X 43000 (a and b) and X 36000 (c)

which the microvilli-like processes of the cell membrane project. The basal cell membrane is mostly smooth and shows invaginations only in isolated cases. The basement membrane is regular in structure focally with varying width but maintained continuity.

Fig. 14a and b. a Surface of the duodenal mucosa with regularly arranged villi, manification X 84; **b** surface of several enterocytes *ec* and a centrally situated goblet cell *gc*. Inset: Individual enterocytes with detached surface coat and therefore visible brush border *bb*, magnification X 6000, inset: X 6000

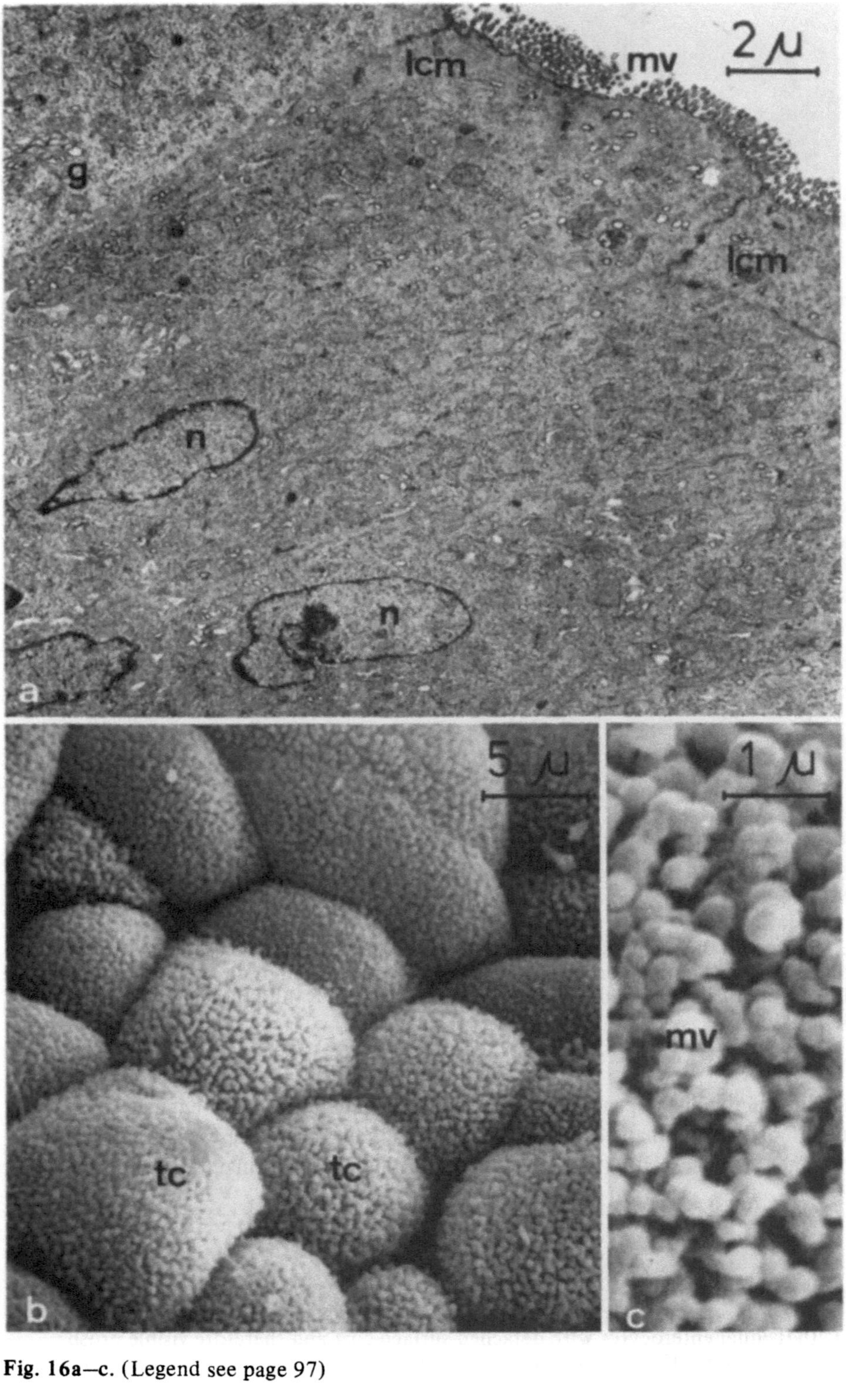

Fig. 16a–c. (Legend see page 97)

Cell nuclei of the tumor cells are largely basal, but may also be localized in apical cell areas; they are round-oval or elongated. Besides these, one also sees slightly pleomorphic nuclei with lobulated nuclear membrane and occasional demonstrable cytoplasmic pseudoinclusions.

Mitochondria in varying number and size can be detected in all cytoplasmic regions of the tumor cells. In cells without appreciable secretory activity, only a few mitochondria are frequently found, whereas abundant mitochondria may be present in epithelia with mucus production. The latter mitochondria may be partly surrounded by lamellae of the *granular endoplasmic reticulum.* The mitochondria mostly show a regular structure. However, mitochondria with indented outer membrane as well as with homogenization, fragmentation, and reduction of the mitochondrial cristae and formation of intramitochondrial myelin lamellae are also found. In the tumor cells of the enterocyte type, one discerns numerous *free ribosomes* predominantly grouped into polysomes, mostly only a few lamellae of the granular endoplasmic reticulum and a poorly developed *Golgi complex.*

Besides these, there exist tumor cells with *secretory granules* in the apical cytoplasm (Fig. 17b). From these cell forms there result fluid transitions to *mucus-producing tumor cells* which may resemble the oligomucous cells in the crypts of the normal small intestinal mucosa (Fig. 18). In the cytoplasm of mucus-producing cells, membrane-limited *mucus granules* are found to greatly differing extents and also larger mucus droplets which are encountered in the entire supranuclear cytoplasm, but in particular directly at the apex. The abundant cisternae of the *granular endoplasmic reticulum* are, in part, appreciably extended and vesicularized with formation of a labyrinthine system of communicating spaces in which fine flocculent material is sometimes deposited (Fig. 17b). Prominent *Golgi complexes* are situated supranuclearly. They are frequently in contact with individual mucus vacuoles.

Lysosomes are frequently localized in the supranuclear cytoplasm of the tumor cells, but also infranuclearly in varying number and size. Autophagic vacuoles with lamellar and vacuolar contents are also found (Fig. 17a). They are structures with a largely perinuclear location surrounded by a sometimes discontinuous fragmentary membrane and with a diameter of about 5 μ. They contain interior vacuoles and concentrically layered membrane structures which in some cases resemble myelin lamellae. In some of these large vacuoles are distinguishable preserved organelles of the constricted cytoplasmic areas, whereas in others the structures are highly condensed and homogenized (Fig. 19). Acid phosphatase can be detected cytohistochemically in most autophagic vacuoles, so that these structures can be regarded as autolysosomes (cf. *Pfeifer*, 1976).

In some of the adenomas examined electron microscopically tumor cells were found with a dense, high microvillous border such as observed in the cylindrical epithelia of the upper third of the crypts. Remarkable in a few of these highly differentiated tumor

---

Fig. 16a–c. a Tumor cells of enterocyte type in a tubulo-villous adenoma of the duodenum. Microvilli *mv*, lateral cell membrane *lcm*, cell nucleus *n*, Golgi zone *g*, magnification × 6900; **b** and **c** surface of tumor cells of enterocyte type of a tubulo-villous adenoma: differences in size of the tumor cells *tc* with regular microvillous border *mv*, magnification × 3120 (b) and × 15600 (c)

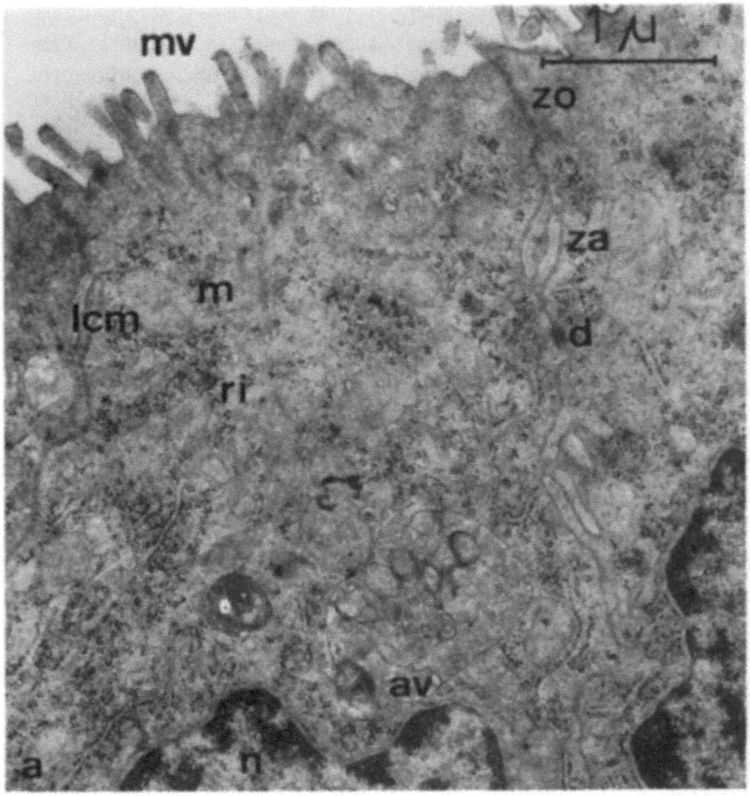

Fig. 17a and b. Tubulo-villous adenoma:
a tumor cells with irregular microvilli border *mv* and an autophagic vacuole *av*. Zonula occludens *zo*, zonula adhaerens *za*, desmosome *d*, lateral cell membrane *lcm*, ribosomes *ri*, cell nucleus *n*, mitochondria *m*, magnification X 23400

cells of enterocyte type are paranuclear and supranuclear glycogen deposits (Fig. 19b) which are not demonstrable in the normal intestinal epithelium of adult rats but which can be observed in the colon epithelium of human fetuses and infant rats (*Lev* and *Weisberg*, 1969; *Mäkelä* et al., 1971; *Bannert*, 1973). Besides these there occur focal epithelial atypias in some adenomas; these are associated with an increase in nuclear polymorphism and a decreasing differentiation of the surface structures.

β) Carcinomas

The tumor cells of *well-differentiated adenocarcinomas* display an ultrastructural picture which is partly similar to that of adenomas. The majority of the tumor cells possess only a few microvilli (e.g. Fig. 20c), whereas some glandular epithelia form a relatively even and high microvillous border (e.g. Fig. 20a) which is covered by a very

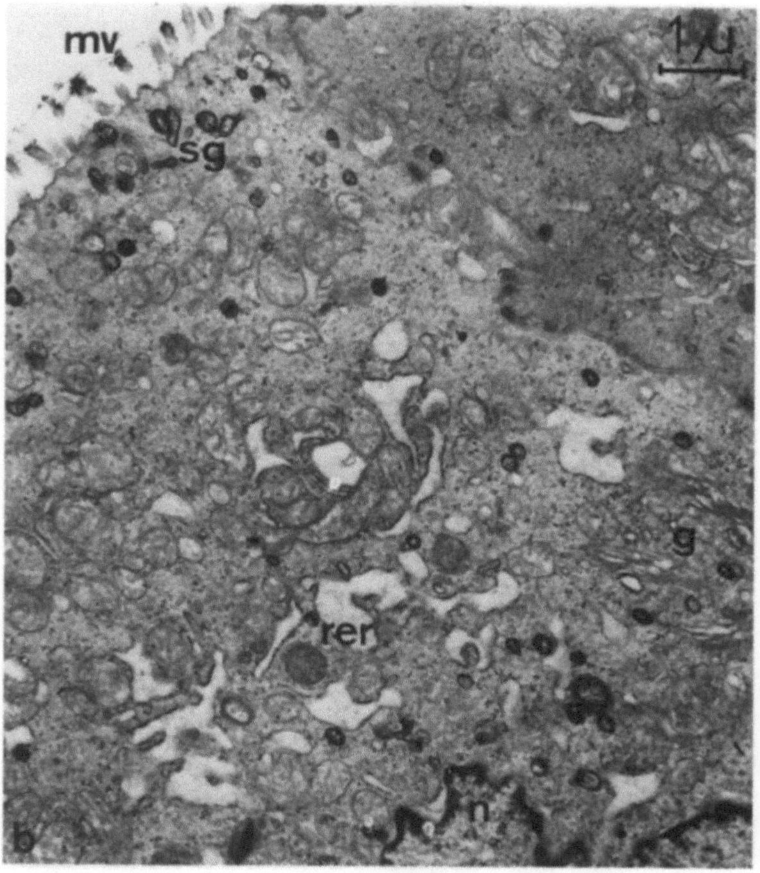

Fig. 17b. Tumor cells with secretory granules *sg*, enlarged cisternae of the rough endoplasmic reticulum *rer* and well-developed Golgi apparatus *g*, microvilli *mv*, cell nucleus *n*, magnification × 11500

thin glycocalyx compared to normal enterocytes (Fig. 15b). The apical portion of tumor cells adjacent to the lateral cell membranes is linked by a zonula occludens of varying length which may be adjoined by a zonula adherens and desmosomes as further adhesive structures (Fig. 20b). In absent or defective development of the adhesive complexes, there arise wide intercellular spaces (Fig. 20c and d). This indicates a reduced coherence of the tumor cells compared to normal epithelial cell cohesion. The basal cell membrane frequently shows irregular, microvilli-like evaginations which come into contact with the subepithelial stroma through gaps in the discontinuous basement membrane. The cell nuclei are still predominantly situated in the basal cytoplasm, even at a differing height from cell to cell.

Just as in the adenomas, two cell forms of varying differentiation can be distinguished among the carcinomas: cells of the enterocyte precursor type and mucus-producing tumor cells. Both cell types show a variable morphological picture. In the

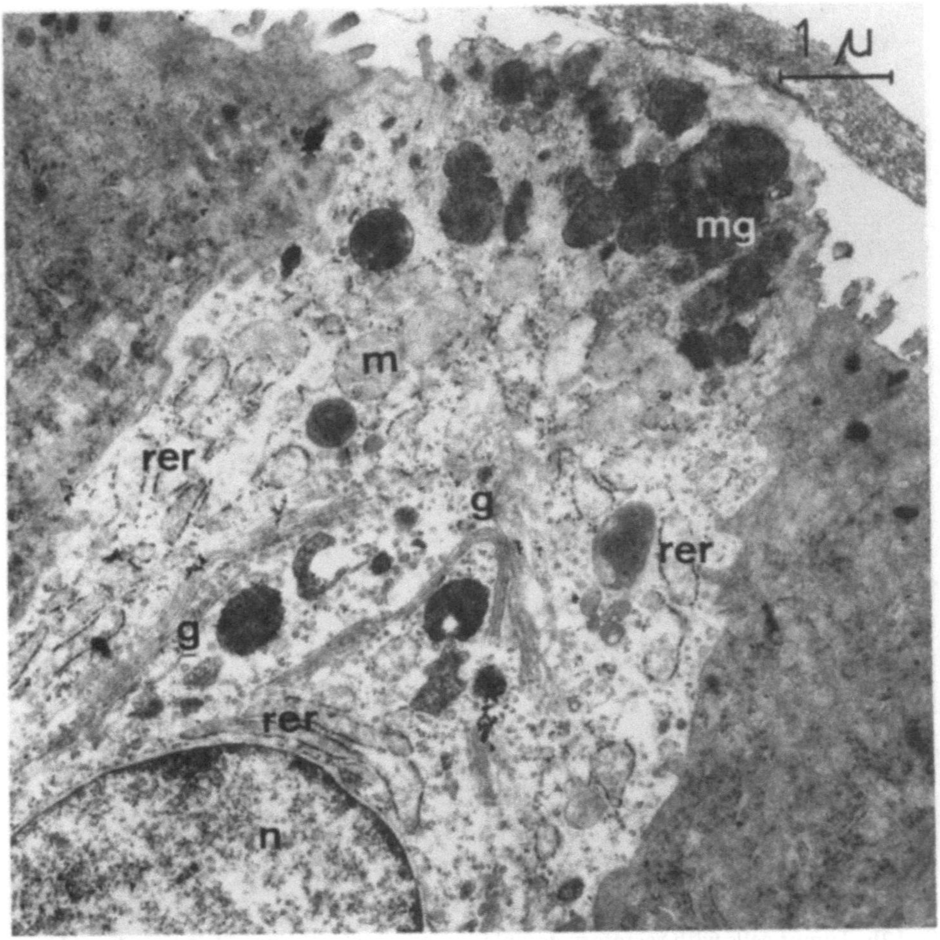

Fig. 18. Mucus-producing tumor cell of a tubulo-villous adenoma. Mucus granules *mg*, rough endoplasmic reticulum *rer*, Golgi complex *g*, mitochondria *m* and cell nucleus *n*, magnification X 14400

majority of the well-differentiated adenocarcinomas, *tumor cells of the enterocyte type* predominate, the individual cells showing a cytoplasm with a varying abundance of organelles. Mitochondria are found in all cytoplasmic regions. In some cases they differ greatly in size, with irregularly arranged intramitochondrial cristae. Between the mitochondria are found numerous free ribosomes, mainly in the form of polysomes, cisternae, and vesicles of the granular endoplasmic reticulum and Golgi complexes,

---

Fig. 19a and b. Tubulo-villous adenoma of the duodenum: **a** early stage of an autophagic vacuole *av*, phase of segregation: accumulation of numerous lysosomes *l* and lipid droplets *ld*, cell nucleus *n*, mitochondria *m*, magnification X 16200; **b** tumor cell with deposition of glycogen *gly*, cell nucleus *n*, mitochondria *m*, Golgi complex *g*, autophagic vacuole *av*, magnification X 23400

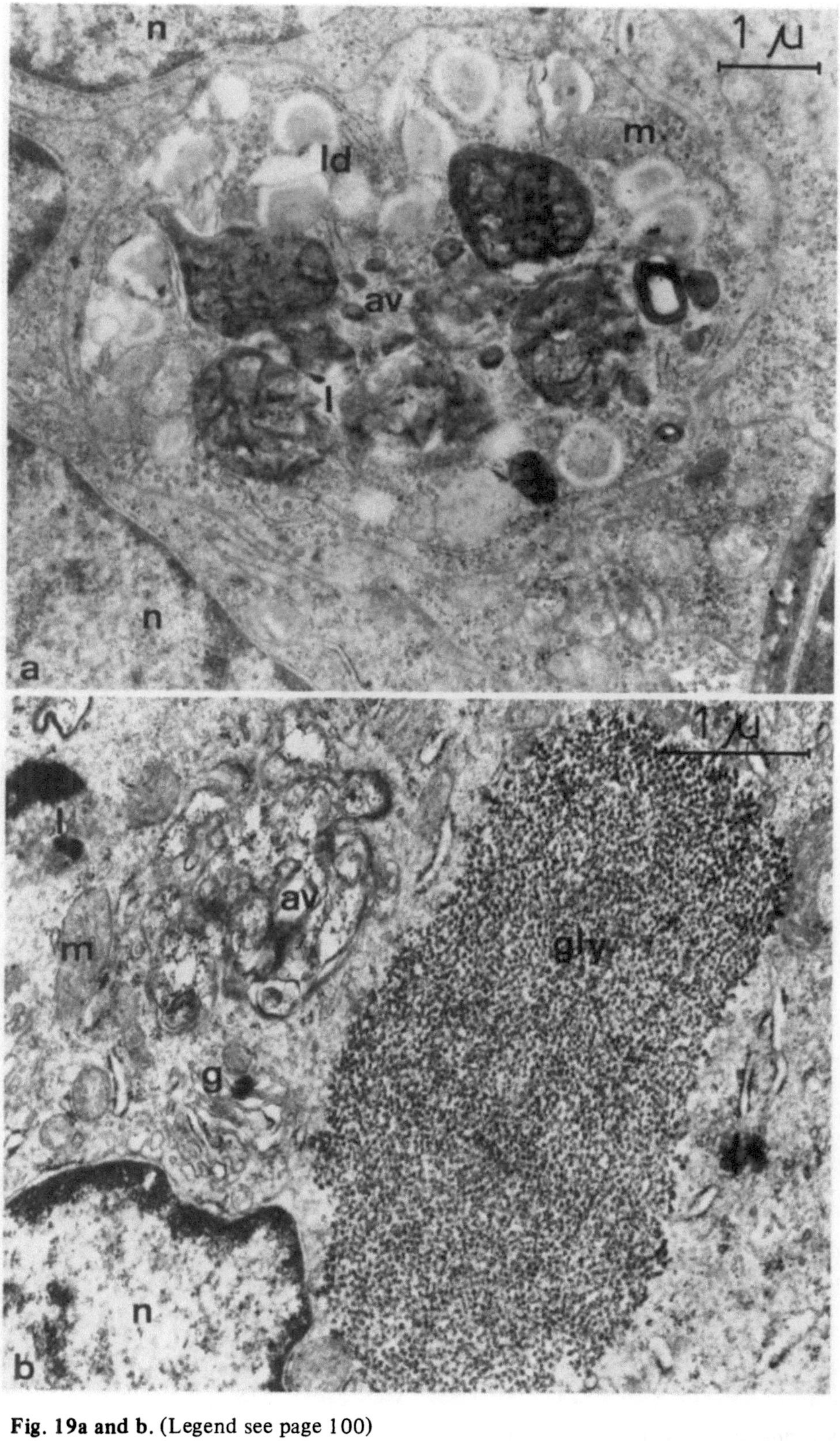

Fig. 19a and b. (Legend see page 100)

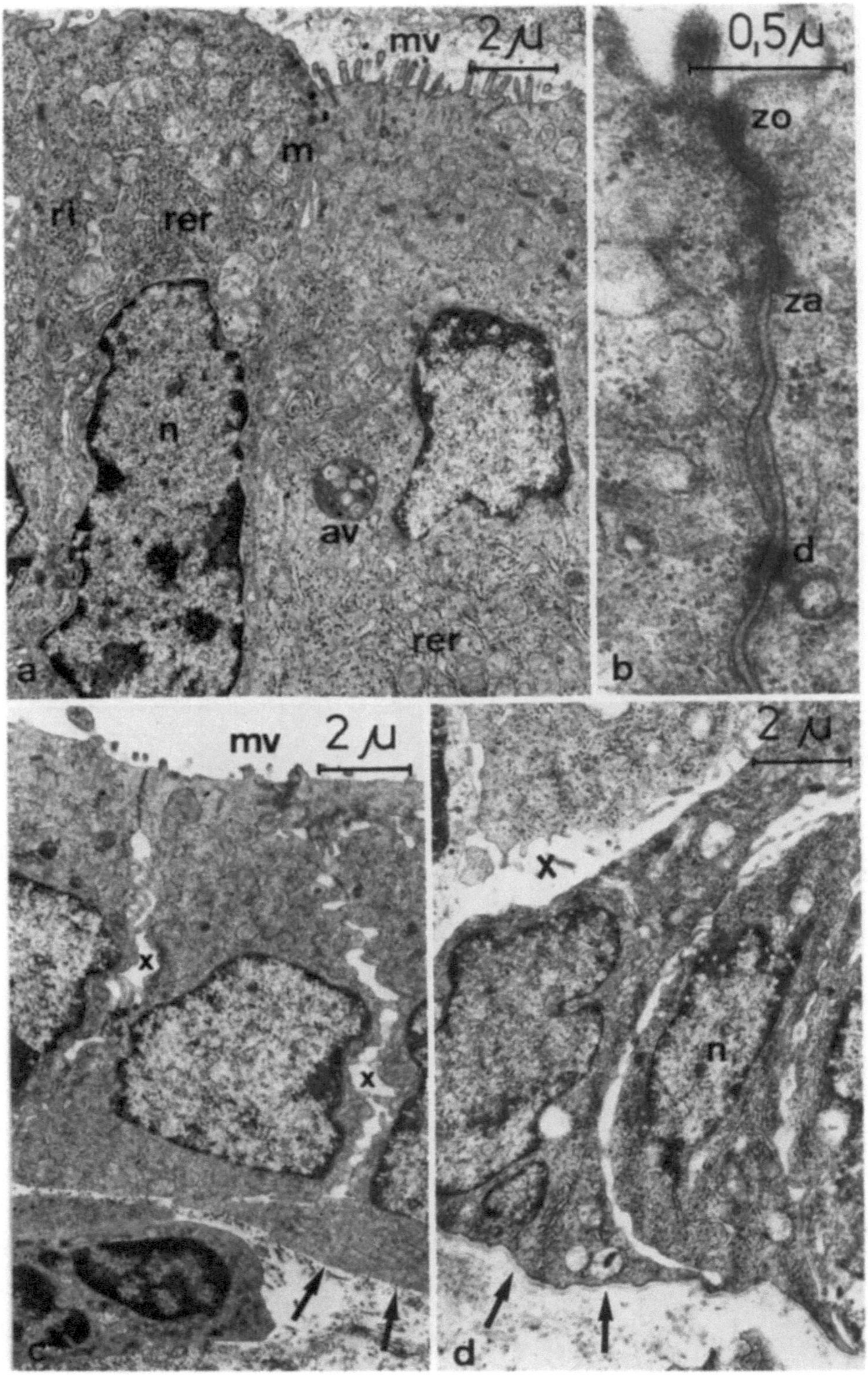

Fig. 20a–d. (Legend see page 103)

which are frequently irregularly distributed in the cytoplasm (Fig. 21). The cytoplasm of some tumor cells of the enterocyte type is poor in organelles; free ribosomes predominate here. In a few tumor cells, supranuclear glycogen deposits can be demonstrated.

The *mucus-producing tumor cells* show a variable ultrastructural picture just as the tumor cells of the enterocyte type. Only one of the electron microscopically examined adenocarcinomas of the small intestine possesses a predominantly mucus-producing epithelial component (Figs. 22 and 23a). Part of the epithelia of this tumor displays a cytoplasmic differentiation which is comparable with the goblet cells of the normal mucosa (Fig. 23a). The entire supranuclear cytoplasm is filled by mucus droplets which push the cell organelles into the cell periphery. Only a few mucus droplets are surrounded by a membrane, the rest flows together into larger accumulations of mucus. Situated in the vicinity of the lateral cell membrane and directly supranuclearly are mitochondria, granular endoplasmic reticulum, and the Golgi complex in close functional association. Besides these apparently mature, mucus-producing epithelial cells, tumor cells are discerned in the majority of adenocarcinomas which are comparable with the immature, mucus-producing epithelia of the basal crypt zone of the normal intestinal mucosa. These tumor cells produce only a few mucus droplets which are partly surrounded by membranes; these are distributed either only in the apical cytoplasm or loosely in the entire supranuclear cytoplasm. They often possess a wide, labyrinthine ramified or even vesicular granular endoplasmic reticulum and a well-differentiated Golgi complex in the vicinity of the cell nucleus. Autophagic vacuoles are found in numerous tumor cells of the adenocarcinomas, mainly in the infranucelar and paranuclear cytoplasm.

Fig. 20a–d. Tumor cells of adenocarcinomas of the duodenum: **a** tumor cells with organelle-rich cytoplasm; mitochondria *m*, rough endoplasmic reticulum *rer*, ribosomes *ri*, autophagic vacuoles *av*, cell nucleus *n*, microvilli *mv*, magnification X 6900; **b** well-differentiated junctional complex of a lateral cell membrane: zonula occludens *zo*, zonula adherens *za* and desmosome *d*, magnification X 46000; **c** tumor cells with scanty formation of microvilli *mv* , large intercellular spaces *x* and absence of basement membrane *arrows*, magnification X 6440; **d** tumor cells with large intercellular spaces *x* and with a basement membrane *arrows*, cell nucleus *n*, magnification X 7200

Fig. 21a and b. Tumor cells of a well-differentiated adenocarcinoma of the duodenum with organelle-rich cytoplasm; mitochondria *m*, rough endoplasmic reticulum *rer*, free ribosomes *ri*, Golgi complex *g*, cell nucleus *n* and intercellular space *i*, magnification X 27000 (a), X 16000 (b)

Fig. 22a and b. Surface of a mucus-producing adenocarcinoma: **a** survey (*t* = tumor; *v* = normal small intestinal villi), magnification X 24; **b** mucus-producing tumor cells with protruding apical cell membrane *mt* and tumor cells of enterocyte type with microvilli *mv*, magnification X 2220 and X 3600 (inset)

Fig. 23a and b. **a** Mucus-producing adenocarcinoma of the duodenum: mucus-producing tumor cells *mt* and tumor cells of enterocyte type *te*, mucus granules *mg* and microvilli *mv*, magnification X 7440; **b** tumor cells of a poorly differentiated adenocarcinoma surrounding a narrow glandular lumen *lu*; no basement membrane *arrows*, cell nuclei *n* and rough endoplasmic reticulum *rer*, magnification X 9920

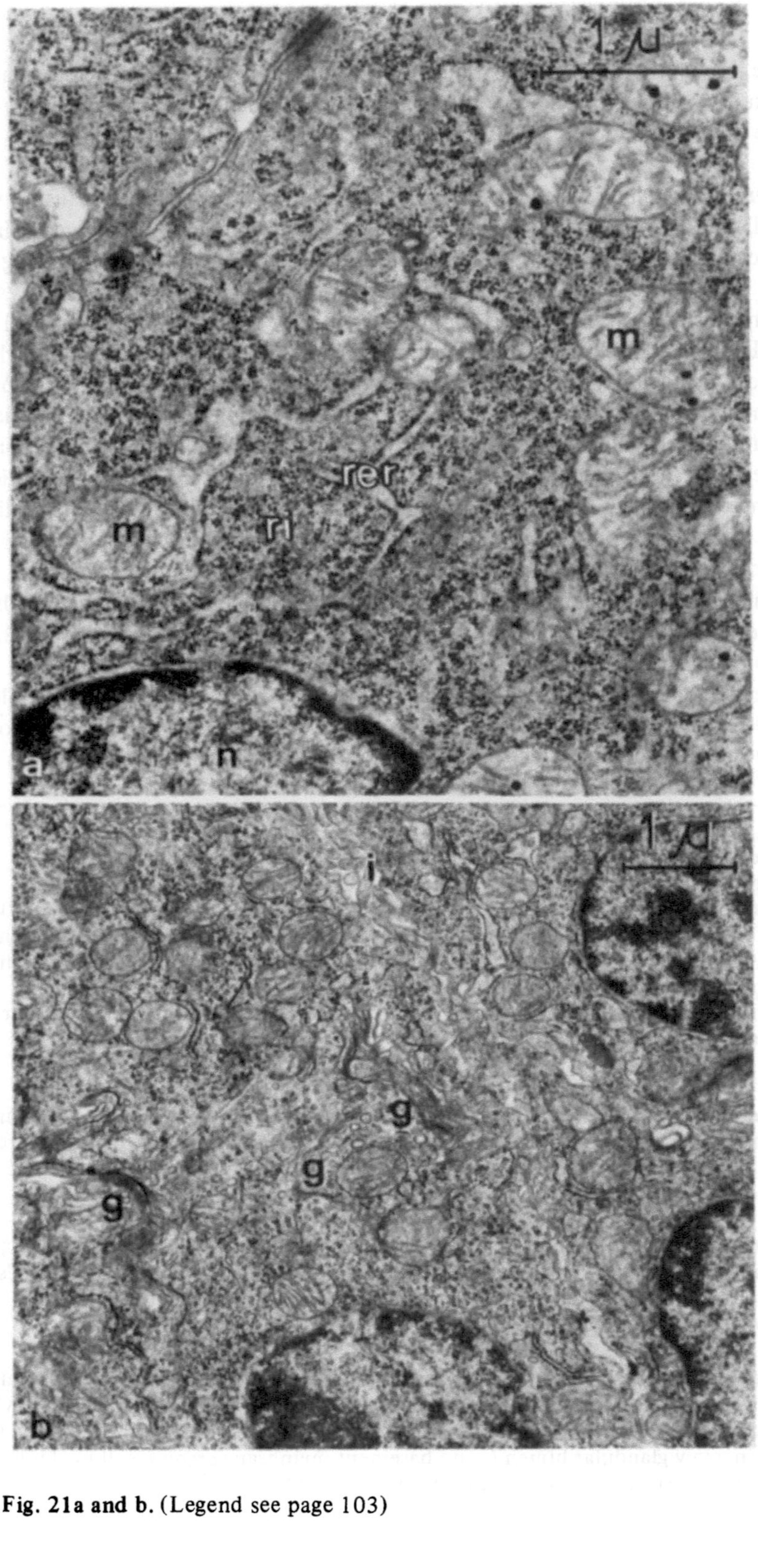

Fig. 21a and b. (Legend see page 103)

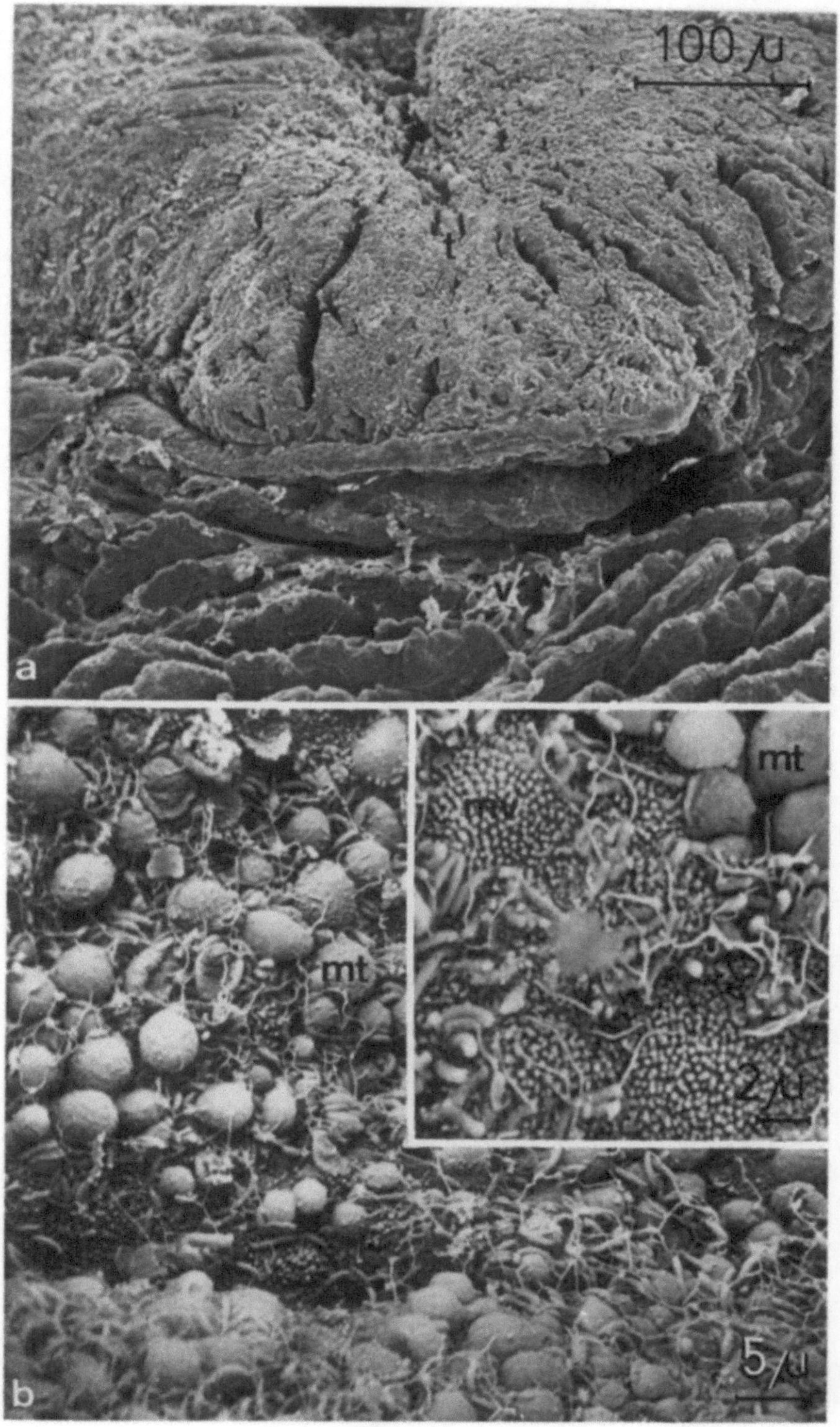

Fig. 22a and b. (Legend see page 103)

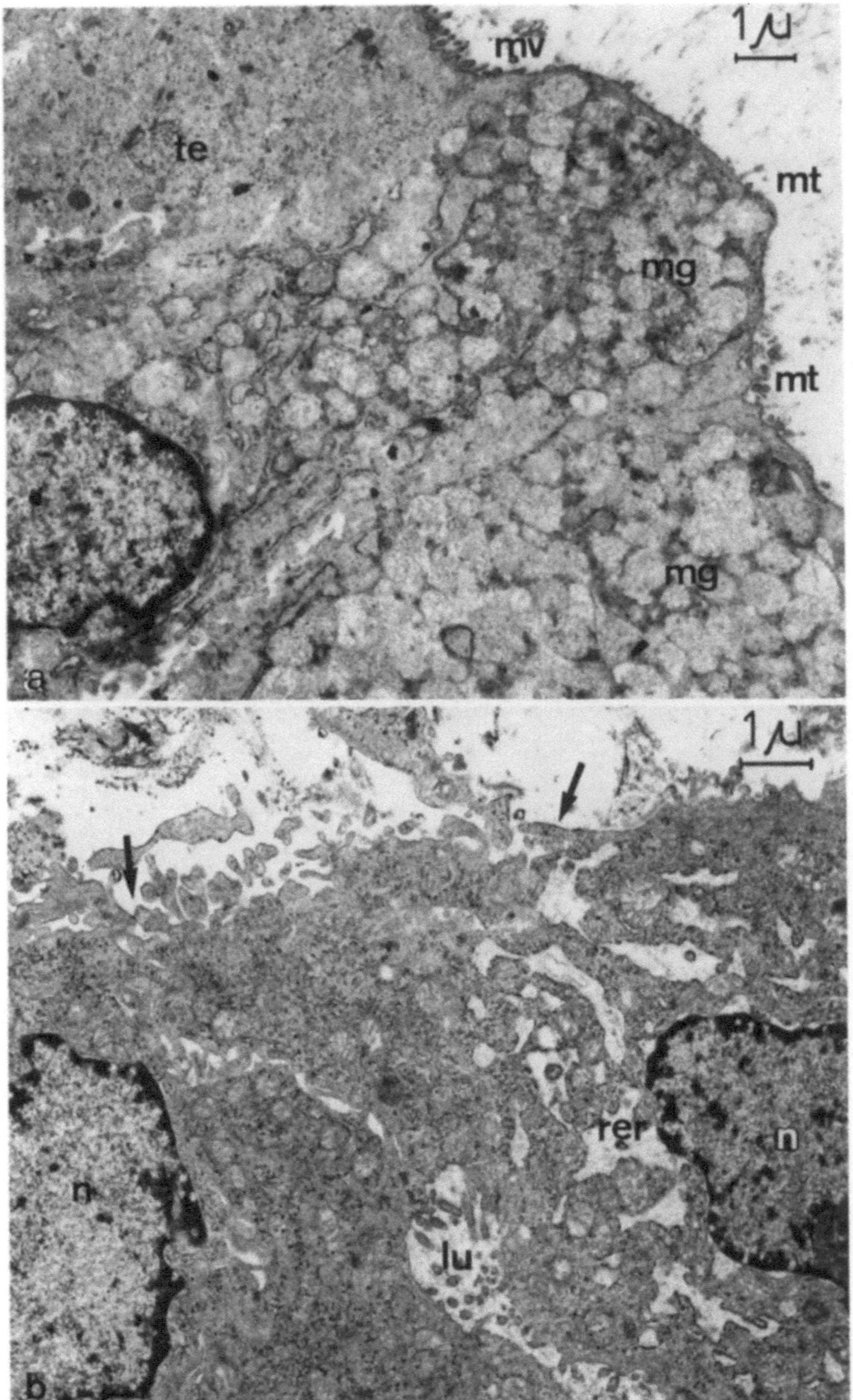

Fig. 23a and b. (Legend see page 103)

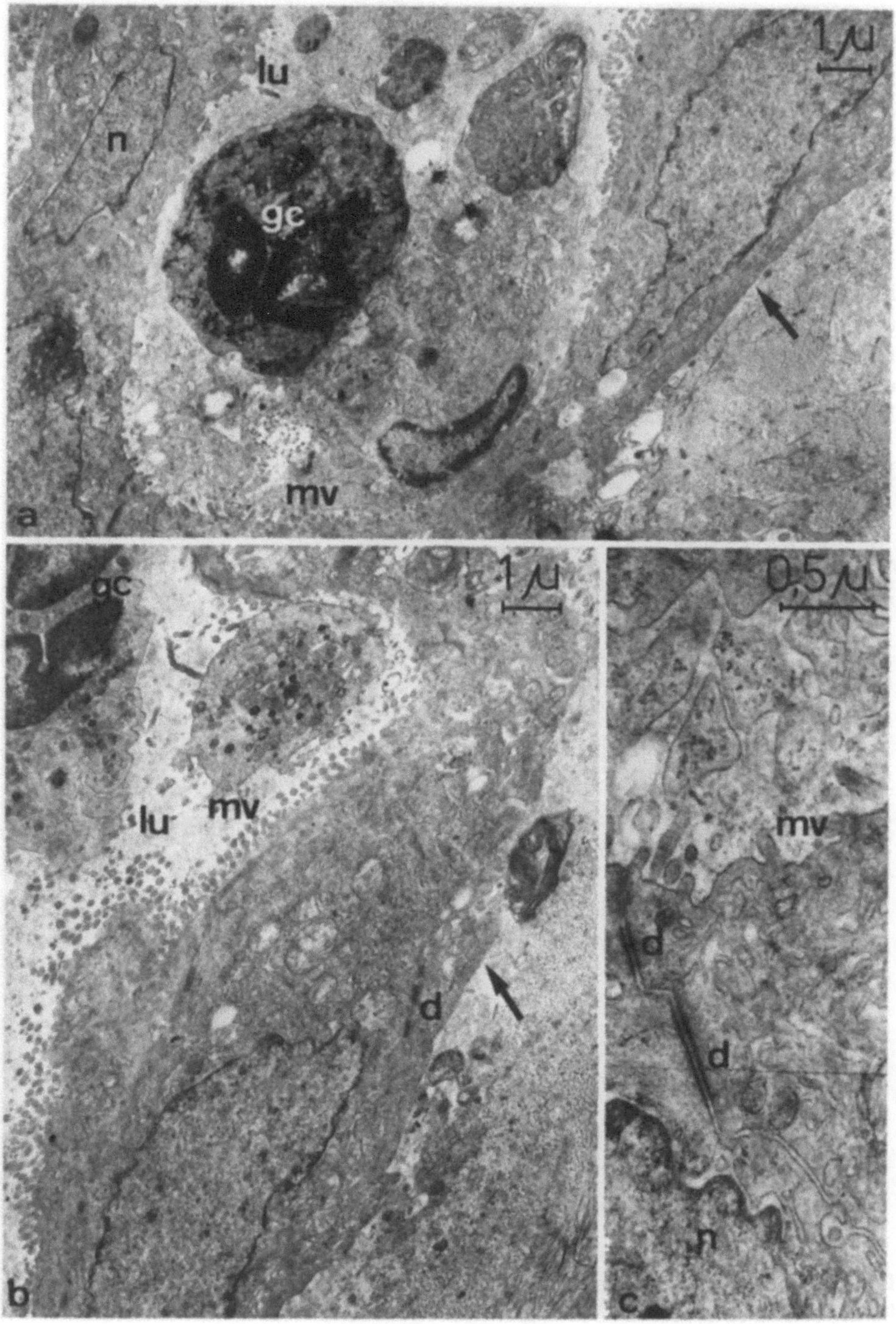

Fig. 24a–c. a and **b** Wide luminal glands of a poorly differentiated adenocarcinoma with flat tumor cells: in the gland lumina *lu* desquamated cells (e.g., granulocytes = *gc*), no basement membrane *arrows,* microvilli *mv*, desmosomes *d*, magnification X 6900 (a) and X 8280 (b); **c** interepithelial junctional complex with elongated desmosomes *d*, microvilli *mv*, cell nuclei *n*, magnification X 27000

The transition from well-differentiated to *poorly differentiated adenocarcinomas* is fluid. The glands of the poorly differentiated adenocarcinomas often consist of only a few tumor cells which in some cases enclose tiny glandular lumina (Fig. 23b). In addition, wide glands formed from elongated, flat tumor cells are also found. In the lumina of these glands, tumor cells and granulocytes in various stages of disintegration are seen (Fig. 24). The structures of the outer cell membrane show a constitution which varies from cell to cell. Individual epithelia have a regular microvillous border, others only coarse membrane protrusions or even a smooth surface (Fig. 25). The structure and arrangement of the interepithelial adhesion structures, which only incompletely link the tumor cells to each other, also vary to the same extent (Fig. 24c). A basement membrane is frequently absent. Compared with the more highly differentiated small intestinal tumors, one notices an increasing disorganization of the cellular organelles, e.g., bizarre deformation of the mitochondria. In addition, one observes filament bundles and secretory vacuoles in numerous tumor cells (Fig. 27b).

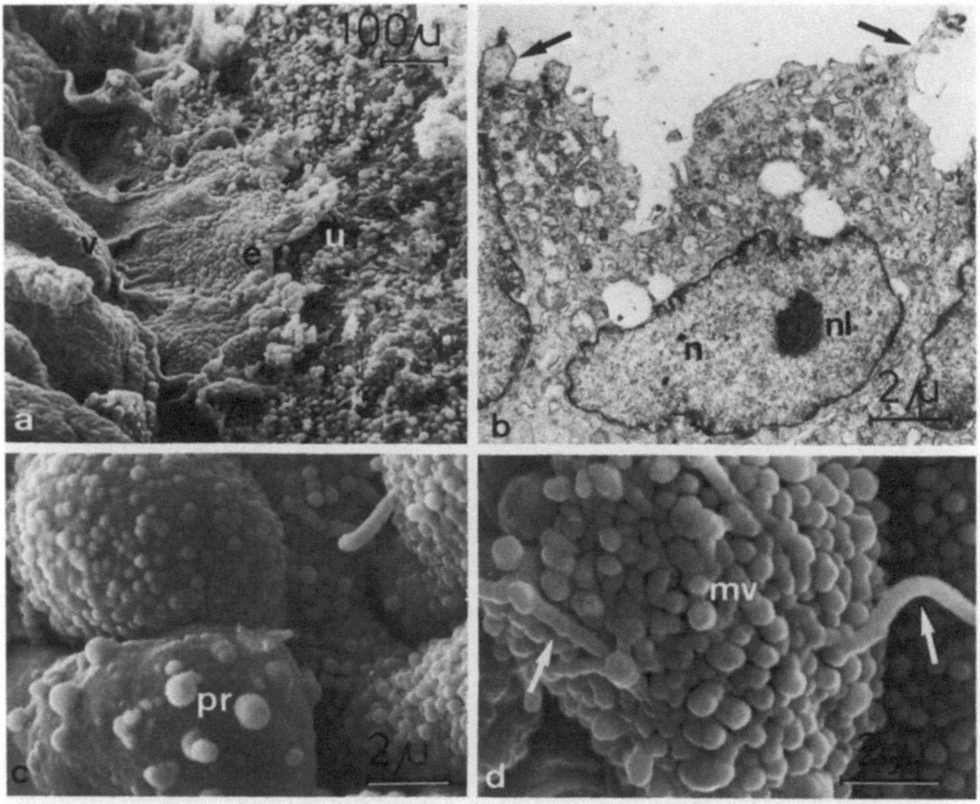

Fig. 25a–d. Surface of a poorly differentiated adenocarcinoma: **a** border zone between tumor and normal small intestinal mucosa (*u = ulcerated tumor surface, e* = epithelialized tumor surface, *v* = small intestinal villi), magnification × 90; **b** tumor cells with coarse protrusions *arrows* of the apical cell membrane, cell nucleus *n*, nucleolus *nl*, magnification × 5500; **c** tumor cells with coarse protrusions *pr* of the apical cell membrane, magnification × 5800; **d** tumor cells with highly regular microvillous border *mv*, scattered long fingerlike microvilli *arrows*, magnification × 6400

Essentially three cell forms can be differentiated in the *solid carcinomas:* anaplastic tumor cells with varying abundance of organelles in the cytoplasm, tumor cells with intracytoplasmic lumina, and mucus-producing tumor cells.

Anaplastic tumor cells may be isolated or occur in the stroma as small cell associations (Fig. 7c and d) which may sometimes be enveloped by a fragmentary basement membrane. These cell groups variously form cohesive epithelial associations with smooth densely packed cell membranes which are linked by irregularly arranged desmosomes. Other tumor cells form loose cell associations with broad intercellular spaces into which project numerous partly interdigitating, microvilli-like cell processes. The anaplastic tumor cells possess large pleomorphic cell nuclei in part with lobulated nuclear membrane and cytoplasmic pseudoinclusions which leave free only narrow cytoplasmic border in numerous cells. There are distinct differences between the various tumor cells with regard to cytoplasmic differentiation. Thus, individual tumor cells possess a cytoplasm having abundant organelles with numerous mitochondria and abundant ergastoplasm (Fig. 26a), whereas in other cells these structures completely recede into the background and the cytological picture is determined by densely packed free ribosomes (Fig. 26b).

Tumor cells with intracytoplasmic lumina may be isolated in the stroma or grouped together into small epithelial associations (Fig. 27a). The intracytoplasmic lumina are delimited by a microvillous border. Hetero- and autophagosomes or autolysosomes can be demonstrated in the cytoplasm.

Mucus-producing tumor cells, the third cell form of the solid carcinomas, show a highly variegated cytological picture. Some of these tumor cells involve typical signet ring cells with one or several large intracytoplasmic mucus droplets which push the flat-concave cell nucleus and the cellular organelles into the narrow cytoplasmic margin (Fig. 28a). Besides these, one recognizes elongated cylindrical cells with numerous small mucus vacuoles delimited in some cases by membranes. In the perinuclear cytoplasm, there are mitochondria, a dilated granular endoplasmic reticulum and Golgi complexes. These tumor cells are probably precursors of typical signet ring cells: numerous morphological transitions between the two cell variants can be observed. For example, elongated cylindrical tumor cells with a few large mucus vacuoles, cells with centrally situated cell nuclei surrounded by individual vacuoles and cells with

---

Fig. 26a and b. Solid (anaplastic) carcinoma: **a** tumor cells with organelle-rich cytoplasm and microvilli-like evagination of the outer membrane *arrows*, magnification × 15000; **b** tumor cell with few intracytoplasmic organelles, rough endoplasmic reticulum *rer*, mitochondria *m*, ribosomes *ri*, magnification × 16800

Fig. 27a and b. **a** Two tumor cells of a solid carcinoma with intracytoplasmic lumina *icl* surrounded by microvilli *arrows*, autophagic vacuole *av*, magnification × 9000; **b** tumor cells with intracytoplasmic filament bundles *arrows*, microvilli *mv*, desmosomes *d*, lysosomes *l* and cell nucleus *n*, magnification × 28750

Fig. 28a and b. Tumor cells of a signet ring cell carcinoma: mucus vacuoles *mv*, cell nuclei *n*, magnification × 7500 (a) and × 6440 (b)

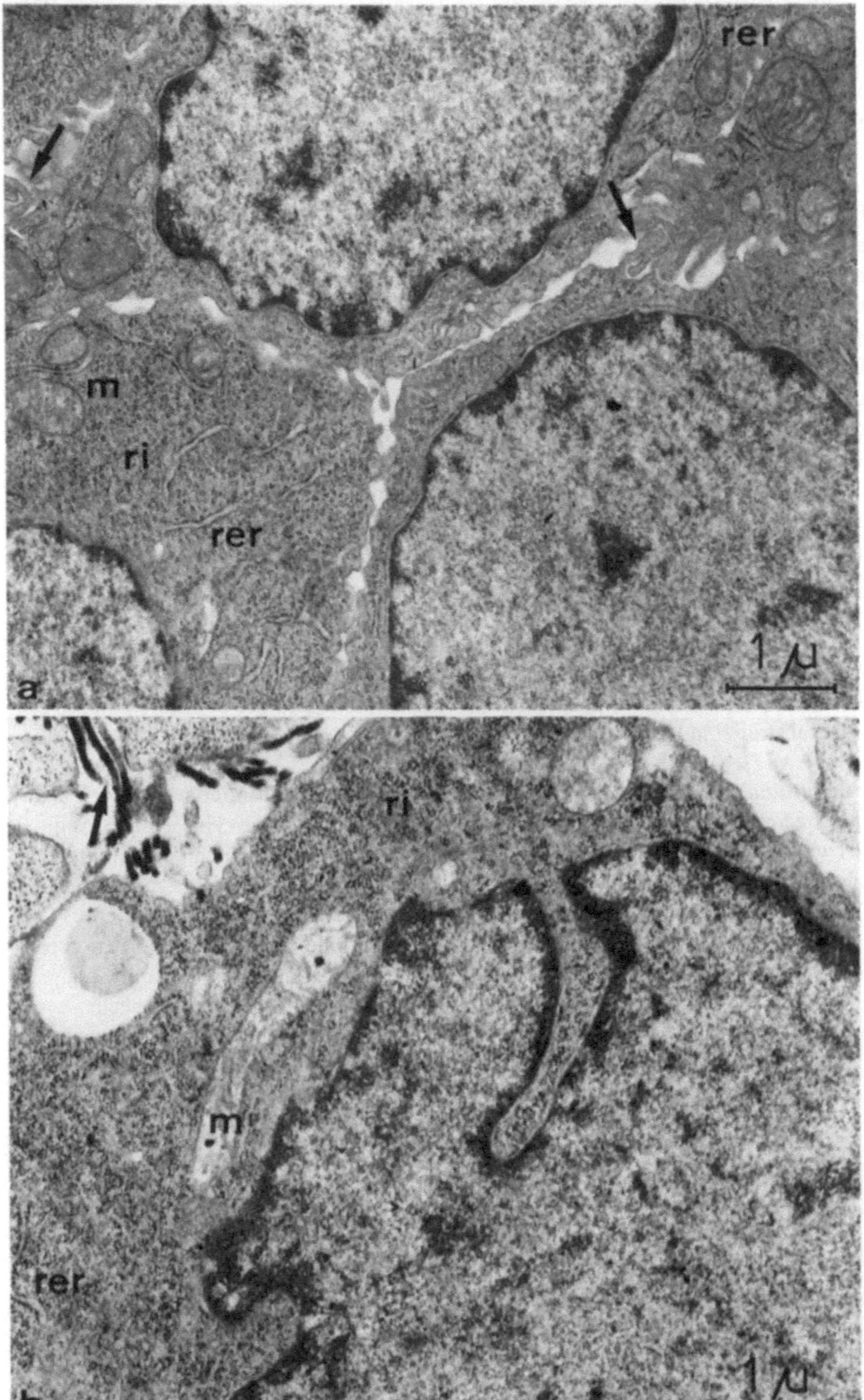

Fig. 26a and b. (Legend see page 109)

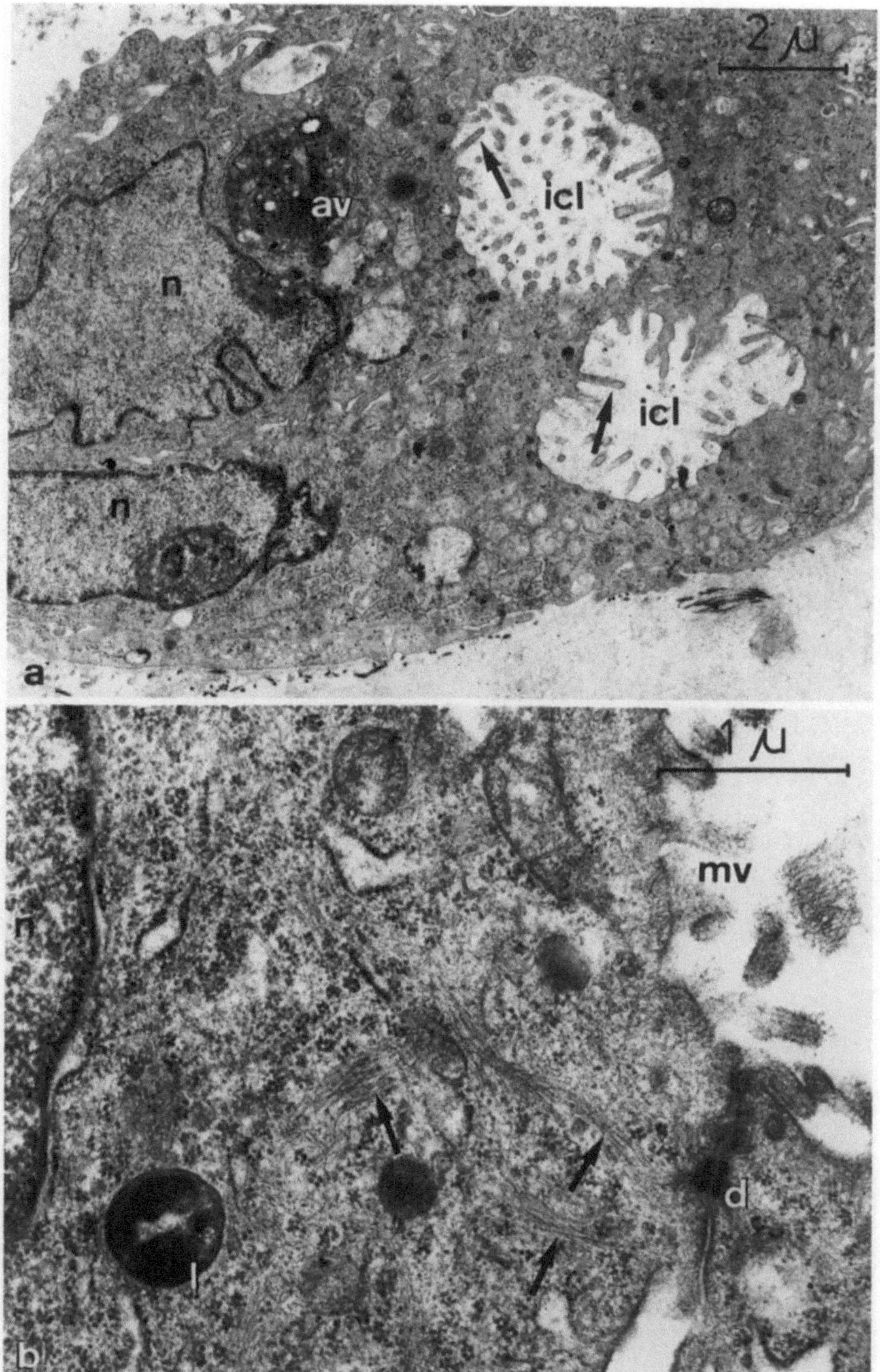

Fig. 27a and b. (Legend see page 109)

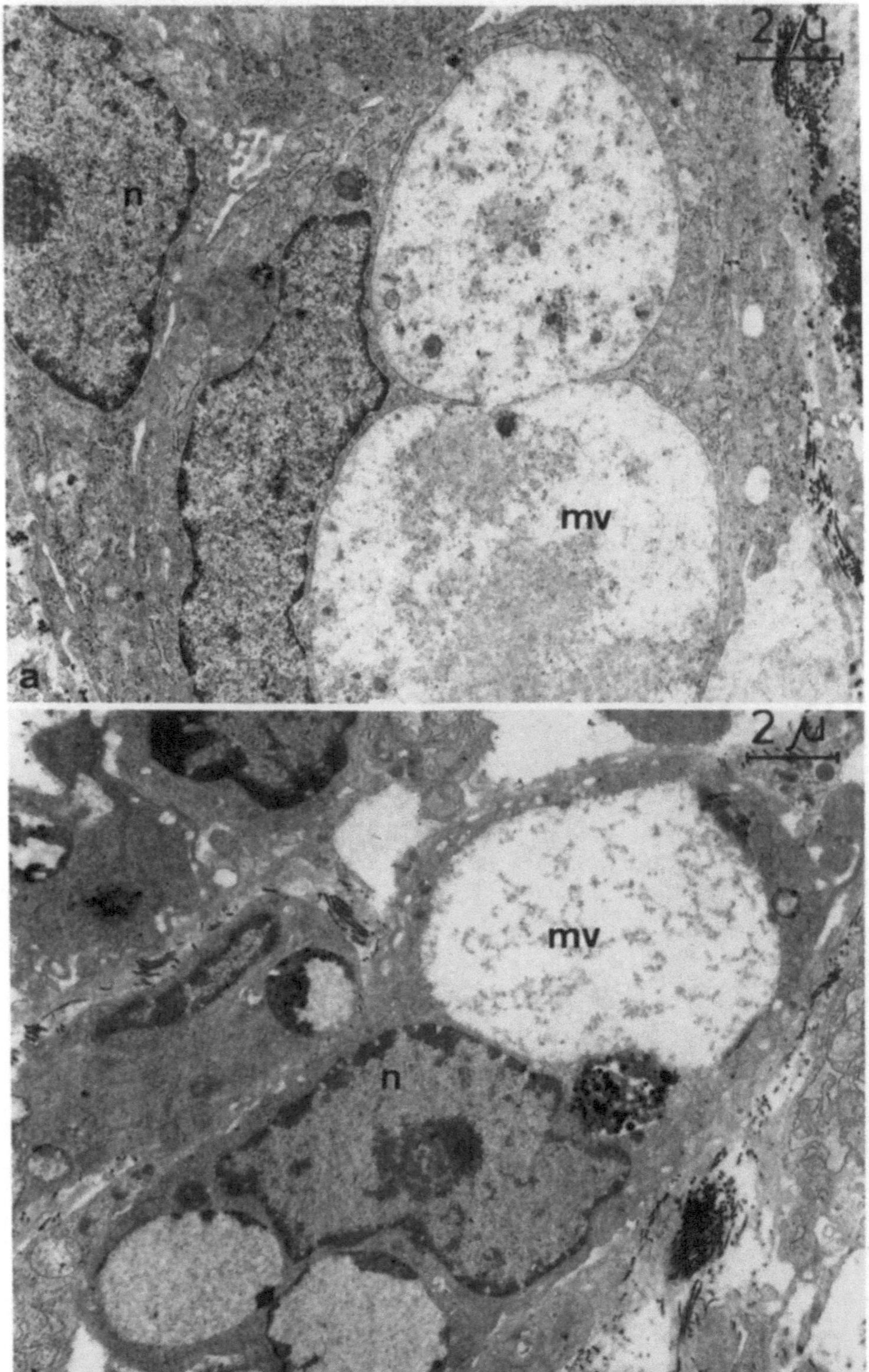

Fig. 28a and b. (Legend see page 109)

incipient displacement of the cell nuclei and the cellular organelles into the cytoplasmic periphery are found (Fig. 28b).

5. Enzyme Histochemical Findings

A description of the enzyme histochemical findings in the normal small intestinal mucosa can be dispensed with at this point since there are already a large number of appropriate investigations (*Pearse* and *Riecken*, 1967; *Lojda* et al., 1970; *Riecken*, 1975; *Gossrau*, 1975a, b; *Schäfer* and *Höhn*, 1975; *Höhn* et al., 1977, 1978).

a) Enzyme Patterns in Experimentally Induced Small Intestinal Tumors

In accordance with the largely normal cytological appearance of the epithelial cells in the *hyperplastic mucosal areas*, this shows the same kind of enzyme histochemical picture as in the normal small intestinal mucosa.

α) Adenomas

In comparison with the enterocytes of the proximal small intestine, the abrupt fall in activity of some of the histochemically investigated *hydrolases* is noticeable in the tumor cells of the adenomas. This finding is correlated with the histologically sharp boundary between normal mucosa and tumor. Histochemically, glucose-6-phosphatase, 5'-nucleotidase, neutral α-glucosidase, and leucyl-β-naphthylamidase can no longer be detected in the tumors. In the histochemical demonstration of nonspecific esterase, only a few granules of dye are found in the supranuclear cytoplasm. Alkaline phosphatase, on the other hand, reacts positively to very different extents in individual tumor cells. The majority of tumor cells do not possess any alkaline phosphatase activity, whereas in a few glandular epithelia the apical cell membrane shows intense positive staining and the lateral cell membrane is also stained occasionally. There is a similar histochemical finding with ATPase. The capillaries between the glands frequently show a positive alkaline phosphatase reaction.

Acid phosphatase activity is not much less in the epithelia of the adenomas than in the crypt epithelial of a normal small intestinal mucosa. There is a fine granular reaction in the supranuclear cytoplasm of tumor cells but a coarser precipitation of dye is infranuclearly in individual epithelial cells. The specific reaction of acid phosphatase can be demonstrated ultrahistochemically in lysosomes. Some macrophages between the glandular sacs also show a positive acid phosphatase reaction.

The activity of all histochemically investigated *oxidoreductases* mostly decreases markedly in tumor cells compared to the villous epithelia of normal small intestinal mucosa. This applies especially to G-6-PD, HBDH, IDH, GDH, and MAO, whereas LDH, SDH, and MDH only show a slight or no loss of activity. In tumor cells, the activity decreases in the apical cytoplasm, whereas perinuclearly it remains largely stable or decreases only slightly.

β) Carcinomas

Adenocarcinomas: Most *hydrolases* (G-6-P, 5'nucleotidase, neutral α-glucosidase, leucyl-β-naphthylamidase, nonspecific esterase, and acid phosphatase; Fig. 29a) in adenocarcinomas of the small intestine show a histochemical behavior similar to adenoma hydrolases. In contrast to adenomas, alkaline phosphatase and ATPase can also be demonstrated in individual larger epithelial cell associations of adenocarcinomas. The activity of these enzyems is mainly localized in the outer cell membrane; membrane-positive and membrane-negative tumor cells cannot be distinguished from each other morphologically (Fig. 29b and c).

The *oxidoreductases* of the adenocarcinomas (without mucus formation) display a reaction pattern comparable to that seen in adenomas, but the enzyme activities are still irregularly distributed within the tumors. The intra-epithelial localization and concentration of the formazan granules may differ without any discernible systematics even within a single gland. LDH, MDH, and SDH activities are attenuated compared with the normal mucosa but still pronounced in almost all adenocarcinomas. MAO reacts to a varying extent in the carcinomas. In a few tumors, MAO activity can no longer be demonstrated, whereas other carcinomas show a reaction comparable to that of normal mucosa. The remainder of the oxidoreductases investigated display only a weak positive reaction. In the mucus-producing tumor cells, the formazan granules are pushed out into the cell periphery by the intracytoplasmic accumulation of mucus. As a whole, the activity of oxidoreductases is lower in these tumor cells than in tumor cells which do not form mucus.

Solid Carcinomas: Alkaline phosphatase shows a high activity in solid carcinomas; tumor cells and tumor stroma are stained to a different extent and in varying relation to each other. An intensive reaction can be demonstrated in some carcinomas in almost all tumor cells in the outer cell membrane and its microvilli-like evaginations (Fig. 30). On the other hand, only a few tumor cells are stained in other tumors. Furthermore, alkaline phosphatase shows a histochemically detectable activity in the Golgi apparatus and in individual profiles of the endoplasmic reticulum in some of the membrane-positive cells.

Large, round intracytoplasmic areas with specific dye precipitates are sometimes found light microscopically in tumor cells. These may involve the stained structures around the membrane, occupied by microvilli, which surrounds the intracytoplasmic lumina. In the material embedded for ultrahistochemistry, cells reacting in this way cannot be found. The ATPase in solid carcinomas shows a histochemical reaction comparable to that of alkaline phosphatase.

In solid carcinomas, no G-6-P, 5'nucleotidase, neutral α-glucosidase, or LNA can be detected using histochemical methods. The nonspecific esterase only shows a slight E600-resistant activity in the majority of solid carcinomas. On the other hand, in individual carcinomas there is an intensive reaction of the E600-sensitive nonspecific esterase in the cytoplasm of tumor cells.

Fig. 29a–c. Tumor cells of an adenocarcinoma: **a** positive reaction of acid phosphatase in lysosomes, magnification ×29600; **b** and **c** positive reaction of alkaline phosphatase in the microvilli *mv* of the apical cell membrane *acm, arrows* of tumor cells, magnification × 13800 (b) and × 34500 (c)

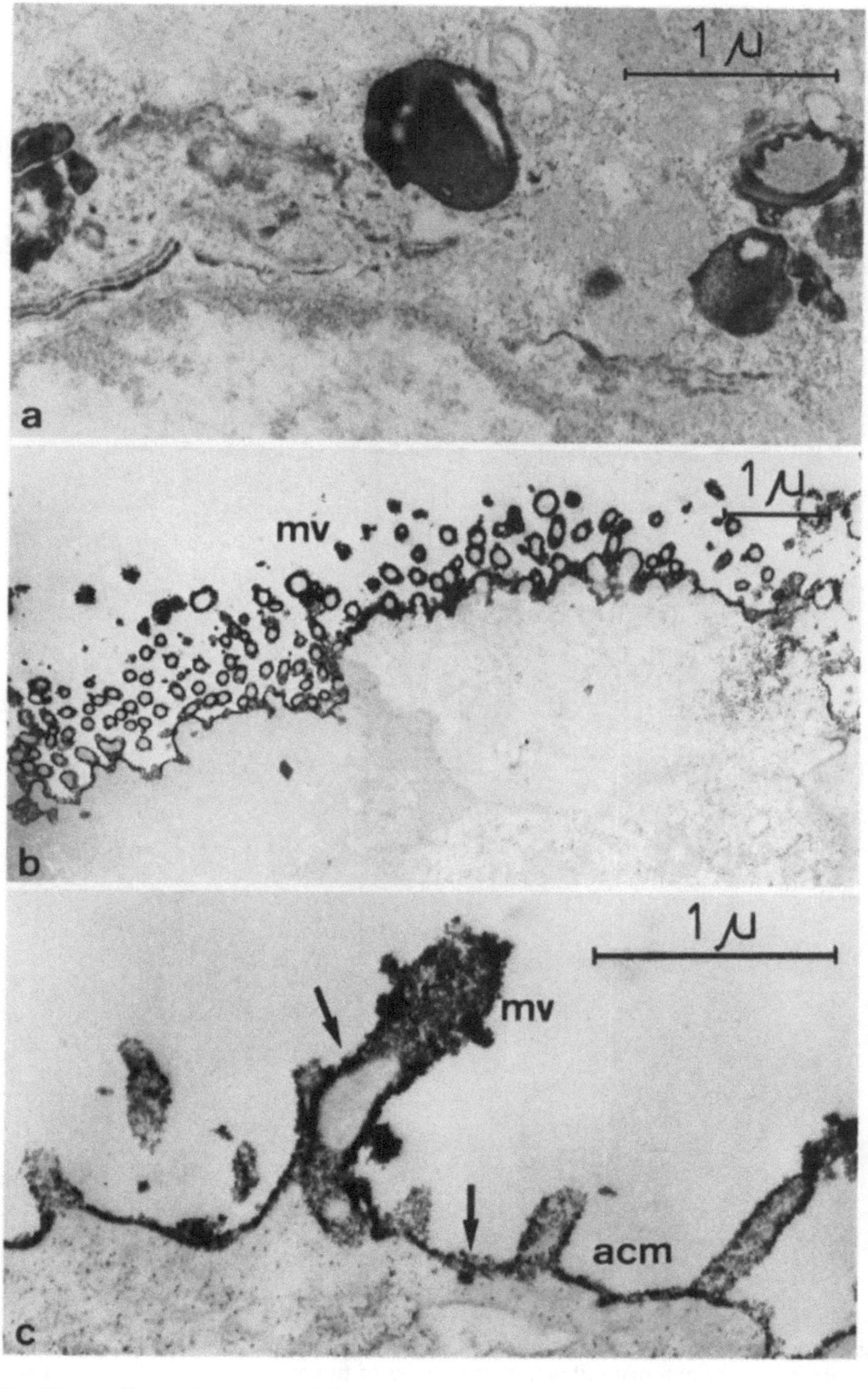

Fig. 29a–c. (Legend see page 114)

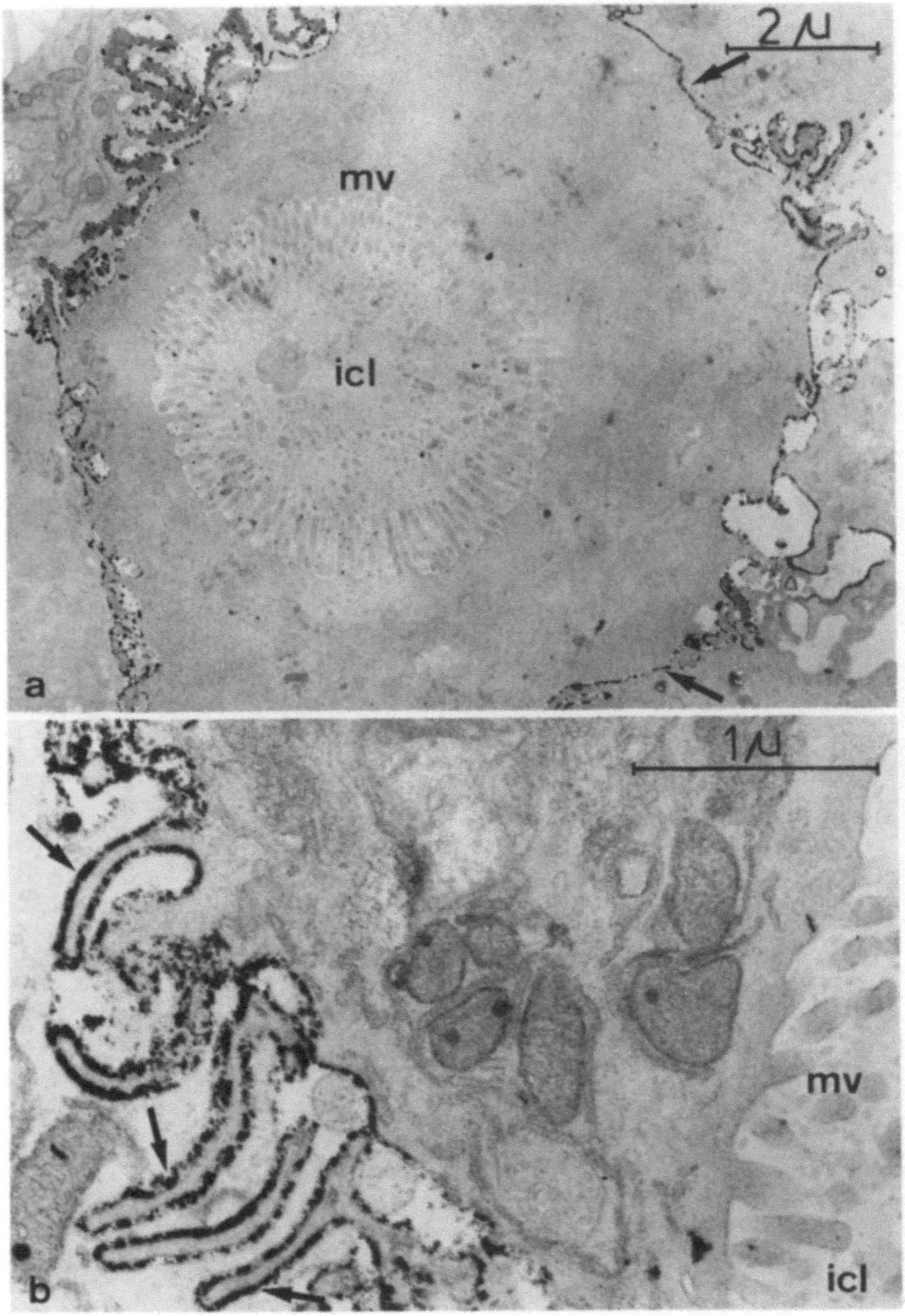

Fig. 30a and b. Tumor cell with intracytoplasmic lumen *icl*: positive reaction of alkaline phosphatase in the external cell membrane *arrows* of tumor cells, microvilli *mv*, magnification × 10580 (a) and × 34500 (b)

Corresponding to the low degree of differentiation of solid carcinomas, the activity of *oxidoreductases* is even lower in solid tumors than in gland-forming tumors. This applies particularly to G-6-PD, HBDH, and MAO. MDH and SDH, but mainly LDH, still show a marked activity in most solid carcinomas. The intracellular localization and concentration of formazan granules does not only vary from tumor to tumor in the assay of all oxidoreductases investigated, but also in the tumor cells of one and the same carcinoma. Some tumor cells or cell groups with very high enzyme activities are stained, whereas neighboring tumor areas only display a slight reaction or none at all. In mucus-forming tumor cells, the granules of dye become confluent around the accumulations of mucus. As a whole, the activity of the oxidoreductases is lower in signet ring cell carcinomas than in solid carcinomas which do not produce mucus.

6. Disc Electrophoretic Findings

a) LDH and MDH Isoenzymes in the Normal Small Intestinal Mucosa of Fetal, Neonatal, and Adult Rats

Lactate dehydrogenase: The European nomenclature is used to designate the isoenzymes of LDH serially as LDH_1 through to LDH_5, where LDH_1 is the form that migrates fastest towards the cathode during electrophoresis and LDH_5 migrates slowest.

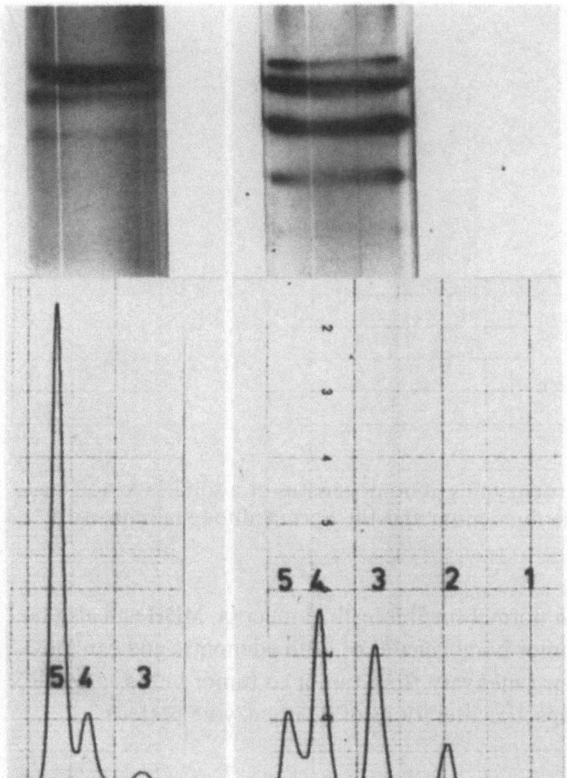

Fig. 31a and b. Electropherograms and densitograms of the LDH isoenzymes of the duodenal mucosa of a fetal **a** and a four month old rat **b**

Largely similar isoenzyme pictures in the duodenum and ileum are revealed in the disc electrophoretic separation of LDH. A pronounced predominance of LDH_4 and LDH_5 is found prenatally and on the first day of life, whereas LDH_1 and LDH_2 do not show any appreciable activity and LDH_3 only a very slight activity (Fig. 31a). On the 10th day of life, an isoenzyme pattern such as can be observed in adult animals is already manifested; there is a fall in activity of LDH_5 and predominance of LDH_4 and LDH_3 as well as an acitivity of LDH_1 and LDH_2 demonstrable in all electropherograms (Fig. 31b).

Malate dehydrogenase: Two isoenzymes can always be demonstrated in the duodenum and ileum in fetal, neonatal, and adult rats. In contrast to LDH, an appreciable age-dependent differentiation with regard to isoenzyme pattern and enzyme activity is not observed for MDH.

b) LDH and MDH Isoenzymes in Experimentally Induced Small Intestinal Tumors

Lactate dehydrogenase: The total activity of LDH in zymograms shows a pronounced variation in adenocarcinomas, particularly in solid carcinomas. Irrespective of their differentiation, LDH_1 cannot be demonstrated in the electropherograms and LDH_2/LDH_3 mostly only at low acitivity in all small intestinal tumors; the acitivity of LDH_5 increases in the same proportion as the decrease in the other isoenzymes (Fig. 32).

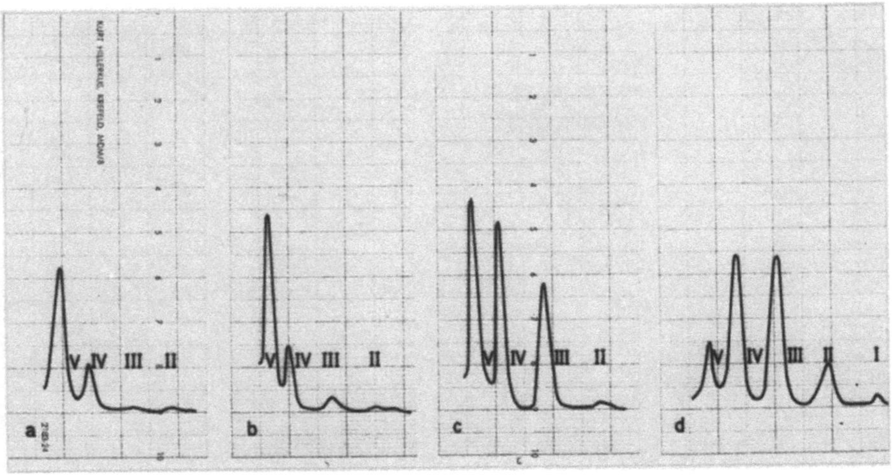

Fig. 32a–d. Densitograms of LDH isoenzymes in homogenates of a solid carcinoma **a**, adenocarcinoma **b**, adenoma **c** of the duodenum and the normal duodenal mucosa **d**

Malate dehydrogenase: Just as in the normal small intestinal mucosa, MDH can also be separated into two isoenzymes in tumor homogenates of both adenomas and carcinomas. The activities of these two isoenzymes vary from tumor to tumor but, as a whole, MDH does not undergo any tumor-specific alterations of its isoenzyme pattern.

IV. Discussion of the Results

1. Experimental Induction of Small Intestinal Epithelial Tumors

The present experimental study shows that benign and malignant epithelial tumors can be induced in rat intestine by subcutaneous injections of 1,2-dimethylhydrazine (DMH). In morphology and biologic behavior, these tumors are very similar to tumors of epithelial origin in human small and large intestines. After administration of low amounts of DMH (less than 14 mg DMH per week/kg body weight), a distribution pattern of the induced tumors results which is similar to that observed in the human intestinal tract: the colon is almost exclusively affected (mainly the rectum and distal regions of the colon) (*Wiebecke* et al., 1973). When the carcinogen dose is raised (e.g., to 21 mg DMH per week/kg body weight), apart from colon tumors, a high percentage of the experimental animals develop tumors in the small intestine (in the present study in 106 of a total of 250 rats treated with DMH). As in man, these are mainly localized in the duodenum and their number falls steeply in the distal regions of the small intestine. This high incidence of tumors of the small intestine in the rat is evidently closely related to the total dose of carcinogenic substance applied. The dose-dependent carcinogenic effect of DMH on the mucosa of the small intestine, in particular that of the duodenum, is attributed to increased (unconjugated?) DMH degradation products reaching the duodenum with the bile when the carcinogen dose is elevated (*Laqueur* and *Spatz,* 1968; *Weisburger,* 1971; *Gennaro* et al., 1973; *Ward,* 1973).

Histologically, the induced benign epithelial tumors mainly involve tubulo-villous adenomas and the malignant tumors mainly involve adenocarcinomas with varying differentiation. Solid carcinomas (signet ring cell carcinomas and anaplastic carcinomas) are observed more rarely (cf. *Pozharisskij,* 1975). Adenoacanthomas and squamous epithelial carcinomas such as demonstrated by *Schauer* et al. (1969) in the intestine of an experimental animal were not found in the present material.

2. Formal Genesis of Small Intestinal Tumors

Aspects of the causal genesis of both human intestinal tumors and DMH-induced intestinal tumors were described in the introduction. At this point, we shall first follow the genesis of tumors in the intestinal mucosa mainly in terms of formal genetic criteria, giving particular attention to the small intestine. The primary process of carcinogenesis (the morphologically undetectable intracellular transformation by the "terminal" carcinogen) takes place in the proliferating stem cells at the base of the crypts in the intestinal mucosa. According to *Nakahara* (1975), this is a stepwise process ("mutation-like genetic alterations") in which an excess growth of the transformed cells follows in a further course of oncogenesis. This growth is more or less able to escape the control of the body's own or organ-specific regulatory mechanisms and, thus, shows a largely autonomous proliferative behavior (cf. *Grundmann,* 1972).

According to some reports, epithelial necroses in the regeneration zone of the small and large intestinal crypts of mice occur a few hours after application of a single dose of DMH (*Löhrs* et al., 1969). This means that DMH (similar to numerous other carcinogenic substances) possesses a cytotoxic effect as well as a tumor-inducing effect. The toxic effect of DMH is more pronounced in the proliferation zone of the large intestinal mucosa than in the small intestine and the duration of the repair phase is also increased (*Löhrs* et al., 1969). These findings indicate a raised "sensitivity" of the large intestinal mucosa to the toxic effect of DMH compared to that of the small intestinal mucosa. In our own investigation material, only focal inflammatory cellular infiltrates, a consequence of the toxic properties of DMH, could be observed to the same extent in the small and large intestinal mucosa, but there were no epithelial necroses. In analogy to the findings made by *Bannasch* (1975) with further references, during experimental cancerization of the liver, the joint occurrence of regressive alterations (i.e., epithelial necroses with inflammatory cell infiltrates in the intestinal mucosa) on the one hand and carcinogenetic alterations on the other probably depends on the DMH dose. The higher the DMH dose, the more likely are the regressive and carcinogenetic alterations in the intestinal mucosa to occur jointly. This means that toxic and carcinogenic effects occur jointly only when DMH is applied in relatively high concentration. On the other hand, if the DMH dose is reduced, probably only the carcinogenic action remains. Such a nonspecific toxic action of DMH which constitutes only a facultative but not an obligatory concomitant manifestation of intestinal carcinogenesis would first have to be proved by experiments with application of varying doses of DMH.

It was not possible to detect "preneoplastic" alterations of the epithelial cells in the small intestinal mucosa as they are manifested as loss of various enzymes and can be demonstrated histochemically during cancerization of the urinary bladder mucosa (*Kunze* et al., 1975) and liver. Evidently, independent of the nature of the hepatotropic carcinogenic substances, a few weeks after commencement of application there occurs a cytochemically demonstrable decrease in activity of glucose-6-phosphatase as a concomitant and/or secondary manifestation of a carcinogen-induced glycogenosis of the hepatocytes (*Bannasch* and *Angerer,* 1974; *Bannasch,* 1975).

The first alterations which can be seen during intestinal carcinogenesis, are localized hyperplasias of the intestinal mucosa which do not show any light microscopic or histochemical difference from the normal cell picture. In contrast to the conditions in the normal small intestinal mucosa, proliferating epithelial cells can be demonstrated in the hyperplastic areas, even in the apical parts of the crypts (see Fig. 9a and b). There are differing views on the biologic importance of the mucosal hyperplasias in the course of carcinogenesis. Whereas some authors believe that mucosal hyperplasias frequently precede manifestation of tumors in the intestine (small intestine of the rat: *Wiebecke* et al., 1973; *Wiebecke,* 1974; colon of the mouse: *Thurnherr* et al., 1973; *Thurnherr* and *Reinhard,* 1975), *Pozharisskij* (1975) was not able to observe a "hyperplasia-tumor sequence" in rats treated with DMH. After DMH application, *Tutton* and *Barkla* (1976) were able to demonstrate in the crypts of the colon mucosa of rats an extension of the zone of proliferation as well as an absolute increase in the number of the crypt epithelia by about 25%–30%. In our own material, crypts are frequently found on careful examination of the hyperplastic areas and their surroundings which are characterized by a loss or a diminution of the goblet cells (see Fig. 9c and d). The crypt epithelia possess a remarkably basophilic cytoplasm and show a high proliferative activity. A further extension of the zone of proliferation and the resulting limitation of the differentiation zone bring about a defective resupply of differentiated enterocytes. This results in a disordered architecture of the mucosal surface with fusions of villi, formation of bridges between individual villi, villous atrophy, and erosions.

Extension of the zone of proliferation does not occur only during cancerization, however, but also during repair processes, e.g., in the regeneration phase after X-irradiation of the intestine (small intestine: *Withers,* 1970; *de Both* et al., 1974; *de Both* and *Plaisier,* 1974; *van Dongen* et al., 1976; colon: *Arenz* and *Oehlert,* 1969). The raised epithelial proliferation is also linked with an increasing diminution of the goblet cells. As an expression of these alterations, the epithelial cells situated in the apical sections of the crypt manifest a [^{3}H]-thymidine incorporation and at the same time a lack of [^{35}S]-sulfate incorporation (cf. *Springer* et al., 1970). These findings point to the close functional relationship and the interplay between the proliferative activity of the crypt epithelia and the maturation of the goblet cells. An epithelial proliferation which also persists in the differentiation compartment and which is linked to a limited ability of the epithelial cells to differentiate can be demonstrated in macroscopically unremarkable areas of the large intestinal mucosa in patients with familial polyposis coli (*Bleiberg* et al., 1972; *Deschner* and *Lipkin,* 1975 inter alia), colitis ulcerosa (*Eastwood* and *Trier*, 1973; and others), and in animal studies involving DMH application.

On the basis of studies of the large intestine, *Lipkin* (1974) designates the proliferative stage of oncogenesis as "phase I of the proliferative lesion." This is characterized by an equilibrium between the rate of epithelial regeneration and the rate of desquamation, so there is as yet no polypous folding of the mucosa despite an increase in the proliferating epithelial cells. As shown by the present study, an identical stage in the course of carcinogenesis is found in the small intestinal mucosa of rats after DMH application (cf. Fig. 9c). The tumor development occurs after a latency period, which cannot be exactly fixed in time, at a stage which is characterized by a higher regeneration rate of the transformed epithelial cells than the desquamation rate in the mucosal surface ("phase II of the proliferative lesion," according to *Lipkin,* 1974). The transition from proliferation phase I into phase II can be accelerated or slowed down in animal experiments by alteration of the total dose of DMH applied (*Thurnherr* and *Reinhart,* 1975). The transformed epithelial cells now escape the influence of the organ-specific proliferation controls and show a largely autonomous proliferation behavior with formation of manifest tumors. They thus deviate from the regulatory mechanism of epithelial proliferation in the normal small intestinal mucosa in which the proliferative activity of the crypt epithelia is thought to be controlled by the functional state of the villous epithelia (*Withers,* 1970). This hypothesis of the interplay between epithelial proliferation and differentiation of the villous epithelia could be confirmed in recent years by the demonstration of tissue-specific, but species-independent, intestinal chalones (*Brugal,* 1976).

The position of the tumor-forming proliferation center in the crypts determines the initial and the further growth behavior of the tumors. If the maximum of [^{3}H]-thymidine labeling is in the apical crypt zone, exophytic tumors develop; when the proliferation center of the transformed epithelial cells is localized in the middle of the crypt, exophytic-endophytic tumors are formed. Histologically, these involve adenomas (in the small intestine, largely tubulo-villous adenomas) and well-differentiated adenocarcinomas. Fluid transitions between adenomas and adenocarcinomas are found in the small intestine; e.g., adenomas with focal epithelial atypias and adenocarcinomas with incipient infiltration of the muscularis mucosae. Since the entire spectrum of these tumor forms develop at the same time in experimental carcinogenesis, it is not possible to express a definite opinion on the problem of the so-called "polyp-carcinoma sequence" which has been much discussed in recent years. In connection with the question as to whether the adenocarcinomas of the large intestine arise from adenomas or whether such carcinomas develop without adenomatous precursors (so-called "de novo carcinomas"), contraversial opinions have been existent for a long time. In particular *Spratt* and *Ackerman* (1960 and 1962) as well as *Spiro* (1970) expressed the opinion that tubular adenomas do not transform or only become malignant in rare cases ("once a polyp always a polyp"). The study group led by *Morson* (*Morson* and *Bussey,* 1970; *Morson,* 1974; *Muto* et al., 1975) were able to demonstrate by means of subtile histologic studies on human biopsy and resection preparations that at least 50% of the adenocarcinomas of the large intestine develop from adenomas. The evidence of a "polyp-carcinoma sequence" is additionally supported by the experimental studies of *Otto* et al. (1976), who induced large intestinal carcinomas by rectal application of N-methyl-N'nitro-N-nitroguanidine; their manifestation was always preceded by a "polyp-stage."

Histologic comparison of the tubular adenomas induced with DMH (which occur almost exclusively in the colon of experimental animals) with the predominantly tubulovillous adenomas of the small intestine, shows that focal epithelial atypias and an earlier transition into an adenocarcinoma is observed more frequently in the latter than in the tubular adenomas of the colon. This finding corresponds to the observations on human colon polyps which indicate that the frequency of malignant transformation of polyps is partly determined by the extent of the villous tumor components (*Kurzon* et al., 1974; *Muto* et al., 1975). The high frequency of transformation of adenomas with villous components, together with the rapid onset of carcinomatous transformation, is probably the reason why experimental benign and malignant adenomatous tumors occur synchronously in the small intestine; thus, a polyp-carcinoma sequence can no longer be proved with certainty. However, a polyp stage can probably be detected as a prestage of the adenocarcinomas (i.e., a positive polyp-carcinoma sequence) in the small intestine by a modification of the experimental arrangement, since there is a strict dependence on time between the rate of genesis of precancerous changes and of manifest carcinomas, on the one hand, and the total dose of carcinogen on the other (cf. *Wiebecke* et al., 1973; *Bannasch,* 1975). This means that adenomas can probably be observed at an early time in the study and a predominance of adenocarcinomas at a later time by a slowing of carcinogensis, e.g., by application of the total DMH dose required for tumor induction over a longer period of time. However, such a connection between the level of the carcinogen dose and the separate appearance of benign and malignant small intestinal tumors in time would still have to be proved by an appropriate experimental study (a low weekly DMH dose distributed over a longer period of induction).

In contrast to the adenomas and well-differentiated adenocarcinomas, the solid carcinomas (signet ring cell carcinomas and anaplastic carcinomas) appear frequently to develop directly from the transformed basal crypt epithelia (de novo carcinomas) with development of the proliferation maximum of the tumor cells at the base of the tumor (see Fig. 11). They show an aggressive behavior, rapidly penetrate all wall layers of the intestine to spread in the loose connective tissue of the submucosa and the subserosa, and tend to metastasis. The proliferative behavior of the tumor cells of solid carcinomas differs from that of the well-differentiated, gland-forming and predominantly exophytic tumors not only in the localization of the center of proliferation, but also with regard to the proliferative activity. Integrated over the entire tumor area, the latter show a mean value for the [^{3}H]-thymidine labeling index of 25%–30%, which is comparable with that of the proliferation compartment of the normal small intestinal mucosa, whereas in the solid carcinomas only 5%–10% of the tumor cells are labeled.

In the center of solid carcinomas, frequently only a few tumor cells or cell groups, mainly situated in the vicinity of blood vessels, display an incorporation of [^{3}H]-thymidine in the cell nuclei. On the other hand, in the marginal zone of the tumor there is a border of labeled tumor cells of varying width (it must be added that the [^{3}H]-Thymidine labeling index was only determined in tumors without any necrotic alteration); (see Fig. 11d). The main reason for the low proliferation rate of the tumor cells in the center of solid carcinomas appears to be the poor supply of blood vessels compared to the tumor periphery (*Tannock,* 1968; *Tannock* and *Steel,* 1970). *Vaupel* et al. (1976) were able to demonstrate, on the basis of morphometric investigations, that the capillary volume of the tumors and the tumor blood supply continuously decrease in DS carcino-sarcomas. Cellular proliferation does not decrease regularly within solid tumors with increasing tumor size, but regional centers of proliferation develop (*Kligerman* et al., 1962). These are thought to be due to local differences in the nutrient supply (e.g., glucose and oxygen) of the tissue (*Tannock,* 1968). In general, the tumor periphery of solid carcinomas has a better blood supply than the center of the tumor (*Vaupel,* 1974, 1976). These experimental results indicate that a diminution of the vessel supply and the consequent diminished blood flow to the tissue in the center of the tumors is the limiting factor for the proliferative activity of the tumor cells. A regional fall of proliferative activity comparable with the findings in solid carcinomas could not be observed in the center of the DMH-induced adenomas and well-differentiated adenocarcinomas. It can be concluded from this that the development of the vascular network in these tumors keeps pace with tumor growth, despite the high rate of new formation of tumor cells, and that there is an interaction between the differentiation of the epithelial components of the experimental intestinal tumors and the functional differentiation of the blood vessels. In the (rapidly proliferating) adenomas and well-differentiated adenocarcinomas, a dense capillary-rich network of blood vessels can be demonstrated by light and electron microscopy as well as by histochemistry (positive reaction of alkaline phosphatase in the capillary endothelia).

3. Fine Structure of Adenomas

There are no specific ultrastructural characteristics of benign and malignant tumor cells in experimental tumors of the small intestine, as compared with human tumors (*Fasske,* and *Themann,* 1960; *Mercer,* 1962; and others). Depending on their degree of differentiation, the tumor cells display the structural characteristics of native tissue. The DMH-induced adenomas and well-differentiated adenocarcinomas show a cytological relation to the proliferating crypt epithelia which are the target cells of the carcinogen.

The microvillous border (brush border), characteristic for mature enterocytes, is reduced in *tumor cells of enterocyte type,* displays an irregular arrangement, and is even completely absent in some tumor cells. As shown by scanning electron microscopy tumor cells exist whose surface structure can hardly be distinguished from that of mature enterocytes. *Fenoglio* et al. (1975) was able to make the same kind of scanning electron microscopic findings in tubular adenomas and villous adenomas of the human large intestine. A further feature of the enterocyte surface, the "surface coat" (glycocalyx), shows a defective development in the tumor cells. *Isselbacher* (1974) was able to demonstrate in biochemical and immunological studies that fetal epithelial cells of the intestinal mucosa, crypt epithelia of adult individuals, and tumor cells of intestinal tumors synthesize "incomplete surface glycoproteins" which differ from the glycoproteins at the surface of normal enterocytes. The formation of incomplete surface glycoproteins is probably caused by a genetic defect in the process of production of glycoproteins in the tumor cells and a disorder in the differentiation of the Golgi apparatus (cf. *Bennett,* 1970; *van Dongen* et al., 1976). In adenomas, the interepithelial junctional complexes of the lateral cell membrane largely resemble those of the normal crypt epithelia and the continuity of the basement membrane is preserved. A "terminal web" cannot be demonstrated in the apical cytoplasm.

Besides the numerically predominant tumor cells of enterocyte type, there also develop isolated *mucus-producing tumor cells* which in some cases resemble the oligomucous cells in normal small intestinal crypts. An ultrastructural picture largely resembling that in the DMH-induced adenomas in the small intestine of the rat is found in experimentally induced adenomas in the colon of the rat (*Spjut* and *Smith,* 1967), mouse (*Touth* et al., 1976), and in the tubular adenomas of man (*Fisher* and *Sharkey,* 1962; *Imai* et al., 1965; *Spjut* and *Smith,* 1967; *Goldmann* et al., 1970; *Kaye* et al., 1973). There are as yet no corresponding studies on the small intestine.

In contrast to the epithelial cells of the intestinal mucosa of adult rats, predominantly supranuclearly situated glycogen granules can be observed in the tumor cells of individual adenomas and well-differentiated adenocarcinomas of the small intestine. *Korhonen* et al. (1971) also described a similar kind of glycogen storage in the tumor cells of adenocarcinomas of the human colon, but not in tubular adenomas. The phenomenon of glycogenosis in the course of tumor development is manifested especially in the cancerization of the liver (*Bannasch,* 1968, 1975; further literature cited here). *Bannasch* assumes that the hepatocellular glycogenosis develops in the preneoplastic stage, whereas the transformation to the hepatoma cell is characterized by a reduction of glycogen (see also Sect. 4). In the normal mucosa of the small and large intestine of humans and rats, an intra-epithelial storage of glycogen can only be demonstrated during fetal development (*Graumann* and *Neumann,* 1964; *Häkkinen* et al., 1968; *Lev* and *Weisberg,* 1969) and during the first weeks of life (colon of the rat: *Bannert,* 1973). Intestinal glycogenosis in the fetal period of man and other species is attributed to the higher activity of enzymes catalyzing glycogen synthesis in the fetal intestinal mucosa than in the mature organ (*Takeuchi,* 1958). *Lev* and *Weisberg* (1969) suggest that intra-epithelial glycogen may constitute an energy reserve for the metabolism of the rapidly developing organism.

4. Fine Structure of Carcinomas

There are mostly only gradual ultrastructural differences between the tumor cells of the adenomas and the *adenocarcinomas with a high degree of differentiation.* In comparison with the epithelium of origin in the crypts, this could be paraphrased as "attenuation of the isoplasia." An appreciable morphological difference between the tumor cells of the adenomas and the tumor cells of the adenocarcinomas is that in the latter the interepithelial junctional complexes are often only poorly developed. This finding indicates a diminished coherence of the tumor cells amongst themselves. The glands of the adenocarcinomas frequently lack a basement membrane over large distances. Taken as a whole, the ultrastructure of the experimentally induced adenocarcinomas in the small intestine of the rat is largely identical with that of adenocarcinomas in the large intestine of man (*Imai* and *Stein,* 1963; *Birbeck* and *Dukes,* 1963; *Spjut* and *Smith,* 1967).

Within individual adenocarcinomas are found, in places, glandulas containing mucus-producing tumor cells. Ultrastructurally, one recognizes numerous transition forms of immature mucus-producing cells which in some cases, resemble oligomucous cells and in other cases resemble mature goblet cells. These findings largely agree with the data of *Lauren* (1961) who distinguishes five types of mucus-forming tumor cells on the basis of light microscopic criteria. The composition of the mucus substances in the tumor cells and in the epithelial cells from the vicinity of tumors is said to differ histochemically from the mucus synthesized in the goblet cells of the normal intestinal mucosa (*Lauren,* 1961; *Filipe* and *Branfoot,* 1974; *Dawson* and *Filipe,* 1976).

In the perinuclear and basal cytoplasm of numerous tumor cells of the adenomas and adenocarcinomas, as well as to a smaller extent in the cytoplasm of tumor cells of solid carcinomas, are found round-oval structures with a diameter of up to 5 μ in which acid phosphatase can often be demonstrated histochemically. *Ioachim* and co-workers (1974) designate these vacuolar structures "inclusion bodies." They are surrounded by a single or double membrane which sometimes shows a discontinuous, fragmentary structure. Situated within this structure are cellular organelles in various stages of degradation to residual bodies which only contain dense, partly granular, and partly amorphic material. The inclusion bodies were first described by *Leuchtenberger* (1954) in the tumor cells of benign and malignant tumors of the rectum and later in the epithelial cells of the normal mucosa and during various intestinal diseases, e.g., in familial polyposis coli, colitis ulcerosa, diverticulitis etc. (*Helwig,* 1959; *Monis* and *Mendeloff,* 1961; *Guerin,* 1967). The genesis of the vacuolar structures has not yet been completely clarified despite numerous investigations (cf. *Ioachim* et al., 1974). The initial view that these are virus particles (*Leuchtenberger,* 1954; *Helwig,* 1959) was refuted by electron microscopic studies (*Fisher* and *Sharkey,* 1962). Other authors suggest that they are residues of phagocytozed lymphocytes (*Birbeck* and *Dukes,* 1963). In connection with our own studies and those of *Ioachim* et al. (1974), it must be assumed that the majority of the inclusion bodies are to be regarded as autophagic vacuoles or as autolysosomes. On the other hand, in a few vacuoles remains of phagocytozed foreign material can be seen (e.g., remains of leukocytes and possibly also of necrotic tumor cells) so that one would have to refer, in these cases, to heterophagosomes or heterolysosomes (cf. *Allison,* 1974).

The genesis of autophagic vacuoles in the epithelial cells of the small intestinal mucosa may also be induced by experimental interventions on the small intestine of the rat, e.g., in the remaining segment of the intestine after small intestinal resection (*Schäfer* and *Höhn,* 1975), after X-irradiation of the intestine (*Hugon* and *Borgers,* 1966a) etc. The findings indicate that the formation of autophagic vacuoles is triggered by cell damage and by the influence of a more intense functional demand in the course of which the damaged and/or dispensable areas of cytoplasm are separated by membranes from the still-functional cytoplasm and are then degraded by acid hydrolases (cf. *Pfeifer,* 1969, 1976). The appearance of intra-epithelial autophagic vacuoles is, accordingly, the morphological manifestation of a raised "cellular wastage" such as demonstrated during rat fetal development by the conversion of multistratified intestinal epithelium into a monostratified epithelium (*Gossrau,* 1975b).

A marked decrease of specific structural characteristics compared with the initial tissue is observed in the less differentiated adenocarcinomas. These mostly form small glands with narrow lumina. The interepithelial adhesion structures are often only poorly developed and the basement membrane is frequently absent. Bundles of fine filaments with a diameter of 50–60 Å are found in the cytoplasm of numerous tumor cells; these are also demonstrable in the tumor cells of the anaplastic intestinal carcinomas. Such intracytoplasmic filaments are also observed in almost all cell kinds under physiological conditions (*David,* 1970), e.g., in epithelial cells of the gastric and intestinal mucosa ("fibrillovesicular cells": *Toner* et al., 1971). In numerous pathological conditions, in particular in the tumor cells of malignant tumors, an increase of such filaments can be observed (prostate carcinoma: *Kastendieck* et al., 1973; anaplastic bronchial carcinoma: *Stoebner* and *Le Gal,* 1967; etc.). Morphologically, they resemble the filaments found in the epithelial cells of the epidermis (tonofilaments) (*Sandborn,* 1970). The function of the intracytoplasmic filaments has not yet been unequivocally elucidated. It is suggested that they have supporting functions and serve as a cytoskeleton for the inner reinforcement of the cell (*Fawcett,* 1973).

From the poorly differentiated adenocarcinomas there are fluid transitions to the solid carcinomas, which are formed to a varying extent by signet ring cells, tumor cells with intracytoplasmic lumina, and anaplastic tumor cells. These three cell forms may be observed in undifferentiated gastric carcinomas (*Hananouchi* et al., 1974), in mammary carcinomas (*Ahmed,* 1974; *Steinbrecher* and *Silverberg,* 1976; and others), and numerous other human and experimentally induced solid carcinomas. On the other hand, there are no ultrastructural studies of solid carcinomas of the intestinal tract.

Mucus-producing *signet ring cells* have a well developed Golgi apparatus, lamellae of the granular endoplasmic reticulum, and mitochondria. *Tumor cells with intracytoplasmic lumina* mostly have only a few cellular organelles. According to *Caesar* (1973) it has not yet been established with certainty as to whether these lumina (which are often surrounded by a microvillous border) are slices of the extracellular space, i.e., pseudointracytoplasmic formations, or primary cavities which have arisen intracellularly. However, since a connection between the intracytoplasmic lumen and extracellular space could not be demonstrated electronmicroscopically in any solid carcinoma, it must be assumed that these lumina and the membranes with microvilli surrounding them are structures which have arisen intracytoplasmically. Such cells are observed quite frequently in prostate carcinomas (*Kastendieck* et al., 1973) and mammary carcinomas (*Goldenberg* et al., 1969; and others). The *tumor cells of anaplastic small intestinal carcinomas* do not possess any structural characteristic of their starting tissue. In these tumors, free ribosomes predominate in the cytoplasm, but profiles of the granular endoplasmic reticulum and mitochondria can still be demonstrated in varying numbers. However, in individual anaplastic carcinoma cells, the content of rough endoplasmatic reticulum may be raised compared to normal (*Vogel* and *Glatthaar,* 1958).

In the tumor cells of poorly differentiated adenocarcinomas and solid carcinomas, no glycogen deposits could be demonstrated (seel also Sect. 3). A possible explanation for the appearance of glycogenotic tumor cells (e.g., in intestinal adenomas and in well-differentiated adenocarcinomas) and the absence of glycogen-deposits in poorly differentiated tumor cells is provided by the metabolic scheme for glycogen metabolism in formation of kidney carcinomas drawn up by *Thoenes* and *Schneider* and supported by data in the literature (*Thoenes,* 1973). According to this scheme, increased amounts of lactate are produced in the course of cancerification and synchronous with the rise in activity of glycolysis in the tumor cells; in turn, this stimulates gluconeogenesis. Since, at the same time, no activity of glucose-6-phosphatase can be demonstrated histochemically (liver *Gössner* and *Friedrich-Freksa,* 1964), production of glycogen results since the last step of gluconeogenesis cannot be performed. Activity of glucose-6-phosphatase can also no longer be detected in the tumor cells of the DMH-induced intestinal tumors using light microscopic-histochemical methods. The loss of the ability to form glycogen in the tumor cells of poorly differentiated carcinomas may be based on a lack of specific enzyme systems catalyzing the individual synthetic steps of gluconeogenesis and glycogenesis. However, it must be added that, according to data from other authors, glycolysis and gluconeogenesis function alternatively so that they cannot be raised at the same time in one and the same cell (e.g., *Weber,* 1968). Considered as a whole, there is thus no satisfactory explanation for the appearance of glycogenotic tumor cells.

5. Enzyme Histochemistry

Enzyme histochemical studies have revealed that *hydrolases* localized in the brush border (e.g., neutral α-glucosidase, LNA etc.) and endoplasmic reticulum (glucose-6-phosphatase and nonspecific esterase) of normal enterocytes cannot be demonstrated, or only at a very low activity, in tumor cells (both adenomas and carcinomas). On the other hand, lysosomal hydrolases (acid phosphatase and, to a small extent, the E 600-resistant nonspecific esterase) show a positive reaction in almost all tumors. Accordingly, the brush border enzymes manifest a behavior corresponding to the "surface coat" of tumor cells.

In the normal small intestinal mucosa, the brush border enzymes in the epithelial cells of the proliferation compartment of the crypts are not detectable. They may possibly be present as "pro-enzymes" in the epithelia of the differentiation compartment (*Wachsmuth* and *Torhorst,* 1974) and develop their full activity only in the enterocytes at the base of the villi with inception of the resorptive function (*Webster* and *Harrison,* 1969; *Gossrau,* 1975a, b). By expansion of the proliferation compartment with an increase in the proliferative activity of the crypt epithelia (e.g., in the repair phase following X-irradiation of the intestine), there results a diminished activity of individual brush border enzymes in the villous epithelium (*De Both* et al., 1974; *Rijke* et al., 1975) and of the E 600-sensitive nonspecific esterase localized in the endoplasmic reticulum (*De Both* et al., 1974). Since tumor cells, including the highly differentiated adenomas, do not pass through a morphological and functional differentiation phase comparabel to the normal epithelial cells and always remain in the proliferation compartment, most brush border enzymes are not detectable in the apical and outer cell membrane of the tumor cells. However, this only applies with reservations to the behavior of alkaline phosphatase (*Malik* and *Butterworth,* 1976). Whereas activity is not detectable with enzyme histochemical methods in the outer cell membrane of normal crypt epithelia, the apical and lateral cell membrane of individual tumor cells of the gland-forming tumors stain positively as shown by electron microscopic-histochemical studies. A particularly strong reaction is found in the tumor cells of anaplastic carcinomas; as in gland-forming tumors, this reaction can also be inhibited with L-phenylalanine. Corresponding studies on human colon mucosa and colon tumors gave rise to contradictory results. The majority of authors were unable to detect any activity of alkaline phosphatase in tumor cells using light microscopic histochemical methods (*Czernobilsky* and *Tsou,* 1968; *Koudstaal* et al., 1975a), whereas there is an intense histochemical reaction in tumor cells of colon carcinoma according to *Maggi* and *Wyatt* (1970).

Karasaki (1975) studied alkaline phosphatase during the course of experimental cancerization of rat liver. During malignant transformation of the hepatocytes, an alkaline phosphatase can be demonstrated in the external cell membrane which differs from normal hepatocyte alkaline phosphatase in terms of its localization and its behavior towards inhibitors (inhibition by L-phenylalanine, no inhibition by L-homoarginine or by warming to 65°C). The alkaline phosphatase in the cell membrane of hepatoma cells thus possesses some biochemical properties of the so-called carcinoplacental alkaline phosphatase which is detectable in carcinomas and in serum of cancer-patients (positive finding in 7%–53.8% of patients, depending on carcinoma type; *Lehmann,* 1975). This enzyme is thought to be both biochemically and immunologically identical with the alkaline phosphatase of human placenta (*Fishman,* 1974; *Sasaki* and *Fishman,* 1974; reviews: *Lamerz* and *Fatah-Moghadam,* 1975; and others). The carcinoplacental isoenzyme can be separated into subfractions on the basis of its behavior in the presence of inhibitory substances. The most well known of these is the Regan isoenzyme. The synthesis of an "ectopic isoenzyme" of alkaline phosphatase in tumor cells is resulting from a derepression of the genome of the carcinoma cells (*Fishman,* 1969). The Regan isoenzyme could also be detected in the tumor cells of colon carcinomas (*Miyayama* et al., 1976) and in the serum of patients with tumors of the gastrointestinal tract (*Lehmann,* 1976).

Generally, the *oxidoreductases* in the tumor cells of adenomas and carcinomas react approximately as intensly as the crypt epithelia of the normal small intestinal mucosa and, thus, possess a lower histochemically detectable enzyme activity than the villous epithelia. The tumor cells of gland-forming tumors generally stain more strongly than those of solid carcinomas. An intense enzyme histochemical reaction is shown by SDH and MDH (but mainly LDH) even in solid carcinomas, whereas the other oxidoreductases, especially HBDH, G-6-PD, IDH, GDH, and MAO only show a low activity. The histochem ical investigations on human colon tumors yielded similar results, although a rise of G-6-PD compared to the normal mucosa is frequently reported (*Cohen* et al., 1968; *Marsden* and *Dawson,* 1974; *Koudstaal* et al., 1975b; and others); such a rise could not be observed in the present study.

6. Disc Electrophoresis

In agreement with the results of histochemical and biochemical investigations on numerous human tumors and on tumors induced in experimental animals, a high activity of LDH was also found in the experimental small intestinal tumors of the present study. When the LDH in tissue homogenates is separated by disc electrophoresis, it is noticeable that the slowly migrating LDH isoenzymes (LDH_4/LDH_5) predominate in the small intestinal tumors irrespective of the kind of tumor, whereas the isoenzymes LDH_1/LDH_2 only show very low activites or cannot be detected at all. A similar finding was observed in numerous human tumors (colon: *Langvad,* 1968; brain: *Stavrou,* 1975; and others) and in experimentally induced tumors (liver: *Farron* et al., 1972; mamma: *Richards* and *Hilf,* 1972; brain: *Stavrou,* 1975; colon: *Brox,* 1976; and others). During human and experimental ontogenesis, an activity maximum of LDH_4/LDH_5 and an activity minimum of LDH_1/LDH_2 are found in numerous organs (review: *Kowalewski,* 1972). Such an activity behavior is also shown by the LDH isoenzymes in intestinal fetal and neonatal rats (*Paasch,* 1974). The isoenzyme picture observed in adult animals develops a few days after birth with an activity maximum of LDH_3/LDH_4 and a detectable activity of LDH_1/LDH_2. It will not be discussed further at this point whether the isoenzyme pattern in experimental small intestinal tumors resembling the fetal LDH isoenzyme pattern ("fetalism" of the tumors; *Knox,* 1976) is a consequence of the particular metabolic conditions in the tumors or consequence of an altered gene expression (cf. *Criss,* 1971; *Weinhouse,* 1972, 1976; and others; review: *Kowalewski,* 1972).

7. Concluding Reflections

The model for histogenesis of epithelial tumors in the small intestinal mucosa shown in Figure 33 can be derived from the results of the morphological, autoradiographic, and enzyme histochemical studies (cf. *Pierce* et al., 1973; *Pierce,* 1974). According to this model, all small intestinal tumors, i.e., both the well-differentiated tumors (adenomas and adenocarcinomas) and the poorly differentiated or undifferentiated tumors (solid carcinomas), develop from transformed basal crypt epithelia ("tumor stem cells"). A portion of the transformed crypt epithelial cells still possesses the ability to migrate along the crypt wall. During their migration in the direction of the crypt orifice, the transformed epithelial cells undergo a morphological (even if incomplete compared to the normal crypt epithelia) differentiation. At varying levels of the crypt (and thus linked to a different development phase), adenomas and adenocarcinomas may develop from these epithelial cells. The electron microscopic and histochemical picture shows the close relationship of the tumor cells of well-differentiated intestinal tumors with the crypt epithelia of the normal mucosa. In contrast to the mature, gland-forming

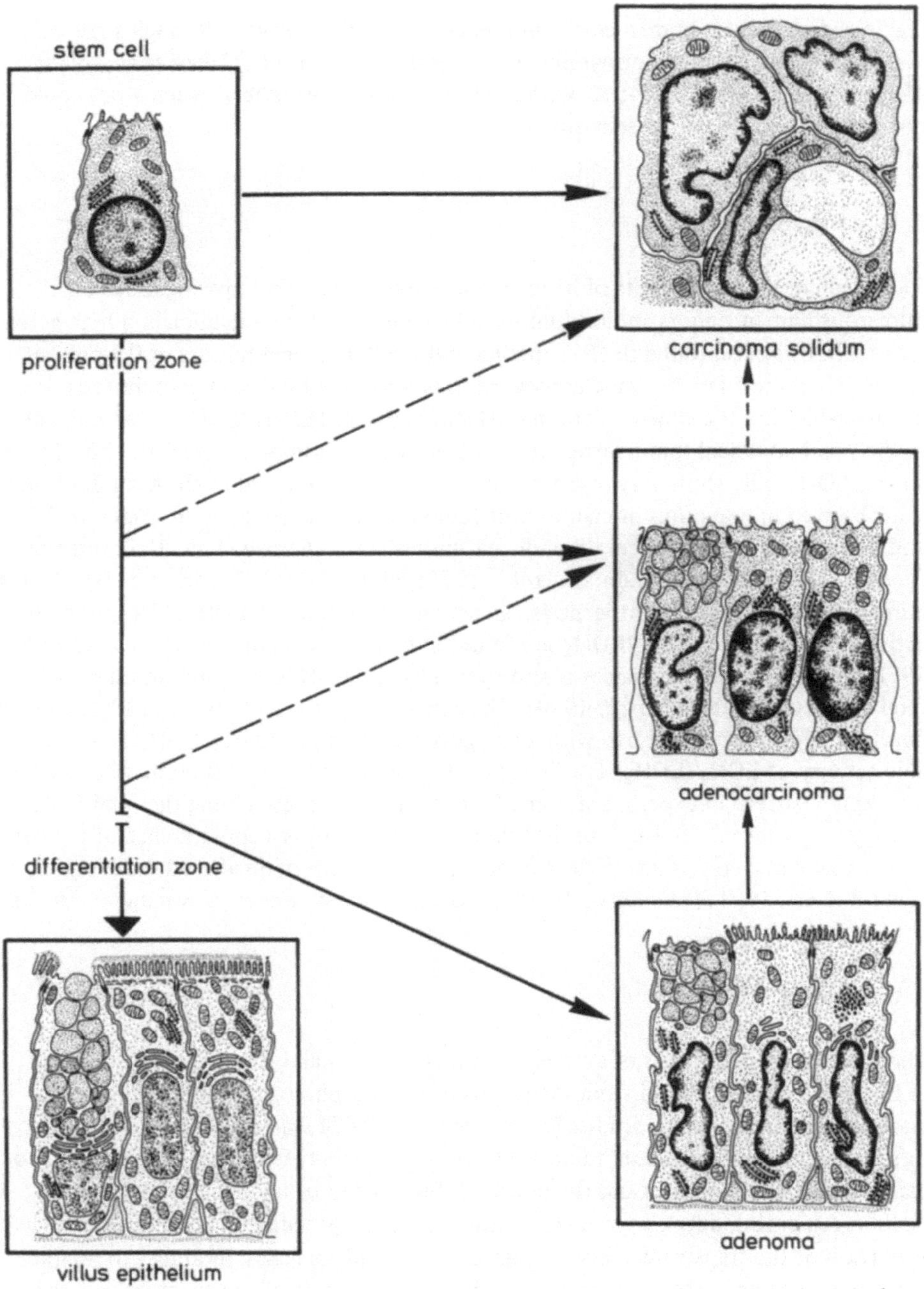

Fig. 33. Hypothesis on the histogenesis of experimentally induced small intestinal tumors: solid carcinomas, adenocarcinomas, and adenomas arise at different differentiation levels from the crypt epithelia capable of proliferation which are transformed by 1,2-dimethylhydrazine

small intestinal tumors, the solid (signet ring cell and anaplastic) carcinomas arise directly from the transformed basal crypt epithelia which have largely lost the ability to migrate along the crypt wall and, thus, the capacity for further differentiation. As indicated in the scheme (Fig. 33), tumors with a low degree of maturation can develop stepwise from well-differentiated tumors. The cellular mechanisms which bring about such a dedifferentiation have not been completely explored. Possible explanations for this would be, e.g., shortening of the postmitotic presynthetic phase of the generation cycle of the tumor cells (cf. *Oehlert,* 1969) as has been demonstrated for experimentally induced adenocarcinomas of the colon (*Schauer* et al., 1971) and/or a "restricted availability of the genetic information" which is probably linked to the process of carcinogenesis (cf. *Harbers* and *Sandritter,* 1968).

The present study shows that, as far as they are derived from precursors of enterocytes and goblet cells, all forms of adenomas and carcinomas that also arise in the small and large intestine of man can be induced by application of DMH in the small intestine of the rat. The conclusion can be drawn from this that the formal genesis of these tumors (which is apparently independent of the nature of the carcinogenic agent) follows the same path in both species. The animal experimental model presented does not only permit a statement on the morphology and morphogenesis of the intestinal tumors, but with appropriate modification (*Schmähl* et al., 1976) is probably also suitable for answering questions on the causal pathogenesis of intestinal tumors. The knowledge of the genesis of human intestinal tumors which could be gained in epidemiological studies might thereby be deepened and extended in animal experiments.

V. Summary

Tumors were induced in the intestinal tract in 250 rats after subcutaneous injection of 1,2-dimethylhydrazine (DMH) after an induction period of 90–200 days (total DMH dose: 200–350 mg/kg body weight). Mostly multiple tumors could be observed in the small intestine of 106 experimental animals. Their site of predilection was in the upper small intestine (the duodenum and the directly adjacent segment of the jejunum was affected in 82 animals). The first detectable alterations in the course of carcinogenesis are manifested in circumscribed mucosal hyperplasias with [^{3}H]-thymidine incorporation in individual epithelial cells of the upper half of the crypts and an extention of the proliferation zone to the entire crypt. The expansion of the proliferation compartment is associated with a far-reaching atrophy of the goblet cells and the loss of the capacity of the enterocyte precursors to differentiate. From these centers of proliferation develop adenomas (mainly tubulo-villous adenomas) and well-differentiated adenocarcinomas (with or without mucus production) with a proliferation maximum in the region of the middle and apical parts of the crypts. The poorly differentiated adenocarcinomas and the solid carcinomas (signet ring cell carcinomas and anaplastic carcinomas) probably arise directly from transformed basal crypt epithelia. The proliferation maximum of the tumor cells of such carcinomas is localized at the base of the tumor. The tumors show a largely endophytic growth and rapidly infiltrate the deeper layers of the intestinal wall. The mean value of the [^{3}H]-thymidine labeling index of the tumor cells of gland-forming tumors integrated over the entire tumor area is between 25% and 30%. The [^{3}H]-thymidine labeling index in the proliferation compartment of the normal mucosa is about 30% and only between 5% and 10% in solid carcinomas.

The tumor cells (tumor cells of the enterocyte precursor type and mucus-producing tumor cells) show an electron microscopic picture which still displays numerous characteristic structures of the crypt epithelia (e.g., polar cell differentiation, formation of microvilli, development of the interepithelial adhesion structures etc.). These differentiation features of the maternal tissue are no longer or only allusively developed in the tumor cells of solid carcinomas. In solid carcinomas, three cell forms can be distinguished cytologically: Anaplastic tumor cells with cytoplasm which is poor in organelles but with a predominance of free ribosomes; tumor cells with intracytoplasmic lumina, and mucus-forming cells which show a variable degree of cytoplasmic differentiation. Autophagic vacuoles, heterophagosomes and heterolysosomes as well as filamentous structures are found in numerous tumor cells of all tumor types. The filamentous structures are almost exclusively detectable in the tumor cells of poorly differentiated carcinomas.

Scanning electron microscopic investigations have revealed that the differentiation of certain structures also decreases with decreasing degree of maturation of the tumors. Numerous tumor cells of adenomas still possess a quite regular microvillous border, whereas malformed villi are frequently observed in adenocarcinomas with a low degree of maturation and solid carcinomas (e.g., long, finger-like villi, crude protrusions of the apical cell membrane).

Light and electron microscopic demonstration of acid glycoproteins (iron-binding reaction after *Hale*) reveals that the slight differentiation of the apical cell membrane of the tumor cells compared with the brush border of normal enterocytes is associated with a markedly diminished development of the glycocalyx.

Enzymes localized mainly in the endoplasmic reticulum (glucose-6-phosphatase, non-specific esterase) and the brush border of the enterocytes (e.g., neutral α-glucosidase, leucyl-β-naphthylamidase) can no longer be demonstrated histochemically in the tumor cells with the exception of alkaline phosphatase, which reacts positively in the outer cell membrane of individual tumor cells. The tumor cells of individual anaplastic carcinomas show an especially intensive histochemical reaction. The high activity of the acid phosphatase in the tumor cells is mainly localized in the autolysosomes and heterolysosomes. The oxidoreductases investigated frequently display a histotopochemical picture in the tumor cells similar to that in the crypt epithelia of the normal intestinal mucosa. The well-differentiated tumors generally manifest a more intense histochemical reaction than the tumors with a low degree of maturation. The highest histochemical activity is possessed by LDH, SDH, and MDH, which sometimes reaches that of normal enterocytes.

After performing electrophoresis, the slowly migrating LDH isoenzymes (LDH_4/LDH_5) stain most intensely in homogenates of the small intestinal mucosa of fetal and neonatal rats, whereas LDH_3/LDH_4 predominate in adult animals; LDH_1/LDH_2 can always be detected. An isoenzyme pattern of LDH such as observed in fetal and neonatal rats can be seen in tumor homogenates.

In conclusion, the morphogenesis and morphology of the small intestinal tumors induced experimentally in rats are largely identical with those of adenomas and carcinomas in the human intestinal tract.

Acknowledgements: Special thanks are due to Prof. Dr. P. Bannasch (Department of Cytopathology at the German Cancer Research Center in Heidelberg) and Prof. Dr. W. Thoenes (Director of the Institute for Pathology of the Johannes Gutenberg University in Mainz) for their valuable advice in the compilation of the manuscript. I thank medical assistant Miss Dorothea Dellee for her reliable help in laboratory work and Mrs. Karin Schulze for making the electron microscopic preparations. Thanks are due to Mr. Winfried Meyer for preparing the drawings and Mrs. Isolde Weitmann for the photographic work.

The animal experiments for autoradiography were performed at the Institute for Radiology of the University of Mainz (Director: Prof. Dr. L. Diethelm). Thanks are due to Dr. W. Sonntag for making the autoradiographic preparations and Prof. Dr. K. Paulini for his expert advice. The scanning electron microscopic preparations were made at the Institute for General and Experimental Pathology of the Federal Army in Mainz (Director: Prof. Dr. H.G. Fassbender). My thanks are due to Dr. R. Wagner for making the preparations and his expert advice.

References

Ahmed, A.: Electron-microscopic observation of scirrhous and mucin-producing carcinomas of the breast. J. Pathol. *112*, 177–181 (1974)

Allison, A.C.: Lysosomes in cancer cells. J. Clin. Pathol. *27*, [Suppl.] (R. Coll. Pathol.) *7*, 43–50 (1974)

Alrich, E.M., Blank, R.H., Fomon, J.J.: Primary tumours of the small intestine. Am. J. Surg. *99*, 33–39 (1960)

Arenz, F., Oehlert, W.: Die Regeneration der Dickdarmschleimhaut der Ratte nach Lokal- und Ganzkörperbestrahlung. Strahlentherapie *138*, 365–374 (1969)

Bannasch, P.: The cytoplasm of hepatocytes during carcinogenesis. In: Recent results in cancer research, *19*. Rentchnick, P. (ed.). Berlin, Heidelberg, New York: Springer 1968

Bannasch, P.: Die Cytologie der Hepatocarcinogenese. In: Handbuch der allgemeinen Pathologie, Vol. VI/6: Geschwülste, Tumors III, pp. 123–276. Grundmann, E. (ed.) Berlin, Heidelberg, New York: Springer 1975

Bannasch, P. Angerer, H.: Glykogen und Glukose-6-Phosphatase während der Kanzerisierung der Rattenleber durch N-Nitrosomorpholin. Arch. Geschwulstforsch. *43*, 105–114 (1974)

Bannert, U.: Postnatale Differenzierung der Colonschleimhaut der Ratte. Medical thesis. Mainz *1973*

Barka, T.: Electron histochemical localization of acid phosphatase activity in the small intestine of the mouse. J. Histochem. Cytochem. *12*, 229–238 (1964)

Barka, T., Anderson, P.J.: Histochemical methods for acid phosphatase using hexazonium pararosanilin as coupler. J. Histochem. Cytochem. *10*, 741–753 (1962)

Bauer, K.-H.: Das Krebsproblem. Berlin, Heidelberg, New York: Springer 1963

Bennett, G.: Migration of glycoproteins from golgi apparatus to cell coat in the columnar cells of the duodenal epithelium. J. Cell. Biol. *45*, 668–673 (1970)

Bennett, H.S.: Morphological aspects of extracellular polysaccharides. J. Histochem. Cytochem. *11*, 14–23 (1963)

Berg, J.W., Howell, M.A.: The geographic pathology of bowel cancer. Cancer *34*, 807–814 (1974)

Birbeck, M.S.C., Dukes, C.E.: Electron microscopy of rectal neoplasms. Proc. R. Soc. Med. *56*, 793–797 (1963)

Bleiberg, H., Mainguet, P., Galand, P.: Cell renewal in familial polyposis. Comparison between polyps and adjacent healthy mucosa. Gastroenterology *63*, 240–245 (1972)

de Both, N.J., van Dongen, J.M., van Hofwegen, B., Keulemans, J., Vissner, W.J., Galjaard, H.: The influence of various cell kinetic conditions on function differentiation in the small intestine of the rat. Dev. Biol. *38,* 119–137 (1974)
de Both, N.J., Plaisier, H.: The influence of changing cell kinetics on functional differentiation in the small intestine of the rat. J. Histochem. Cytochem. *22,* 352–360 (1974)
Broitman, S.A., Vitale, J.J., Vavrousek-Jakuba, E., Gottlieb, L.: Polyunsaturated fat, cholesterol and large bowel tumorgenesis. Cancer *40,* 2455–2463 (1977)
Brox, G.: Disc-elektrophoretische und histochemische Untersuchung der sauren Phosphatase und Lactatdehydrogenase experimenteller Darmtumoren. Medical thesis. Mainz 1976
Brugal, G.: Presence of intestinal chalones. In: Stem cells of renewing cell populations, pp. 41–50. New York, San Francisco, London: Academic Press 1976
Burdette, W.J.: Colorectal carcinogenesis. Cancer *34,* 872–877 (1974)
Burkitt, D.P.: Epidemiology of cancer of the colon and rectum. Cancer *28,* 3–13 (1971)
Burstone, M.S.: Histochemical comparison of naphthol-AS-phosphates for the demonstration of phosphatases. J. Natl. Cancer Inst. *20,* 601–610 (1958)
Busch, W., Wodak, E.: Beitrag zu Klinik der Pathologie des primären Dünndarmkrebses. Z. Gastroenterol. *4,* 315–323 (1966)
Caesar, R.: Die Bedeutung der Ultrastruktur für die Tumordiagnostik. Verh. Dtsch. Ges. Pathol. *57,* 81–84 (1973)
Chang, W.W.L., Leblond, C.P.: Renewal of the epithelium in the descending colon of the mouse. Am. J. Anat. *131,* 73–100 (1971)
Cheng, H., Leblond, C.P.: Origin, differentiation and renewal of the four main epithelial cell types in the mouse small intestine. V. Unitarian theory of the origin of the four epithelial cell types. Am. J. Anat. *141,* 537–562 (1974)
Cheng, H., Leblond, C.P.: Identification of stem cells in the small intestine of the mouse. In: Stem cells of the renewing cell population, Cairnie, A.B., Lala, P.K., Osmond, D.G. (eds.), pp. 7–31. New York, San Francisco, London: Academic Press 1976
Chomchai, C., Bhadrachai, N., Nigro, N.N.: The effect of bile on the induction of experimental intestinal tumors in rats. Dis. Colon Rectum *17,* 310–312 (1974)
Cohen, H.J., Elizalde, A., Miller, S.P.: Cytologic studies of glucose-6-phosphate dehydrogenase in malignancy. Cancer *21,* 1055–1060 (1968)
Coombs, M.M., Bhatt, T.S., Croft, C.J.: Correlation between carcinogenecity and chemical structure in cyclopentaphenanthrene. Cancer Res. *33,* 832 (1973)
Corpron, R.E.: The ultrastructure of the gastric mucosa in normal and hypophysectomized rats. Am. J. Anat. *118,* 53–90 (1966)
Criss, W.E.: A review of isozymes in cancer. Cancer Res. *31,* 1523–1542 (1971)
Czernobilsky, B., Tsou, K.C.: Adenocarcinoma, adenomas and polyps of colon: the histochemical study. Cancer *21,* 165–177 (1968)
David, H.: Zellschädigung und Dysfunktion. In: 1. Pathologie des Protoplasmas. Protoplasmatologica Vol. X. Alfert, M., Bauer, H., Harding, C.V., Sandritter, W., Sitte, P. (eds.) Wien, New York: Springer 1970
Dawson, I., Pryse-Davies, J.: The distribution of certain enzyme systems in the normal gastrointestinal tract. Gastroenterology *44,* 745–760 (1963)
Dawson, P.A., Filipe, M.J.: An ultrastructural and histochemical study of the mucosa membrane adjacent to and remote from carcinoma of the colon. Cancer *37,* 2388–2398 (1976)
Deimling, O.v.: Die Darstellung phosphatfreisetzender Enzyme mittels Schwermetall-Simultan-Methoden. Histochemie *4,* 48–55 (1964)
Deschner, E.E., Lipkin, M.: Proliferative patterns in colonic mucosa in familial polyposis. Cancer *35,*413–418 (1975)
Dietz, A., Lubrano, T.: Separation and quantitation of lactic dehydrogenase isoenzymes by disc-electrophoresis. Anal. Biochem. *20,* 246–257 (1967)

Dongen, J.M. van, Visser, W.J., Daems, W.Th., Galjaard, H.: The relation between cell proliferation, differentiation and ultrastructural development in rat intestinal epithelium. Cell Tissue Res. *174,* 183–199 (1976)

Druckrey, H.: Production of colonic carcinomas by 1,2-dialkylhydrazines and azoxyalkanes. In: Carcinoma of the colon and antecedent epithelium. Burdette, W.J. (ed.), pp. 258–279. Springfield, Ill.: Thomas 1970

Druckrey, H.: Organospecific carcinogenesis in the digestive tract. In: Topics in chemical carcinogenesis. Nakahara, W. (ed.), pp. 73–101. Baltimore: University Park Press 1972

Druckrey, H., Preussmann, R., Ivanković, S., Schmidt, C.H., So, B.T., Thomas, C.: Carcinogene Wirkung von Azoäthan und Azoxyäthan an Ratten. Z. Krebsforsch. *67,* 31–45 (1965)

Druckrey, H., Preussmann, R., Matzkies, F., Ivanković, S.: Selektive Erzeugung von Darmkrebs bei Ratten durch 1,2-Dimethylhydrazin. Naturwissenschaften *48,* 165–166 (1967)

Eastwood, G.L., Trier, J.S.: Epithelial cell renewal in cultured rectal biopsies in ulcerative colitis. Gastroenterology *64,* 383–390 (1973)

Ebert, P.A., Zuidema, G.D.: Primary tumors of the small intestine. Arch. Surg. *91,* 452–455 (1965)

Eder, M.: Die Bedeutung des "Turnover" von Epithelersatz und -differenzierung für die Orthologie und Pathologie der Dünndarmfunktion. Verh. Dtsch. Ges. Pathol. *53,* 45–55 (1969)

Evans, J.T., Luitman, G., Mittelmann, A.: The induction of multiple large bowel neoplasms in mice. J. Med. *3,* 212–215 (1972)

Farron, F., Hsu, H.H.T., Knox, W.E.: Fetal-type isoenzymes in hepatic and nonhepatic rat tumors. Cancer Res. *32,* 302–308 (1972)

Fasske, E., Themann, H.: Die elektronenmikroskopische Struktur menschlicher Carcinome. Beitr. Pathol. Anat. *122,* 313–344 (1960)

Fawcett, D.W.: Atlas zur Elektronenmikroskopie der Zelle. München, Berlin, Wien: Urban & Schwarzenberg 1973

Fenoglio, C.M., Richart, R.M., Kaye, G.J.: Comparative electron-microscopic features of normal, hyperplastic and adenomatous human colonic epithelium. II. Variations in surface architecture found by scanning electron microscopy. Gastroenterology *69,* 100–109 (1975)

Fiala, E.S.: Investigation into the metabolism and mode of action of the colon carcinogen 1,2–Dimethylhydrazine. Cancer *36,*2407–2412 (1975)

Fiala, E.S.: Investigations into the metabolism and mode of action of the colon carcinogens 1,2-dimethylhydrazine and azoxymethane. Cancer *40,* 2436–2445 (1977)

Filipe, M.I., Branfoot, A.C.: Abnormal patterns of mucus secretion in apparently normal mucosa of large intestine with cancer. Cancer *34,* 282–290 (1974)

Fisher, E.R., Sharkey, D.A.: The ultrastructure of colonic polyps and cancer with special reference to the epithelial inclusion bodies of Leuchtenberger. Cancer *15,* 160–170 (1962)

Fishman, W.H.: Immunologic and biochemical approaches to alkaline phosphatase isoenzyme analysis: the Regan isoenzyme. Ann. N.Y. Acad. Sci. *166,* 745–757 (1969)

Fishman, W.H.: Perspectives on alkaline phosphatase isoenzymes. Am. J. Med. *56,* 617–650 (1974)

Gabbert, H.: Disk-elektrophoretische Untersuchungen zur postnatalen Differenzierung des Enzymmusters der alkalischen Phosphatase und Malatdehydrogenase im Darm der Ratte. Medical thesis. Mainz 1973

Garbridge, M.G., Denunzio, A., Legator, M.S.: Cycasin: Detection of associated mutagenic activity in vivo. Science *163,* 689–691 (1969)

Gennaro, A.R., Villanueva, R., Sukonthaman, Y., Vathanophas, V., Rosemond, G.P.: Chemical carcinogenesis in transposed intestinal segments. Cancer Res. *33,* 536–541 (1973)

Glenner, G.G., Burtner, J.H., Brown, G.W.: The histochemical demonstration of monaminoxidase by tetrazolium salts. J. Histochem. Cytochem. *5,* 591–600 (1957)
Gössner, W.: Histochemischer Nachweis hydrolytischer Enzyme mit Hilfe der Azofarbstoffmethode. Untersuchungen zur Methodik und vergleichenden Histotopik der Esterasen und Phosphatasen bei Wirbeltieren. Histochemie *1,* 48–96 (1958)
Gössner, W., Friedrich-Freksa, H.: Histochemische Untersuchungen über die Glukose-6-Phosphatase in der Rattenleber während der Cancerisierung durch Nitrosamine. Z. Naturforsch. *19,* 862–684 (1964)
Goldenberg, V.E., Goldenberg, N.S., Sommers, S.C.: Comparative ultrastructure of atypical ductal hyperplasia, intraductal carcinoma and infiltrating ductal carcinoma of the breast. Cancer *24,* 1152–1169 (1969)
Goldmann, H., Ming, S., Hickok, D.F.: Nature and significance of hyperplastic polyps of the human colon. Arch. Pathol. *89,* 349–354 (1970)
Gomori, G.: An improved histochemical technic for acid phosphatase. Stain. Technol. *25,* 81–85 (1950)
Gossrau, R.: Review: Enzyme histochemistry of the intestinal brush border. Acta Histochem. Cytochem. *8,* 153–163 (1975a)
Gossrau, R.: Die Lysosomen des Darmepithels. Advances in Anatomy, Embryology and Cell Biology, Vol. LI/5, Berlin, Heidelberg, New York: Springer 1975b
Graumann, W., Clauss, W.: Weitere Untersuchungen zur Spezifität der histochemischen Polysaccharid-Eisenreaktion. Acta Histochem. (Jena) *6,* 1–7(1958)
Graumann, W., Neumann, K.: Handbuch der Histochemie, Bd. II/2. Stuttgart: Fischer 1964
Grözinger, K.H., Schüler, H.W.: Dünndarmtumoren. Z. Gastroenterol. *8,* 471–479 (1970)
Grundmann, E.: Mechanismen der Onkogenese. Verh. Dtsch. Ges. Inn. Med. *78,* 34–45 (1972)
Guerin, M.: Le problème des corps d'inclusion dans les tumeurs. II. Chez l'homme. Bull. Cancer (Paris) *54,* 263–284 (1967)
Häkkinen, I., Korhonen, L.K., Saxen, L.: The time of appearance and distribution of sulphoglycoprotein antigens in the human foetal alimentary canal. Int. J. Cancer *3,* 582–592 (1968)
Haenszel, W., Correa, P.: Cancer of the colon and rectum and adenomatous polyps. A review of epidemiological findings. Cancer *28,* 14–24 (1971)
Haenszel, W., Berg, J.W., Kurihara, M., Locke, F.B.: Large-bowel cancer in hawaiian japonese. J. Natl. Cancer Inst. *51,* 1765–1799 (1973)
Hale, C.W.: Histochemical demonstration of acid polysaccharides in animal tissues. Nature *157,* 802 (1946)
Hananouchi, M., Fukushima, S., Takahashi, M.: Electron microscopic studies on experimental undifferentiated adenocarcinomas of the glandular stomach in rats. Gann *65,* 323–330 (1974)
Harbers, E., Sandritter, W.: Gesteigerte Heterochromatisierung als pathogenetisches Prinzip. Dtsch. med. Wochenschr. *93,* 269–271 (1968)
Hawks, A., Swann, P.F., Magee, P.N.: Probable methylation of nucleic acids of mouse colon by 1,2-dimethylhydrazine in vivo. Biochem. Pharmacol. *21,* 432–433 (1972)
Hecker, E.: Aktuelle Probleme der Krebsentstehung. Z. Krebsforsch. *78,* 99–122 (1972)
Hecker, E.: Cocarcinogens and cocarcinogenesis (with a note on synergetic processes in cocarcinogenesis). In: Handbuch der allgemeinen Pathologie. Vol. VI/7: Geschwülste, Tumors II. Grundmann, E. (ed.), pp. 651–676. Berlin, Heidelberg, New York: Springer 1975
Heidelberger, C.: Chemical carcinogenesis. Annu. Rev. Biochem. *44,* 79–121 (1975)
Helwig, F.C.: Epithelial cytoplasmic inclusion bodies of possible viral origin in clinically early ulcerative colitis. Dis. Colon Rectum *2,* 23–26 (1959)

Hess, M.W., Zimmermann, A., Brun del Re, G., Cottier, H.: Immunologische Aspekte gastrointestinaler Neoplasien. Schweiz. Med. Wochenschr. *105*, 570–575 (1975)
Hill, M.J.: Steroid nuclear dehydrogenation and colon cancer. Am. Clin. Nutr. *27*, 1475–1480 (1974)
Hill, M.J.: The role of colon anaerobes in the metabolism of bile acids and steroids, and its relation to colon cancer. Cancer *36*, 2387–2400 (1975)
Höhn, P., Gabbert, H., Wagner, R.: Differentiation and ageing of the rat intestinal mucosa. II. Morphological, enzyme-histochemical and disc-electrophoretic aspects of the aging of the small intestinal mucosa. Mech. Ageing Dev. *7*, 217–226 (1978)
Höhn, P., Schäfer, A., Gabbert, H.: Differentiation and aging of the intestinal mucosa of the rat. I. Morphological, enzyme-histochemical and disc-electrophoretic aspects of the prenatal and postnatal differentiation of the intestinal mucosa. Mech. Ageing Dev. *6*, 35–51 (1977)
Holt, S.J.: Factors governing the validity staining methods for enzymes and their bearing up on the Gomori acid phosphatase technique. Exp. Cell. Res. (Suppl.) *7*, 1–27 (1959)
Hugon, J., Borgers, M.: Fine structural changes and localization of phosphatases in the epithelium of the duodenal crypt of X-irradiated mice. Histochemie *6*, 209–225 (1966a)
Hugon, J., Borgers, M.: Ultrastructural localization of alkaline phosphatase activity in the absorbing cells of the duodenum of the mouse. J. Histochem. Cytochem. *14*, 629–640 (1966b)
Imai, H., Saito, S., Stein, A.A.: Ultrastructure of adenomatous polyps and villous adenomas of the large intestine. Gastroenterology *48*, 188–197 (1965)
Imai, H., Stein, A.A.: Ultrastructure of adenocarcinoma of the colon. Gastroenterology *44*, 410–418 (1963)
Ioachim, N.-J., Delaney, W.E., Madrazo, A.: Villous adenoma of the colon and rectum: an ultrastructural study. Cancer *34*, 586–596 (1974)
Isselbacher, K.J.: The intestinal cell surface: some properties of the normal, undifferentiated and malignant cells. Ann. Intern. Med. *81*, 681–686 (1974)
Ito, S.: The enteric surface coat on cat intestinal microvilli. J. Cell Biol. *27*, 475–491 (1965)
Kanagalingam, K., Balis, M.E.: In vivo repair of rat intestinal DNA damage by alkylating agents. Cancer *36*, 2364–2372 (1975)
Karasaki, S.: Cell proliferation and subcellular localization of alkaline phosphatase activity in rat liver parenchyma during azo dye carcinogenesis. Cancer Res. *35*, 482–491 (1975)
Kastendieck, H., Altenähr, E., Burchardt, P.: Elektronenmikroskopische Untersuchungen zur Zelldifferenzierung in Prostata-Carcinomen. Virchows Arch. (Pathol. Anat.) *361*, 241–256 (1973)
Kaye, G.I., Fenoglio, C.M., Pascal, R.R., Lane, N.: Comparative electron microscopic features of normal, hyperplastic and adenomatous human colonic epithelium. Gastroenterology *64*, 926–945 (1973)
Keeley, A.F., Gottlieb, L.S.: Villous adenoma of the small bowel: an unusual lesion. Gastroenterology *57*, 185–190 (1969)
Kligerman, M.M., Heidenreich, W.F., Greene, S.: Distribution of triated thymidine about a capillary sinusoid in a transplanted mouse tumor. Nature *196*, 282–283 (1962)
Knox, W.E.: Enzyme patterns in fetal, adult and neoplastic rat tissues. Basel, München, Paris: Karger 1976
Korhonen, K., Mäkelä, V., Lilius, G.: Carbohydrate-rich compounds in the colonic mucosa of man. II. Histochemical characteristics of colonic adenocarcinomas. Cancer *27*, 128–133 (1971)

Koudstaal, J., Makkink, B., Overdiep, S.H.: Enzyme histochemical patterns in human tumors. I. Hydrolytic enzymes in carcinoma of the colon and the breast. Eur. J. Cancer *11,* 105–109 (1975a)

Koudstaal, J., Makkink, B., Overdiep, S.H.: Enzyme histochemical patterns in human tumours. II. Oxidoreductases in carcinoma of the colon and the breast. Eur. J. Cancer *11,* 111–115 (1975b)

Kowalewski, S.L.: Die Isoenzyme der Lactatdehydrogenase. Biochemie und Klinik. Stuttgart: Thieme 1972

Kümmerle, F., Schier, J.: Dünndarmtumoren. In: Klinische Gastroenterologie. Demling, L. (ed.), Vol. I, pp. 418–431. Stuttgart: Thieme 1973

Kunze, E., Schauer, A., Krüsmann, G.: Focal loss of alkaline phosphatase and increase of proliferation in preneoplastic areas of the rat urothelium after administration of N-Butyl-N-(4-Hydroxybutyl)-Nitrosamine and N-(4-(5-Nitro-2-Furyl)-2-Thiazolyl) Formamide. Z. Krebsforsch. *84,* 143–160 (1975)

Kurzon, R.M., Ortega, R., Rywlin, A.M.: The significance of papillary features in polyps of the large intestine. Am. J. Clin. Pathol. *62,*447–454 (1974)

Lacassagne, A., Buu-Hoi, N.P., Zajdela, F.: Carcinogenic activity in situ of further steroid compounds. Nature *209,* 1026–1027 (1966)

Lamerz, R., Fateh-Moghadam, A.: Carcinofetale Antigene. III. Andere carcinofetale Antigene. Klin. Wochenschr. *53,* 403–417 (1975)

Langvad, E.: Lactate dehydrogenase isoenzyme patterns in the tumor-bearing colon. Int. J. Cancer *3,* 17–29 (1968)

Laqueur, G.L.: Carcinogenic effects of cycad meal and cycasin, methylazoxymethanol glycoside in rats and effects of cycasin in germfree rats. Fed. Proc. *23,* 1386–1387 (1964)

Laqueur, G.L.: The induction of intestinal neoplasms in rats with the glycoside cycasin and its aglycone. Virchows Arch. (Pathol. Anat.) *340,* 151–163 (1965)

Laqueur, G.L., McDaniel, E.G., Matsumoto, H.: Tumor induction in germfree rats with methylazoxymethanol (MAM) and synthetic MAM acetate. J. Natl. Cancer Inst. *39,* 355–371 (1967)

Laqueur, G.L., Mickelsen, O., Whiting, M.G., Kurland, L.T.: Carcinogenic properties of nuts from Cycas circinalis L. indigenous to Guam. J. Natl. Cancer Inst. *31,* 919–951 (1963)

Laqueur, G.L., Spatz, M.: Toxicology of Cycasin. Cancer Res. *28,* 2262–2267 (1968)

Lauren, P.: The cell structure and secretion in the intestinal cancer. Acta Pathol. Microbiol. Scand. (Suppl.) *152,* 9–151 (1961)

Leblond, C.P., Cheng, H.: Identification of stem cells in the small intestine of the mouse. In: Stem cells of the renewing cell populations. Cairnie, A.B., Lala, P.K., Osmond, D.G. (eds.), pp. 7–31. New York, San Francisco, London: Academic Press 1976

Lehmann, F.G.: Tumorantigene in der gastroenterologischen Diagnostik. Leber Magen Darm *5,* 144–158 (1975)

Lehmann, F.G.: α_1-Fetoprotein und Regan-Isoenzym im Serum bei malignen Tumoren des Gastrointestinaltraktes. Z. Gastroenterol. *14,* 268–269 (1976)

Leuchtenberger, C.: Cytoplasmic 'inclusion bodies' containing desoxyribose nucleic acid (DNA) in cells of human rectal polyps. Lab. Invest. *3,* 132–142 (1954)

Lev, R., Weisberg, H.: Human foetal epithelial glycogen: a histochemical and electron-microscopic study. J. Anat. *105,* 337–349 (1969)

Lipkin, M.: Phase 1 and phase 2 proliferative lesions of colonic epithelial cells in diseases leading to colonic cancer. Cancer *34,* 878–888 (1974)

Löhrs, U., Wiebecke, B., Eder, M.: Morphologische und autoradiographische Untersuchung der Darmschleimhautveränderungen nach einmaliger Injektion von 1,2-Dimethylhydrazin. Z. Gesamte Exp. Med. *151,* 297–307 (1969)

Lojda, Z.: Some remarks concerning the histochemical detection of disaccharidases and glucosidases. Histochemie *5,* 339–360 (1965)

Lojda, Z., Fric, P., Jodl, J., Chmelik, V.: Cytochemistry of the human jejunal mucosa in the norm and malabosrption syndrome. Curr. Top. Pathol. *52,* 1–63 (1970)
Mäkelä, V., Korhonen, L.K., Lilius, G.: Carbohydrate-rich compounds in the colonic mucosa of man. I. Histochemical characteristics of normal and adenomatous colonic mucosa. Cancer *27,* 120–127 (1971)
Magee, P.N., Pegg, A.E., Swann, P.F.: Molecular mechanisms of chemical carcinogenesis. In: Handbuch der allgemeinen Pathologie, Vol. VI/7, Geschwülste, Tumors II. Grundmann, E. (ed.), pp. 329–419. Berlin, Heidelberg, New York: Springer 1975
Maggi, V., Wyatt, A.P.: Observations on an unusual enzyme distribution pattern in the colon of a case of familial polyposis with malignant changes. Gut *11,* 319–322 (1970)
Malik, N., Butterworth, P.J.: Rat intestinal alkaline phosphatase: a heterogenous dimeric glycoprotein. Biochem. Soc. Trans. *4,* 646–649 (1976)
Marsden, J.R., Dawson, I.M.P.: An investigation into the enzyme histochemistry of adenocarcinomas of human large intestine and of the transitional epithelium immediately adjacent to them. Gut *15,* 783–787 (1974)
Matsumoto, H., Nagawama, T., Larson, H.O.: Studies on methylazoxymethanol, the aglycon of cycasin: a synthesis of methylazoxymethyl acetate. Biochem. J. *95,* 130–140 (1965)
Matsumoto, H., Strong, F.M.: The occurrence of methylazoxymethanol in Cycas circinalis L. Arch. Biochem. *101,* 299–310 (1963)
Mercer, E.H.: The cancer cell. Br. Med. Bull. *18,* 187–192 (1962)
Merzel, J., Leblond, C.P.: Origin and renewal of goblet cells in the epithelium of the mouse small intestine. Am. J. Anat. *124,* 281–306 (1969)
Mir-Madjlessi, S.-H., Farmer, R.G., Hawk, W.A.: Villous tumours of the duodenum and jejunum. Report of four cases and review of the literature. Am. J. Dig. Dis. *18,* 467–476 (1973)
Miyayama, H., Doellgast, G.J., Memoli, V., Gandbhir, L., Fishman, W.H.: Direct immunoperoxidase staining for Regan isoenzyme of alkaline phosphatase in human tumour tissues. Cancer *38,* 1237–1246 (1976)
Moersch, R.N., Woolner, L.B., Clagett, O.T.: Villous adenoma of the duodenum. Surgery *51,* 574–577 (1962)
Monis, B., Mendeloff, A.: Observations on inclusion bodies in normal and pathologic mucosa of the colon in man. J. Natl. Cancer Inst. *26,* 1429–1443 (1961)
Morson, B.C.: Evolution of cancer of the colon and rectum. Cancer *34,* 845–849 (1974)
Morson, B.C., Bussey, H.J.R.: Predisposing causes of intestinal cancer. In: Curr. Probl. Surg. Chicago: Yearbook Medical Publishers 1970
Morson, B.C., Dawson, I.M.P.: Gastrointestinal pathology. Second printing. Oxford, London: Blackwell 1974
Muto, T., Bussey, H.J.R., Morson, B.C.: The evolution of cancer of the colon and rectum. Cancer *36,* 2251–2270 (1975)
Nachlas, M., Crawford, D., Seligman, A.: The histochemical demonstration of leucine aminopeptidase. J. Histochem. Cytochem. *5,* 264–276 (1975)
Nachlas, M., Seligman, A.M.: The comparative distribution of esterase in the tissue of five mammals by a histochemical technique. Anat. Rec. *105,* 677–695 (1949)
Nachlas, M., Walker, D., Seligman, A.: A histochemical method for the demonstration of diphosphopyridine nucleotide diaphorase. J. Biophys. Biochem. Cytol. *4,* 29–38 (1958)
Nakahara, W.: Pharmacodynamic mechanism in carcinogenesis. In: Handbuch der allgemeinen Pathologie, Bd. VI/7: Geschwülste, Tumors II, Grundmann, E. (ed.), pp. 595–650. Berlin, Heidelberg, New York: Springer 1975
Narisawa, T., Magadia, N.E., Weisburger, J.H., Wynder, E.L.: Promoting effect of bile acid on colon carcinogenesis after intrarectal instillation of N-methyl-N'-nitrosoguanidine in rats. J. Natl. Cancer Inst. *53,* 1093–1097 (1974)

Oehlert, W.: Regeneration, Hyperplasie und Cancerisierung am Beispiel der epithelialen Wechselgewebe. In: Handbuch der allgemeinen Pathologie, Vol. VI/2, Büchner, F. (ed.), pp. 244–374. Berlin, Heidelberg, New York: Springer 1969
Osswald, H., Krüger, F.W.: Die cancerogene Wirkung von 1,2-DMH beim Goldhamster, Arzneim. Forsch. *19*, 1891–1892 (1969)
Otto, H.F., Wanke, M., Zeitlhofer, J.: Darm und Peritoneoum. In: Spezielle pathologische Anatomie, Bd. II/2. Berlin, Heidelberg, New York: Springer 1976
Otto, H.F., Winkler, R., Heitmann, C.: Tierexperimentelle Untersuchungen zur Morphogenese Nitrosamin-induzierter colorectaler Tumoren. Z. Krebsforsch. *87*, 333–342 (1976)
Paasch, W.: Disk-elektrophoretische Untersuchungen zur postnatalen Differenzierung der Laktatdehydrogenase und der sauren Phosphatase im Darm der Ratte. Medical thesis, Mainz 1974
Padykula, H.A.: Recent functional interpretation of intestinal morphology. Fed. Proc. *21*, 873–879 (1962)
Pearse, A.G.E.: Histochemistry. Theoretical and Applied, 3rd ed., Vol. I and II. London: Churchill Livingstone 1968 and 1972
Pearse, A.G.E., Riecken, E.O.: Histology and cytochemistry of the cells of the small intestine, in relation to absorption. Br. Med. Bull. *23*, 217–222 (1967)
Pfeifer, U.: Kombinierte elektronenmikroskopische Darstellung der Arylsulfatase und der sauren Phosphatase in Lysosomen des Nierentubulus. Histochemie *17*, 284–292 (1969)
Pfeifer, U.: Lysosomen und Autophagie. Verh. Dtsch. Pathol. *60*, 28–64 (1976)
Pierce, G.B.: Neoplasms, differentiations and mutations. Am. J. Pathol. *77*, 103–118 (1974)
Pierce, G.B., Nakane, P.K., Mazurkiewicz, J.E.: The natural history of the malignant stem cells. 4th Int. Symp. Princess Takamatsu. Cancer Res. Fund pp. 453–469. Tokio 1973
Pozharisskij, K.M.: Intestinal tumors induced in the rats with 1,2-Dimethylhydrazine. Vop. Onkol. N.S. *18*, 1, 64–71 (1972)
Pozharisskij, K.M.: Morphology and morphogenesis of experimental epithelial tumors of the intestine. J. Natl. Cancer Inst. *54*, 1115–1135 (1975)
Pozharisskij, K.M., Shaposhnikov, J.D., Petrov, A.S., Likhachev, A.J.: Distribution and carcinogenic action of 1,2-Dimethylhydrazine (SDMH) in rats. Z. Krebsforsch. *87*, 67–80 (1976)
Preussmann, R.: Chemische Carcinogene in der menschlichen Umwelt. In: Handbuch der allgemeinen Pathologie, Vol. VI/7: Geschwülste, Tumors II. Grundmann, E. (ed.), pp. 421–594. Berlin, Heidelberg, New York: Springer 1975
Preussmann, R., Druckrey, H., Ivanković, S., Hodenberg, A.v.: Chemical structure and carcinogenicity of aliphatic hydrazo, azo and azoxy compounds and of triazenes, potential in vivo alkylating agents. In: Biological effects of alkylating agents. Ann. N.Y. Acad. Sci. *163*, 697–716 (1969)
Reddy, B.S.: Role of bile metabolites in colon carcinogenesis. Animal models. Cancer *36*, 2401–2406 (1975)
Reddy, B.S., Narisawa, T., Vukusich, D., Mangat, S., Wynder, E.L., Weisburger, J.H.: Effect of quality and quantity of dietary fat on sensitivity of colon to carcinogenic effects of 1,2-dimethylhydrazine in rats. Fed. Proc. *34*, 900 (1975)
Richards, A.H., Hilf, R.: Effect of estrogen administration on glucose-6-phosphatase dehydrogenase and lactate dehydrogenase isoenzymes in rodent mammary tumors and normal mammary gland. Cancer Res. *32*, 611–616 (1972)
Riecken, E.O.: Enzymhistochemie der menschlichen Dünndarmschleimhaut unter normalen und pathologischen Bedingungen. Z. Gastroenterol. *13*, 210–222 (1975)
Rijke, R.P.C., Plaisier, H., Hoogeveen, A.T., Lamerton, L.F., Galjaard, H.: The effect of continous irradiation on cell proliferation and maturation in small intestine epithelium. Cell Tissue Kinet. *8*, 441–453 (1975)

River, L., Silverstein, J., Tope, J.W.: Benign neoplasms of the small intestine. A critical comprehensive review with reports of 20 new cases. Int. Abstr. Surg. *102,* 1–33 (1956)

Rubin, W., Ross, L.L., Sleisenger, M., Jeffries, G.H.: The normal human gastric epithelia. A fine structural study. Lab. Invest. *19,* 598–626 (1968)

Sandborn, E.B.: Stratified squamous epithelium. In: Cells and tissues by light and electron microscopy, pp. 175–187. New York, London: Academic Press 1970

Sasaki, M., Fishman, W.H.: Ultrastructural studies on Regan and non-Regan isoenzymes of alkaline phosphatase in human tumours. In: Electron microscopy and cytochemistry, pp. 59–62. Amsterdam, London, New York: North Holland and American Elsevier 1974

Schäfer, A., Höhn, P.: Funktionelle Morphologie der Darmschleimhaut. Struktur und Enzymmuster bei der Ratte. Gastroenterologie und Stoffwechsel, Bd. VIII. Stuttgart: Thieme 1975

Schauer, A., Kunze, E., Boxler, K.: Generationszeitzyklus von 1,2-Dimethylhydrazin-induzierten Adenocarcinomen des Rattencolon. Naturwissenschaften *58,* 221 (1971)

Schauer, A., Völlnagel, Th., Wildanger, F.: Morphologische und histochemische Untersuchungen bei der Cancerisierung der Darmschleimhaut der Ratte durch 1,2-Dimethylhydrazin. Verh. Dtsch. Ges. Pathol. *53,* 234–236 (1969)

Schipp, R., Höhn, P., Schäfer, A.: Elektronenmikroskopische und histochemische Untersuchungen zur Funktion des Kiemenherzanhanges (Pericardialdrüse) von Sepia officinalis. Z. Zellforsch. *117,* 252–274 (1971)

Schmähl, D.: Entstehung, Wachstum und Chemotherapie maligner Tumoren. Aulendorf: Editio Cantor 1970

Schmähl, D.: Zur kausalen Genese maligner Tumoren. Wien. Med. Wochenschr. *125,* 637 (1975)

Schmähl, D., Danisman, A., Habs, M., Diehl, B.: Experimental investigations on the influence upon chemical carcinogenesis. Z. Krebsforsch. *86,* 89–94 (1976)

Silberman, H., Crichlow, R.W., Caplan, H.S.: Neoplasms of the small bowel. Ann. Surg. *180,* 157–161 (1974)

Sonntag, W., Arnold, M.: Funktionsentwicklung der Lunge des Goldhamsters. Elektronenmikroskopische und histochemische Untersuchungen der Lungenalveolen. Acta Histochem. (Jena) *45,* 21–36 (1973)

Spatz, M., Laqueur, G.: Transplacental induction of tumors in Sprague Dawley rats with crude cycad material. J. Natl. Cancer Inst. *38,* 233–239 (1967)

Sperry, J.F., Salyers, A.A., Wilkins, T.D.: Fecal long chain fatty acids and colon cancer risk. Lipids *11,* 637–639 (1976)

Spiro, H.M.: Clinical gastroenterology. London: Collier-MacMillan 1970

Spjut, H.J.: Newer concepts of cancer of the colon and rectum. Dis. Colon Rectum *15,* 94–99 (1972)

Spjut, H.J., Smith, M.N.: A comparative electron microscopy study of human and rat colonic polyps and carcinomas. Exp. Mol. Pathol. *6,* 11–24 (1967)

Spjut, H.J., Spratt, J.S.: Endemic and morphologic similarities existing between spontaneous neoplasms in man and 3:2'-Dimethyl-4-aminobiphenyl induced colonic neoplasms in rats. Ann. Surg. *161,* 309–324 (1965)

Spratt, J.S., Ackermann, L.V.: Pathologic significance of polyps of the rectum and colon. Dis. Colon Rectum *3,* 330–335 (1960)

Spratt, J.S., Ackermann, L.V.: Small primary adenocarcinomas of the colon and rectum. J. Amer. Med. Assoc. *179,* 337–346 (1962)

Springer, P., Springer, J., Oehlert, W.: Die Vorstufen des 1,2-Dimethylhydrazin-induzierten Dick- und Dünndarmcarcinoms der Ratte. Z. Krebsforsch. *74,* 236–240 (1970)

Stavrou, D.: Biochemie und Histochemie experimenteller Hirntumoren. In: Handbuch der allgemeinen Pathologie, Bd. VI/6. Geschwülste, Tumors III. Grundmann, E. (ed.) pp. 94–103. Berlin, Heidelberg, New York: Springer 1975

Steinberg, L.S., Shieber, W.: Villous adenomas of the small intestine. Surgery *71,* 423–428 (1972)
Steinbrecher, J.S., Silverberg, S.G.: Signet-ring cell carcinoma of the breast. Cancer *37,* 828–840 (1976)
Stier, A.: Zur Bedeutung der Biotransformation von Fremdstoffen: Primäre Giftwirkung durch kovalente Bindung. Internist (Berlin) *14,* 202–211 (1973)
Stoebner, P., Le Gal, Y.: Ultrastructure of anaplastic bronchial carcinomas. Cancer *20,* 286–294 (1967)
Swift, J.G., Mukherjee, T.M.: Demonstration of the fuzzy surface coat of rat intestinal microvilli by freeze-etching. J. Cell Biol. *69,* 491–494 (1976)
Takeuchi, T.: Histochemical demonstration of branching enzyme (Amylo-1,4 → 1,6-transglucosidase) in animal tissues. J. Histochem. Cytochem. *6,* 208–216 (1958)
Tannock, I.F.: The relation between cell proliferation and the vascular system in a transplanted mouse mammary tumor. Br. J. Cancer *22,* 258–273 (1968)
Tannock, I.F., Steel, G.G.: Tumor growth and cell kinetics in chronically hypoxic animals. J. Natl. Cancer Inst. *45,* 123–133 (1970)
Thoenes, W.: Zytoplasmatische Aspekte der Onkozytologie. Verh. Dtsch. Ges. Pathol. *57,* 61–81 (1973)
Thoenes, W., Langer, K.H.: Die Endocytose-Phase der Eiweißresorption im proximalen Nierentubulus. Untersuchungen am Ferritin-resorbierenden Einzeltubulus der Rattenniere. Virchows Archiv (Cell Pathol.) *2,* 361–379 (1969)
Thurnherr, N., Reinhart, K.: Induktion von Kolonkarzinomen mit 1,2-Dimethylhydrazin-hydrochlorid bei der Maus. Schweiz. Med. Wochenschr. *105,* 585–586 (1975)
Thurnherr, N., Deschner, E.E., Stonehill, E.H., Lipkin, M.: Induction of adenocarcinomas of the colon in mice by weekly injections of 1,2-dimethylhydrazine. Cancer Res. *33,* 940–945 (1973)
Toner, P.G.: Cytology of intestinal epithelial cells. Int. Rev. Cytol. *24,* 233–343 (1968)
Toner, P.G., Carr, K.E., Wyburn, G.M.: The digestive system. – An ultrastructural atlas and review. London: Butterworth 1971
Toth, B.: Tumorgenesis studies with 1,2-Dimethylhydrazine dihydrochloride, hydrazine sulfate and isonicotinic acid in golden hamsters. Cancer Res. *32,* 804–807 (1972)
Toth, B., Malnick, L., Shimizu, H.: Production of intestinal and other tumors by 1,2-dimethylhydrazine dihydrochloride in mice. Am. J. Pathol. *84,* 69–80 (1976)
Trasher, J.D., Greulich, R.C.: The duodenal progenitor population. II. The progenitor cell cycle of principal, goblet and paneth cells. J. Exp. Zool. *161,* 9–20 (1966)
Trier, J.S.: Studies on small intestinal crypt epithelium. I. The fine structure of the crypt epithelium of the proximal small intestine of fasting humans. J. Cell Biol. *18,* 599–620 (1963)
Trier, J.S.: Studies on the small intestine crypt epithelium. II. Evidence for a mechanism of secretory activity by undifferentiated crypt cells of the human small intestine. Gastroenterology *47,* 480–495 (1964)
Trier, J.S.: Morphology of the epithelium of the small intestine. In: Handbook of Physiology, Section VI: Alimentary Canal. Code, C.F. (ed.), Vol. III, pp. 1125–1175. Washington: American Physiolgical Society 1968
Trier, J.S., Rubin, C.E.: Electron microscopy of the small intestine: a review. Gastroenterology *49,* 574–603 (1965)
Tutton, P.J.M., Barkla, D.H.: Cell proliferation in the descending colon of dimethylhydrazine treated rats and in dimethylhydrazine induced adenocarcinomata. Virchows Arch. (Cell Pathol.) *21,* 147–160 (1976)
Vaupel, P.: Atemgaswechsel und Glucosestoffwechsel von Implantationstumoren (DS-Carcinosarkom) in vivo. In: Funktionsanalyse biologischer Systeme. Thews, G. (ed.), Vol. I. Wiesbaden: Steiner 1974
Vaupel, P., Thews, G., Wendling, P.: Kritische Sauerstoff- und Glucoseversorgung maligner Tumoren. Dtsch. Med. Wochenschr. *101,* 1810–1816 (1976)

Vogel, A., Glatthaar, E.: Weitere elektronenmikroskopische Untersuchungen am Portiokarzinom. Oncologia *11,* 138–147 (1958)
Wachsmuth, E.D., Torhorst, A.: Possible precursors of aminopeptidase and alkaline phosphatase in the proximal tubules of kidney and the crypts of small intestine of mice. Histochemistry *38,* 43–56 (1974)
Ward, J.M.: Morphogenesis of chemically induced neoplasms of the colon and small intestine in rats. Lab. Invest. *30,* 505–513 (1974)
Ward, J.M., Yamamoto, R.S., Weisburger, J.H.: Cellulose dietary bulk and azoxymethane-induced intestinal cancer. J. Natl. Cancer Inst. *51,* 713–715 (1973)
Watson, A.J., Wright, N.A.: Morphology and cell kinetics of the jejunal mucosa in untreated patient. Clin. Gastroenterol. *3,* 11–31 (1974)
Weber, G.: Carbohydrate metabolism in cancer cells and the molecular correlation concept. Naturwissenschaften *55,* 418–429 (1968)
Webster, H.L., Harrison, D.D.: Enzymic activities during the transformation of crypt to columnar intestinal cells. Exp. Cell Res. *56,* 245–253 (1969)
Weinhouse, S.: Glycolysis, respiration and anomalous gene expression in experimental hepatomas. G.H.A. Clowes memorial lecture. Cancer Res. *32,* 2007–2016 (1972)
Weinhouse, S.: The Warburg hypothesis fifty years later. Z. Krebsforsch. *87,* 115–126 (1976)
Weisburger, J.H.: Colon carcinogens: their metabolism and mode of action. Cancer *28,* 60–70 (1971)
Weisburger, J.H.: Model studies on the etiology of colon cancer. In: Topics in chemical carcinogenesis, pp. 159–174. Baltimore: University Park Press 1972
Weiser, M.M.: Intestinal epithelial cell surface membrane glycoprotein synthesis. I. An indicator of cellular differentiation. J. Biol. Chem. *298,* 2536–2541 (1973)
Wiebecke, B.: Experimental intestinal carcinogenesis and polyp development in rats and mice. In: Special topics in carcinogenesis. Recent Results in Cancer Research *44,* 127–129 (1974)
Wiebecke, B.: Experimentelle Cancerogenese des Magen-Darm-Kanals. B. Darm. In: Handbuch der allgemeinen Patholige, Bd. VI/7. Geschwülste, Tumors III. Grundmann, E. (ed.), pp. 731–767. Berlin, Heidelberg, New York: Springer 1975
Wiebecke, B., Krey, U., Löhrs, U., Eder, M.: Morphological and autoradiographical investigations on experimental carcinogenesis and polyp development in the intestinal tract of rats and mice. Virchows Arch. (Pathol. Anat.)*360,* 179–193 (1973)
Wiebecke, B., Löhrs, U., Gimmy, J., Eder, M.: Erzeugung von Darmtumoren bei Mäusen durch 1,2-Dimethylhydrazin. Z. Gesamte Exp. Med. *149,* 277–278 (1969)
Withers, H.R.: Cellular kinetics of intestinal mucosa after radiation. In: Carcinoma of the colon and antecedent epithelium. Burdette, W.J. (ed.). Springfield/Ill.: Thomas 1970
Wittig, G., Wildner, G.P.: Experimentelle Grundlagen zur Ätiologie des Dickdarm-Neoplasmas. Zentralbl. Chir. *101,* 395–401 (1976)
Wittig, G., Wildner, G.P., Zierbarth, P.: Der Einfluß der Ingesta auf die Cancerisierung des Rattendarmes mit Dimethylhydrazin. Arch. Geschwulstforsch. *37,* 105–115 (1971)
Wood, D.A.: Tumors of the intestines. Atlas of Tumor pathology; Sect. VI. Fasc. 22. Washington: Armed Forces Institute of Pathology 1967
Wynder, E.L., Reddy, B.S.: Studies of large bowel cancer: human leads to experimental application. J. Natl. Cancer Inst. *50,* 1099–1106 (1973)
Wynder, E.L., Reddy, B.S.: The epidemiology of cancer of the large bowel. Am. J. Dig. Dis. *19,* 937–946 (1974)
Wynder, E.L., Shigematsu, T.: Environmental factors of cancer of the colon and rectum. Cancer *20,* 1520–1560 (1967)

Zaldivar, R., Wetterstrand, W.H.: High-fibre, low-saturated-fat diet and the etiology of colo-rectal carcinomata in a low-risk population. Z. Krebsforsch. *87,* 41–45 (1976)

Zedeck, M.S., Brown, G.B.: Methylation of intestinal and hepatic DNA in rats treated with methylazoxymethanol acetate. Cancer *40,* 2580–2583 (1977)

Development of Urinary Bladder Cancer in the Rat *

E. KUNZE

* Supported by the Deutsche Forschungsgemeinschaft (SFB 51) and the Curt Bohnewand-Foundation Munich. The technical assistance of Mrs. R. Schwaiger, R. Polt and V. Vondraceck is gratefully appreciated. The present investigations were awarded the Johann Georg Zimmermann prize for cancer research 1975

I. General Introduction

As early as 1895 – long before any clues to the etiology of tumors in other organs were apparent – *Rehn* reported his observations of the increased occurrence of tumors of the urinary bladder in laborers who had daily contact with basic fuchsin over a long period. He suspected a causal connection between aniline, nitrobenzol, toluidine, and basic fuchsin and the development of the observed tumors. The years immediately following this report did not see confirmation of the suspected carcinogenicity of these substances (for a review of the literature see *Temkin,* 1963; *Sarma,* 1969; *Price,* 1971). Nevertheless, *Rehn*'s observations did initiate an early intensive search for substances that could induce tumors in the human bladder.

At present four chemical substances are known with certainty to cause tumors in the human bladder (*Temkin,* 1963; *Sarma,* 1969; *Price,* 1971). These are β-naphthylamine, benzidine, 4-aminodiphenyl, and chlornaphazine, a substance closely related to β-naphthylamine which has been used to treat polycythemia vera (*Thiede* and *Christensen,* 1969). All these substances, with the exception of chlornaphazine, have proved to be carcinogenic in animal experiments as well, particularly in dogs (*Temkin,* 1963; *Price,* 1971).

In time, other chemical compounds became known that could induce bladder tumors in experimental animals, such as o-aminoazotoluol, 3,2-dimethyl-4-aminodiphenyl, 2-methoxy-3-aminodibenzfurene, and N-2-fluorenylacetamide (for review of the literature see *Temkin,* 1963; and *Price,* 1971). Our knowledge regarding experimental carcinogenesis in the bladder has nevertheless remained quite limited, simply because a carcinogenic substance was not available which induced bladder tumors in a sufficiently high yield in small experimental animals such as rats or mice; therefore it was not possible to draw any conclusions on the basis of a sizable number of animals.

This handicap, however, was overcome with the synthesis of di-N-butylnitrosamine and N-butyl-N-(4-hydroxybutyl)-nitrosamine (*Druckrey* et al., 1962, 1964) and the discovery of the carcinogenic properties of 4-ethylsulphonylnaphthalene-1-sulphonamide (*Bonser* and *Clayson,* 1964) and of N-[4-(5-nitro-2-furyl)-2-thiazolyl] formamide (*Ertürk* et al., 1967), which opened up new opportunities for the study of carcinogenesis in larger experimental series.

Di-N-Butylnitrosamine (DBN)

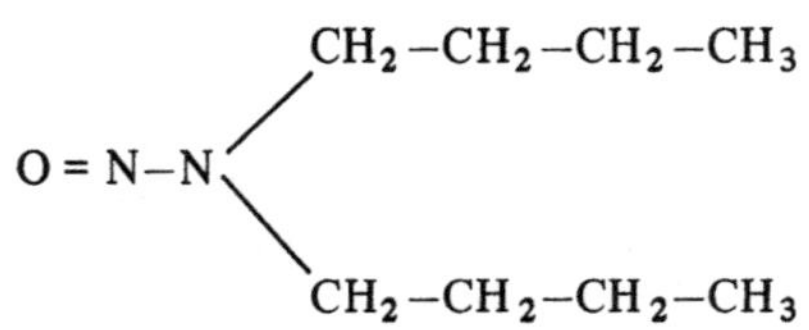

N-Butyl-N-(4-hydroxybutyl)-nitrosamine (BBN)

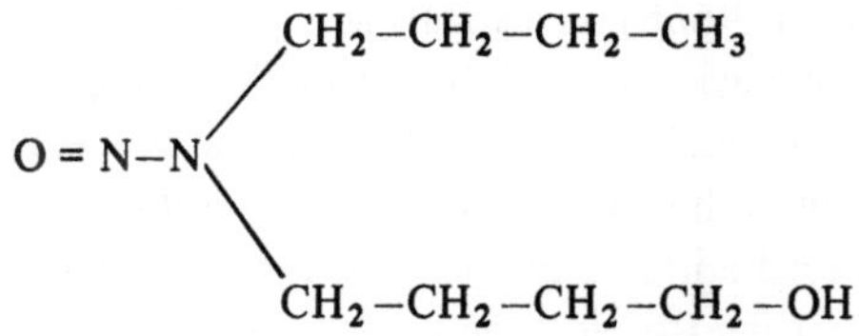

N-[4-(5-nitro-2-furyl)-2-thiazolyl] formamide (FANFT)

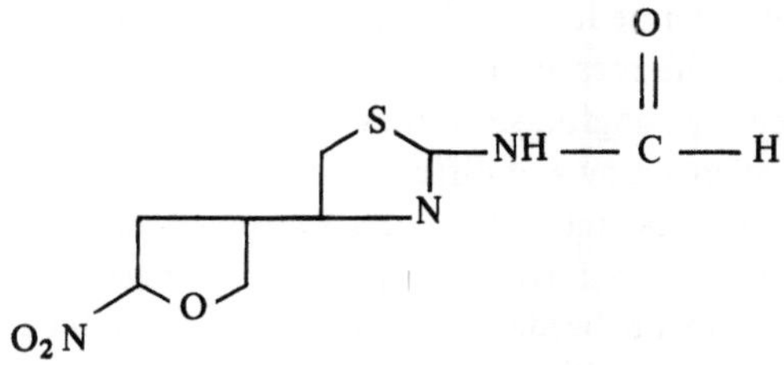

The aim of the present project was to investigate carcinogenesis in the bladder mucosa in the rat up to the development of tumors, by means of morphological, enzyme histochemical, and autoradiographic methods. Particular attention has been paid to the histogenesis of transitional cell carcinomas. The investigations were carried out with various carcinogenic substances, in order to determine whether proven changes have general significance for carcinogenesis in the rat bladder. Di-N-butylnitrosamine and N-butyl-N-(4-hydroxybutyl)-nitrosamine and N-[4-(5-nitro-2-furyl)-2-thiazolyl] formamide seemed particularly relevant as carcinogens due to their different molecular mechanisms.

II. The Normal Mucosa of the Urinary Bladder

1. Histology

In the second half of the 19th century numerous morphological investigations dealt with the normal bladder mucosa of various animal species (for review of the older literature see *Burckhardt*, 1859; *Oberdick*, 1884; *Beltzow*, 1884; *Dogiel*, 1890; *Poljakoff*, 1914; *Danini*, 1924; *Lezava*, 1934; *Fleroff*, 1936; *Petry* and *Amon*, 1966a). A basic similarity in structure was apparent in the bladder mucosa or urothelium (*Melicow*, 1945) of various laboratory animals such as mouse, rat, rabbit, cat, and dog. No agreement, however, has been reached regarding the number of cell layers of the urinary bladder. Some authors consider the urothelium as a single layer of cells (*Poljakoff*, 1914) others believe it to consist of two (*Lendorf*, 1901; *Danini*, 1924; *Gauer*, 1949), three (*Burckhardt*, 1859; *Oberdick*, 1884; *Lezava*, 1934), or even of four layers of cells (*Beltzow*, 1884; *Dogiel*, 1890). These differing views can be traced to the variously distended mucosa, simulating the claimed number of cell layers. In 1859 *Burckhardt* described cytoplasmic processes which connected the urothelial cells with the underlying connective tissue. Similar "foot cells" were observed after this by other investigators (*Oberdick,* 1884; *Danini,* 1924; *Lezava,* 1934; *Fleroff,* 1936; *Martin,* 1962). More recently *Petry* and *Amon* (1966b), investigating this problem with the electron microscope, have come to the conclusion that all the urothelial cells, including superficial cells, are connected with the basal lamina by cytoplasmic processes. On the basis of these findings one must conclude that the urothelium represents a pseudostratified rather than a truly multilayered epithelium. Nevertheless, this assumption has been doubted by other investigators using the electron microscope, since they could not confirm the presence of cytoplasmic processes (*Walker,* 1960; *Richter* and *Moize,* 1963; *Hicks,* 1965, 1966; *Koss,* 1969; *Clayson* and *Cooper,* 1970). The majority of authors therefore currently consider the urothelium as a multilayered cell system, which can be divided into a basal, an intermediate, and a superficial cell layer in a nondistended bladder. For the purpose of the present investigations the distinction between basal and suprabasal cells seemed meaningful, since they can be definitely distinguished from one another by light microscopy and differ in their grade of differentiation, their enzyme-histochemical properties, and their kinetics of proliferation.

The basal cells of the rat bladder mucosa are relatively small and are arranged close to each other. Sometimes they are lined up in a palisade-like manner. They contain a centrally or basally placed round to oval nucleus with dense chromatin structures and one, not always clearly visible, nucleolus. The cytoplasm is abundant and slightly eosinophilic. The superficial or luminal cells are particularly outstanding among the suprabasal cells. As a rule they are polygonal and appear significantly larger than the underlying cells. They consistently contain either one large nucleus or two smaller ones. The average DNA content of the superficial cell nuclei is 16 n, and that of the basal cell nuclei 2 n (*Walker,* 1958; *Levi* et al., 1969b, 1971). Superficial giant cells were observed quite frequently, and contained numerous nuclei (*Oberdick,* 1884; *Dogiel,* 1890; *Danini,* 1924; *Lezava,* 1934; *Fleroff,* 1936; *Gauer,* 1949; *Bucher* and *Délèze,* 1955; *Petry* and *Amon,* 1966). *Dogiel* (1890) considered them to be among the largest within the mammalian organism.

Mechanisms of development of such multinucleated giant cells that have been suggested are amitotic division and nuclear fusion (*Beltzow,* 1884; *Dogiel,* 1890; *Lezava,* 1934; *Gauer,* 1949; *Bucher* and *Délèze,* 1955). The explanation of *Fleroff* (1936) seems more plausible, however, namely, that multinucleated superficial cells develop via endomitosis. Because of their size, the superficial cells cover several underlying cells in an umbrella-like fashion. The numerical ratio between superficial cells and the remaining cells of the urothelium of the rat bladder was estimated to be 1:9 (*Leblond* et al., 1955; *Schreiber* et al., 1969).

The ultrastructure of the rat and mouse urothelium demonstrates an increase in the degree of cell differentiation from the basal to the superficial layer. The outstanding feature of the most highly differentiated superficial cells are numerous fusiform, discoid or spherical cytoplasmic vesicles (*Walker,* 1960; *Leeson,* 1962; *Hicks,* 1965, 1966; *Koss,* 1969; *Levi* et al., 1971), which are bordered by an asymmetrically thickened membrane (*Hicks,* 1965, 1966; *Koss,* 1969). This membrane consists of a component lining the lumen of the vesicles and a thinner component forming the outer envelope. The structure of the vesicular membrane is identical with that of the luminal membrane of the superficial cells. Keratin is considered an important component of the membrane

(*Hicks*, 1965, 1966). The Golgi apparatus is very probably the site of origin of the vesicles (*Hicks*, 1965, 1966; *Koss*, 1969). Numerous communicating vesicles forming long narrow canals are incorporated into the luminal plasma membrane to become part of it. For this reason the vesicle membrane is considered a sort of reserve luminal membrane, required during distension of the bladder. *Richter* and *Moize* (1963) and *Petry* and *Amon* (1966) considered the interdigitations of the cell membrane of the contracted bladder to be reserve folds, which disappear when the bladder is distended. In particular, *Amon* and *Petry* suggested that in addition to the reserve fold mechanism a displacement of the more luminally situated cells, including the superficial cells, in a basal direction is necessary during distention of the bladder. Besides the vesicles, the superficial cells contain numerous mitochondria, lysosomes, polyribosomes and an extensively developed smooth endoplasmatic reticulum. Tonofilaments have also been demonstrated (*Hicks*, 1965, 1966; *Levi* et al., 1971). The superficial cells are said to be bound to each other via desmosomes in various laboratory animals (*Leeson*, 1962; *Richter* and *Moize*, 1963; *Hicks*, 1965).

In summary, the urinary bladder mucosa of the rat can be considered as a multilayered epithelium, which is properly designated a transitional cell epithelium. The great flexibility of each urothelial cell and the particular histological structure of the mucosa permit the bladder to adapt to rapid changes in its capacity.

2. Enzyme Histochemistry

Gomori (1941) inititated enzyme histochemical investigations of the normal bladder mucosa of various laboratory animals. He found a high alkaline phosphatase activity in the urothelium of various animal species such as rat, guinea-pig, rabbit, cat, dog, and pig. This finding was confirmed by other investigators who used techniques based on metallic salts and azo-dyes (Table 1). The results of such testing showed that the reaction pattern of alkaline phosphatase in the urothelium of various laboratory animals was quite uniform. The basal and intermediate cells demonstrated a strong precipitation. The superficial cells, by comparison, showed only apically or at times entirely a negative enzyme reaction. *Vacek* and *Schück* (1960) were the only investigators to report high activity in the luminal cells and a negative reaction in the basal cells. Using the method of *Stutte* (1967), our own investigations demonstrated uniformly strong alkaline phosphatase activity in the cytoplasm of the basal and intermediate cells in the urothelium of Wistar and Sprague-Dawley rats. Occasionally the reaction precipitate was found to be particularly marked in the apical parts of the cytoplasm. The superficial cells showed strong enzyme activity in their basal parts, their lumen-oriented parts were negative. Occasionally completely negative enzyme reactions were found in individual superficial cells or superficial cell formations. Desquamated superficial cells always reacted negatively. There was no demonstrable difference in the reaction intensity in the mucosa of Wistar or Sprague-Dawley rats, or between females and males.

Other hydrolases besides the alkaline phsophatase elicited a positive histochemical reaction, which was consistently weaker in intensity (Table 2). Phosphoamidase (*Meyer* and *Weinmann*, 1957) produced the weakest reaction, even after several hours' incuba-

Table 1. Activity of alkaline phosphatase in the normal bladder urothelium of various experimental animals

Animal species	Authors
Mouse	*Kabat* and *Furth*, 1941
	Bern, 1949
	Martin, 1958
	Levi et al., 1971
	Highman et al., 1975
Rat	*Gomori*, 1941
	Bern, 1949
	Mende and *Chambers*, 1957
	Martin, 1958
	Vacek and *Schück*, 1960
	Amon and *Petry*, 1962
	Leeson, 1962
	Kunze and *Schauer*, 1971
	Stiller and *Rauscher*, 1971
	Kunze et al., 1975
Guinea pig	*Gomori*, 1941
	Bourne, 1943
	Bern, 1949
	Göldi, 1952
	Mende and *Chambers*, 1957
	Martin, 1958
	Amon and *Petry*, 1962
	Martin, 1962
	Kagawa, 1965
Rabbit	*Gomori*, 1941
	Bern, 1949
	Mende and *Chambers*, 1957
	Martin, 1958
Cat	*Gomori*, 1941
	Martin, 1958
Dog	*Gomori*, 1941
	Mende and *Chambers*, 1957
Monkey	*Gomori*, 1941
	Amon and *Petry*, 1962
Pig	*Gomori*, 1941

tion, the weak reaction precipitate being limited to the superficial cells and in part to the intermediate cells. Observations regarding the activity of nonspecific esterases differ among various investigators: *Leeson* (1962) reports no enzyme activity and *Vacek* and *Schück* (1960) only a weak enzyme activity; *Amon* and *Petry* (1962) observed high activity with the nonspecific esterase in the intermediate cells. Acid phosphatase

Table 2. Occurrence of various enzymes in the normal bladder urothelium of laboratory animals

Enzymes	Authors
Hydrolases	
Alkaline phosphatase	cf. Table 1
Acid phosphatase	*Göldi*, 1952 *Amon* and *Petry*, 2962 *Kagawa*, 1965
Nonspecific esterase	*Nachlas* and *Seligman*, 1949 *Vacek* and *Schück*, 1960 *Amon* and *Petry*, 1962 *Kagawa*, 1965
Phosphoamidase	*Meyer* and *Weinmann*, 1957
Aminopeptidase	*Kagawa*, 1965
β-Glucuronidase	*Kagawa*, 1965
Oxidoreductases	
NADH-diaphorase	*Kunze* and *Schauer*, 1971
Succinate dehydrogenase	*Amon* and *Petry*, *Kagawa*, 1965 *Kunze* et al., 1971
Lactate dehydrogenase	*Kagawa*, 1965 *Kunze* and *Schauer*, 1971
Glucose-6-phosphatedehydrogenase	*Kunze* and *Schauer*, 1971
Malate-dehydrogenase	*Kagawa*, 1965
Glutamate-dehydrogenase	*Kagawa*, 1965
1-Glycerophosphatedehydrogenase	*Kagawa*, 1965
Cytochrome-oxidase	*Kunze* et al., 1971
Transferases	
Amylophosphorylase	*Takeuchi* and *Kuriaki*, 1955 *Amon* and *Petry*, 1962
Amylo-1,2–1,6-transglucosidase	*Takeuchi*, 1958

showed a uniformly weak reaction in all the cell layers in the various animal species. *Kagawa* (1965) reported the activity of β-glucuronidase in guinea-pigs as weak only in the intermediate cells; the activity of aminopeptidase showed a slight positive reaction in the basal and intermediate cells.

Among the oxidoreductases, NADH-diaphorase and also succinate and lactate dehydrogenase demonstrated high activity in the urothelium. The precipitates of cytochrome oxidase and glucose-6-phosphatedehydrogenase were moderately strong. The other dehydrogenases were only weakly demonstrable. The precipitates, in the form of blue-black formazan granules, occurred in the cells of the various layers, including the superficial cells, with approximately the same degree of intensity.

As a rule the reaction products were distributed evenly within the cytoplasm, but quite frequently the granules were concentrated in the perinuclear area.

The transferases tested in the urothelium showed moderate activity. However, the authors (*Takeuchi,* 1958; *Takeuchi* and *Kuriaki,* 1955; *Amon* and *Petry,* 1962) made no mention to their occurrence in the various cell layers or their intracellular distribution.

The intracellular distribution of hydrolases, particularly of alkaline phosphatase in the bladder mucosa is largely unknown. Only *Martin* (1958) has pursued this problem. He was of the opinion that alkaline phosphatase was predominantly located in the area of the Golgi apparatus. There have been no conclusive electron-microscopic investigations delineating the intracellular localization of alkaline phosphatase in the urothelial cells. By analogy with findings of alkaline phosphtase in the kidney and intestine, where alkaline phosphatase occurred not only in the brush border but also in the microsomes, it may be assumed that alkaline phosphatase is bound to the microsomes in the urothelial cells.

No details are known regarding the biological significance or function of alkaline phosphatase in the urothelium It may be supposed that its biochemical role consists in dephosphorylation and possibly phosphorylation reactions (*Hoffmann-Ostendorf,* 1954) in the metabolism of carbohydrates, nucleic acids, and proteins. It has been demonstrated biochemically that alkaline phsophtase not only functions as a phosphomono-esterase, but also is capable of breaking pyrophosphate bonds (*Eaton* and *Moss,* 1967; *Cox* et al., 1967).

The intracellular location and the function of oxidoreductases in intermediary metabolism have been known for some time. They are bound predominantly in the mitochondria because of their importance for the respiratory chain and citric acid cycle. Statements about the biochemical importance of NADH diaphorase have limited meaning, because the histochemical demonstrable "diaphorase activity" probably comprises several hydrogen transfer enzymes, whose biochemical identity is largely unknown (*Pearse,* 1972).

One of these enzymes was identified by *Straub* (1939), and later by *Massey* (1958, 1960), as a lipoamide dehydrogenase. Recently *Seidler* (1973) succeeded in identifying the lipoamide dehydrogenase as a NADH diaphorase with enzyme histochemical methods. During the histochemical reaction the NADH diaphorase transfers the hydrogen to an artificial electron acceptor, the tetrazolium salt. The reduction of the tetrazolium salt visualizes the enzyme activity by forming blue black formazan granula. For this reason several authors designated NADH diaphorase a NADH tetrazolium reductase.

In summary, the normal urothelium of small laboratory animals can be said to exhibit a number of enzymes, which are histochemically demonstrable. Because of their high activity, alkaline phosphatase and NADH diaphorase appeared to be particularly suitable as indicator enzymes for the projected investigations concerning the early phases of carcinogenesis in the urinary bladder.

3. Regeneration

Under normal conditions the bladder mucosa of man and of small laboratory animals such as mouse, rat, hamster, and guinea-pig demonstrates a very low cell turnover. With the introduction of autoradiographic techniques it was possible to gain new information regarding the physiological regeneration of the urothelium. The statements in the literature dealing with this problem are quite limited. The ^{3}H-thymidine labeling index (^{3}H-TdR index) of the urothelium of rat was determined at between 0.06% and 0.5%, and the average labeling index determined for the bladder mucosa of mouse is 0.2% to 1.0% (Table 3). The values for the individual animals vary widely, as *Levi* et al. (1969) have shown, with extreme values of 0.1% to 2.1%. The only testing to date in the human urothelium showed an average ^{3}H-TdR index of 0.3% (*Battifora* et al., 1965). Correspondingly low values have been obtained for the mitosis index, which in the case of the mouse is 0.01% (*Levi* et al., 1969b, 1971) or 0.05% (*Campobasso* and *Berrino,* 1972).

Table 3. ^{3}H-thymidine labeling index (^{3}H-TdR index as %) of the normal bladder urothelium of rat, mouse and man

Species	^{3}H-TdR index (%)	Authors
Rat	0.06	*Miyakawa* and *Yoshida,* 1973
	0.12	*Schreiber* et al., 1969
	0.20	*Locher* and *Cooper,* 1970
	0.50	*Messier* and *Leblond,* 1960
	0.26	*Kunze* et al., 1975
Mouse	0.20	*Nettesheim* and *Oehlert,* 1962
	0.80	*Campobasso* and *Berrino,* 1972
	1.00	*Levi* et al., 1969a
Man	0.30	*Battifora* et al., 1965

The author's own investigations on a total of 10 untreated Sprague-Dawley rats (inbred strain of the Institute of Pathology of the University of Munich, Munich, West Germany) yielded a mean ^{3}H-TdR index of 0.26% over the entire urothelium (Table 4) after injection of 6-^{3}H-thymidine (Radiochemical Centre, Amersham, England; specific activity 5 Ci/m mol) and a radioactive exposure time of one hour (details are presented in Section III.2).

The basal cell layer exhibited an index of 0.49% and the suprabasal cells one of 0.09%. Of the DNA-synthesizing cells, 80.9% were located basally. The largest number of labeled cells was found in the lower third of the organ, particularly in the trigone area. After 54 h of intermittent labeling with 6-^{3}H-thymidine, a mean ^{3}H-TdR index of 1.22% (individual values: 0.26%; 0.27%; 0.39%; 2.09%; 3.1%) was determined, which is about twice as high as that obtained by *Levi* et al. (1969) after 36 h of continuous labeling in the bladder mucosa of the mouse.

Tabelle 4. ^{3}H-TdR index (%) of the entire urothelium of control animals and the basal and suprabasal cells, respectively (mean values ± S.E.)

Rat no.	Total urothelium	Basal layer	Suprabasal layers
1	0.44 ± 0.22	0.97 ± 0.40	0.12 ± 0.22
2	0.25 ± 0.34	0.51 ± 0.69	0.00
3	0.21 ± 0.22	0.47 ± 0.67	0.05 ± 0.17
4	0.17 ± 0.28	0.30 ± 0.57	0.06 ± 0.14
5	0.13 ± 0.15	0.23 ± 0.23	0.05 ± 0.06
6	0.15 ± 0.17	0.37 ± 0.34	0.03 ± 0.06
7	0.38 ± 0.48	0.79 ± 1.09	0.12 ± 0.21
8	0.15 ± 0.18	0.32 ± 0.31	0.00
9	0.54 ± 0.30	0.71 ± 0.43	0.39 ± 0.23
10	0.13 ± 0.08	0.18 ± 0.15	0.08 ± 0.16
Average	0.26	0.49	0.09

The high percentage of DNA-synthesizing cells in the basal cell layer demonstrates that the physiological cell regeneration takes place essentially from this layer. *Lezava* (1934) came to this conclusion as early as 1934, when he found mitoses almost exclusively in the basal cell layer, and described it as a "cambium." A similar situation was found in the human bladder mucosa following in vitro labeling of DNA-synthesizing cells (*Lunglmayr* et al., 1972). Mitotic activity limited exclusively to a basal indifferent zone, i.e. as known in the skin and intestine, however, does not occur in the urothelium; the suprabasal cells, although to a limited extent, are still capable of mitosis. However, the regeneration of desquamated superficial cells takes place essentially via advancing of basal cells towards the lumen, undergoing differentiation at the same time. *Schreiber* et al. (1969) followed the process of urothelial regeneration after radiation; they were able to demonstrate a general luminal advancement of the more basally situated cells after 36 and 46 h with a 55- to 45-fold increase of labeled superficial cells. They could not substantiate the findings of *Leblond* et al. (1955) and *Walker* (1956), who claimed that the sloughed-off superficial cells were primarily replaced by the mitotic activity in the superficial cell layer itself.

Although the bladder mucosa is considered to be a tissue with a normally low cell renewal rate, its proliferative capacity and regenerative potential can be markedly increased by suitable stimuli. For example, excision or removal of a strip of mucosa initiates prompt regeneration, which leads to repair of the defect within short time (*McMinn* and *Johnson,* 1955; *Walker,* 1969; *McMinn,* 1967; *Conally* et al., 1971). After total bladder resection in dog a completely new and adequately functioning bladder, including the musculature, can develop within 14–16 weeks (*Tizzoni* and *Poggi,* 1888; *Bohne* et al., 1955). Similar findings have been recorded with other animal species and with the human bladder (for reviews of the literature see *Tucci* and *Haralambidis,* 1963; *Vahlensiek,* 1971). A marked increase in the labeling index in the urothelium of rats and mice was demonstrable also after exposure to X-ray irradiation (*Schreiber* et al., 1969) or chemical agents such as high doses of 4-ethylsulphonylaphthalene-1-sulphonamide (*Levi* et al., 1969) or cyclophosphamide (*Koss,* 1967; *Campobasso* and *Berrini,*

1972; *Locher* and *Cooper*, 1970). In these cases increased numbers of DNA-synthesizing cells were found not only in the basal layer, but also in the suprabasal cell layers.

It may be concluded from the foregoing that the normal bladder urothelium of small laboratory animals can be classified among the tissues with a low cell turnover. The physiological regeneration proceeds primarily from the basal cells. After various adequate stimuli the urothelium is capable of displaying a high proliferative capacity and regenerative potential.

III. Carcinogenesis in the Bladder Mucosa

1. Enzyme-Histochemical Investigations

a) Introduction

Hyperplasia of the urotehlium has been considered the earliest microscopically detectable stage of tumor development reproducible experimentally in the bladder of rats, mice, hamsters, rabbits and dogs after the application of various carcinogens (Table 7). The aim of the present enzyme-histochemical investigations was to determine whether a change in enzyme pattern emerged prior to tumor development. This was prompted by enzyme-histochemical studies in the rat liver treated with diethylnitrosamine. In this study we had found precancerous areas which exhibited a focal loss of nucleoside-5'-triphosphatases (*Schauer* and *Kunze,* 1968) and glucose-6-phosphatase activity (*Gössner* and *Friedrich-Freksa,* 1964; *Schauer* and *Kunze,* 1968) and occurred long before the appearance of tumor development.

b) Material and Methdos

α) Animals

Series I: 25 female and 13 male Sprague-Dawley rats, weighing between 180 and 200 g received 20 mg/kg of N-butyl-N-(4-hydroxybutyl)-nitrosamine (BBN: Chemische Fabrik Dr. Theodor Schuchardt, Munich, West Germany) in their drinking water daily for a period of 50 to 180 days. The object of the study was to detect as many sequential stages of carcinogenesis as possible, rather than to establish any correlation between exposure or induction time and tumor development. The animals were therefore killed at intervals between days 150 and 350. In order to test the irreversibility of the changes observed, administration of the carcinogen was stopped 100–240 days before sacrifice.

Series II: 30 female Wistar rats, initially weighing between 200 and 250 g, received 20 mg/kg of di-N-butylnitrosamine (DBN; Chemische Fabrik Dr. Theodor Schuchardt, Munich, West Germany) daily in their drinking water. All 30 animals were sacrificed, after continuous application of the carcinogen, between days 120 and 300 of the experiment.

Series III: 70 female Wistar rats, with an initial weight of 200 to 250 g, were given 2o mg/kg of di-N-butylnitrosaime daily in their drinking water. These animals were divided into seven groups; each group received the carcinogen for from 50 to 270 days (Table. 5).

Table 5. Groups of the series III, with various duration of exposure and discontinuation

Group	Number of animals	Duration of exposure (days)	Duration of discontinuation (days)	Total dose/animal (mg)
1	10	50	300–350	200
2	14	80	220–320	320
3	9	100	200–270	400
4	9	150	100–120	600
5	8	190	50–120	760
6	8	240	30– 80	960
7	12	200–270	0	800–1080

The time of discontinuation varied between 30 to 350 days. The rats in group 7 received the carcinogen continuously up to the time of sacrifice. The total dose of carcinogen applied amounted to approximately 200–1080 mg/animal.

Series IV: 21 female Wistar rats with an initial weight of between 180 and 200 g received 0.2% N-[4-(5-Nitro-2-furyl)-2-thiazolyl]- formamide (FANFT; Saber Laboratories, Morton Grove, USA) in a powdered standardized feed (Altromin) for 75 to 140 days. The carcinogen was than discontinued for 10 to 135 days. Four animals were sacrified before day 130, the remaining 17 animals at intervals between days 150 and 175.

A group of 30 female and male Wistar and Sprague Dawley rats served as untreated controls. All the animals used were inbred animals (Institute of Pathology of the University of Munich, Munich, West Germany). The rats were kept in macrolon cages in groups of five to each cage, with free access to their drinking water, and fed with a standardized compressed feed (Altromin).

β) Enzyme-Histochemical Methods

Serial sections 5 μm thick and cut with a cryostat were used for the enzyme-histochemical tests; 80 sections were cut from each bladder. All animals used were tested routinely for alkaline phosphatase and NADH diaphorase activity. The animals in series II and III were tested additionally for succinate dehydrogenase and lactate dehydrogenase activity. Only the animals in series II were tested for glucose-6-phosphate dehydrogenase activity.

A. Alkaline phosphatase (method according to *Stutte*, 1967).

Reagents: Solution a: 20 ml 0.2 M tris HCl buffer solution, pH of 8.8
5 mg naphthol AS biphosphate
0.2 ml dimethylformamide

Solution b: 0.2 ml 4% sodium nitrite
0.2 ml 4% basic fuchsin

Procedure: Mix solutions a and b. Incubate sections for 15 min at 37°C.

B. NADH diaphorase (method according to *Scarpelli* et al., 1958).

Reagents: Solution a: 2 mg NADH in 0.5 ml aqua bidestillata.

Solution b: 1.25 ml 0.2% NBT.
0.5 ml 0.2 M phosphate buffer, pH 7.3
0.4 ml Ringer solution

Procedure: Mix solutions a and b. Incubate sections for 30 min at room temperature.

C. Succinate dehydrogenase (method according to *Rosa* and *Tsou*, 1961).

Reagents: Solution a: 15 mg TNBT dissolved in 2 ml dimethylformamide.

Solution b: 10 ml 0.2 M phosphate buffer, pH 7.6
10 ml 0.2 M sodium succinate

Procedure: Mix solutions a and b. Incubate sections for 30 min at 37°C.

D. Lactate dehydrogenase (method according to *Hess* et al., 1958).

Reagents: Solution a: 24 mg NAD dissovled in 2.4 ml 0.1 M phosphate buffer

Solution b: 0.8 ml 1.0 M sodium lactate
0.2 ml NBT
0.8 ml 0.1 M sodiumacid
8.0 ml aqua bidestillata

Procedure: Mix solutions a and b. Incubate sections for 30 min at 37°C.

E. Glucose-6-phosphate dehydrogenase (method according to *Hess* et al., 1958; modified by *Rudolph* and *Klein*, 1964).

Reagenst: Solution a: 10 mg glucose-6-phosphate dissolved in 10 ml aqua bidestillata
10 mg NBT dissolved in 10 ml aqua bidestillata

Solution b: 0.6 ml 0.2 M Tris HCL buffer, pH 7.2
7.5 mg TPN

Procedure: Mix solutions a and b. Incubate sections for 30 min at 37°C.

c) Results

α) Activity of Alkaline Phosphatase and NADH-diaphorase in the Urothelium During Early Stages of Carcinogenesis

Alkaline phosphatase: After application of BBN, DBN, and FANFT a focal, well-defined total loss of alkaline phosphatase activity was consistently observed in an otherwise histologically and cytologicall normal-seeming, nonhyperplastic urothelium. This change developed long before the appearance of tumors and is the earliest lesion in the urothelium due to carcinogens that is detectable by light microscopy (Fig. 1). Single cells with a positive reaction were observed only rarely within these regions. Areas with a gradual attenuation of alkaline phosphatase activity were not demonstrable. The earliest enzyme-deficient area that occurred was observed on day 75 of the experiment after application of FANFT. Multiple enzyme-deficient areas were often found in animals that had received the carcinogen over a relatively long experimental period. Such foci devoid of alkaline phosphatase activity were demonstrable even 11 months after discontinuation of DBN, 8 months after withdrawal of BBN, and 4 1/2 months after withdrawal of FANFT. In H.E. sections the enzyme-deficient urothelial cells were inconspicuous and did not differ in any way from the cells in the adjacent enzyme-positive mucosa.

Simple and papillary hyperplasias of varying thickness developing from enzyme-deficient regions of the urothelium were, as a rule, also devoid of alkaline phosphatase activity (Figs. 2 and 3). Only rarely was alkaline phosphatase activity retained in hyperplastic regions.

NADH-diaphorase: Approximately two-thirds of the urothelial regions exhibiting a loss of alkaline phosphatase activity also showed a reduction in NADH diaphorase activity. The activity, however, was only rarely completely lost. More frequently the NADH-diaphorase showed a varying diminution of acitivty (Fig. 7). Both simple and papillary hyperplasias also demonstrated a varying attenuation of activity (Fig. 8). Hyperplasias with increased enzyme activity were rarely observed.

Fig. 1. Sharply circumscribed area of the urothelium demonstrating a loss of alkaline phosphatase activitiy and a large number of ^{3}H-thymidine labeled nuclei (black) after 54 h of continuous labeling. Positive enzyme reaction (black) in the opposite and surrounding mucosa. Time of exposure *(BBN):* 90 days. Total experimental period: 190 days. 220 X (Z. Krebsforsch. *84,* 143–160 (1975)

Fig. 2. Advanced simple hyperplasia of the urothelium devoid of alkaline phosphatase activity; retained enzyme activity (black) in neighboring mucosa. Time of exposure (*FANFT*): 140 days. Total experimental period: 165 days. 75 X. (Z. Krebsforsch. *84,* 143–160 (1975)

Fig. 3. Papillary hyperplasia of the urothelium exhibiting loss of alkaline phosphatase activity. Preserved enzyme activity (black) in opposite urothelium and at capillaries. Time of exposure (*FANFT*): 140 days. Total experimental period: 165 days. 190 X

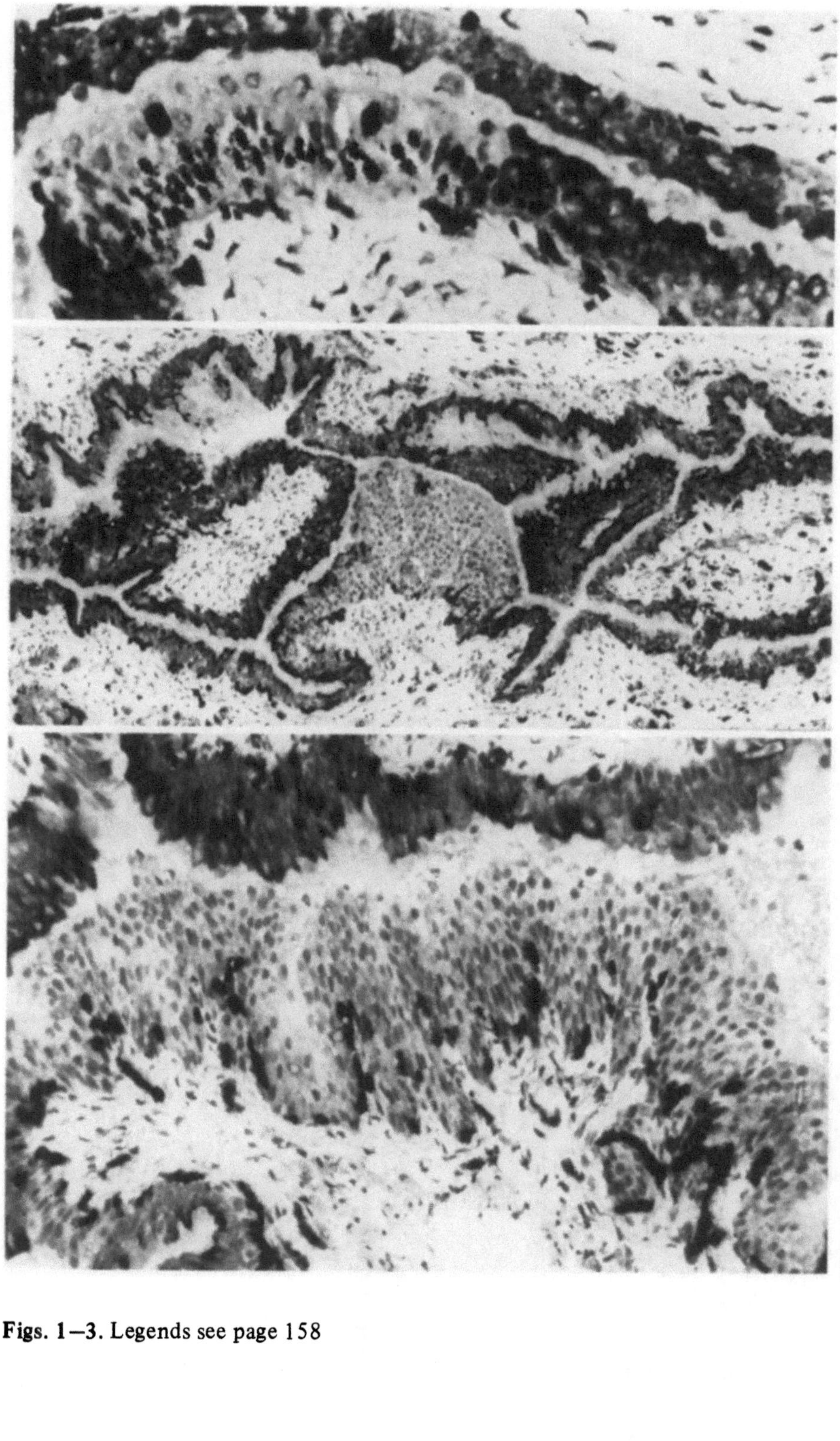

3

Figs. 1–3. Legends see page 158

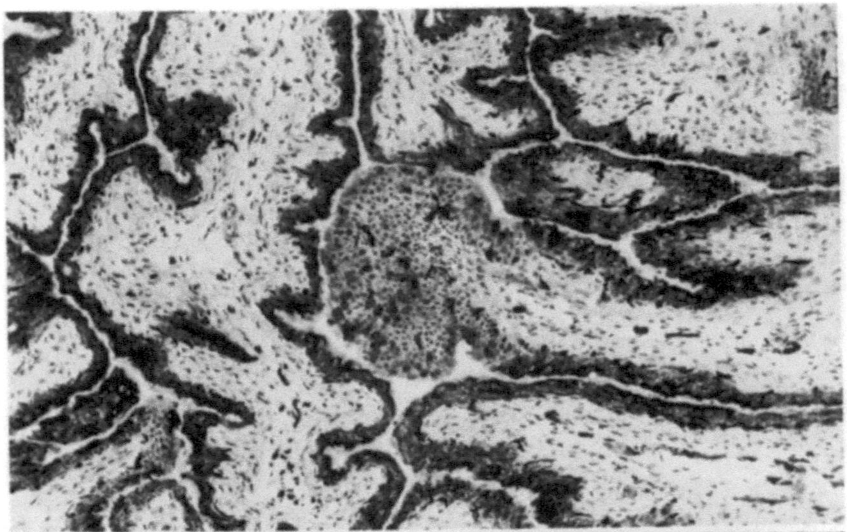

4

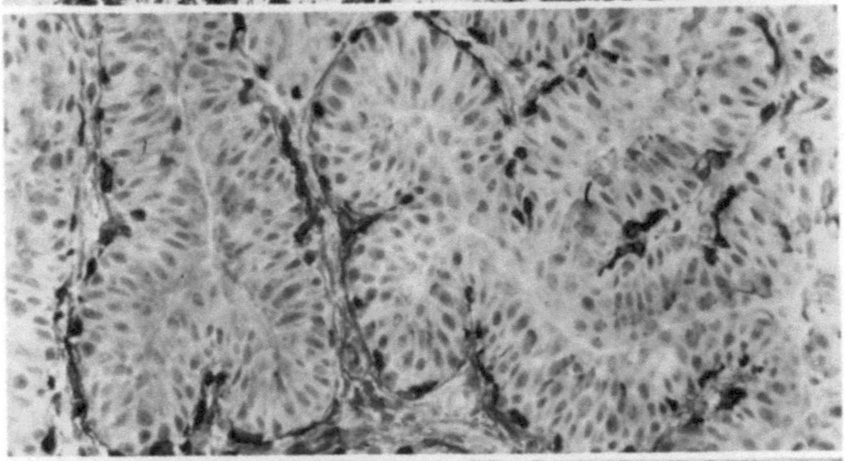

5

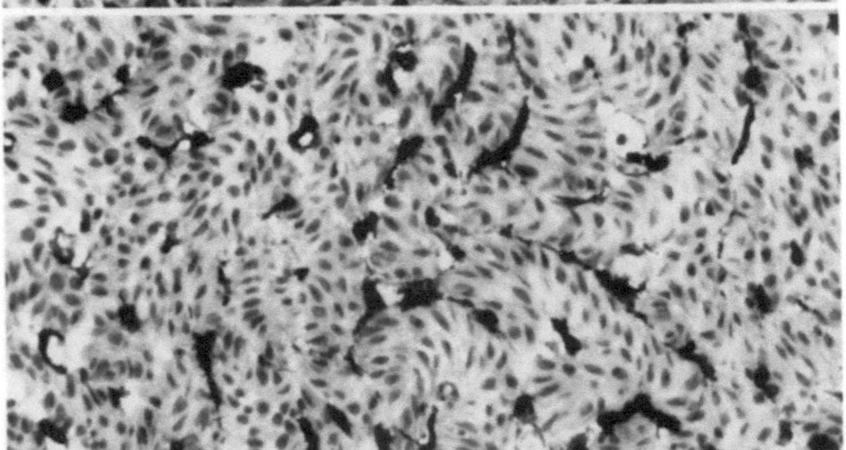

6

Figs. 4–6. Legends see page 161

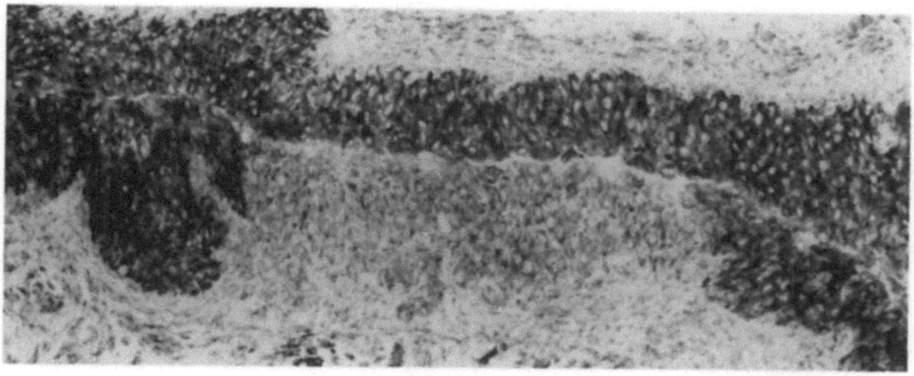

Fig. 7. Markedly diminished activity of NADH-diaphorase within slightly hyperplastic area of urothelium; preserved enzyme activity of adjacent and opposite bladder mucosa. Time of exposure (*FANFT*): 75 days. Total experimental period: 75 days. 190 X (Z. Krebsforsch. *84* , 143–160, 1975)

β) Activity of Alkaline Phosphatase and NADH-Diaphorase in Fully Developed Tumors

Alkaline phosphatase: The great majority of the papillomas induced by BBN, DBN and FANFT also showed an ubiquitous loss of alkaline phosphatase activity (Table 6, Figs. 4 and 5). However, a number of transitional cell papillomas exhibited small areas of partly retained enzyme activtiy (Fig. 9). It was very rare for alkaline phos-

---

Fig. 4. Small papilloma devoid of alkaline phosphatase activity; positive enzyme reaction (black) in surrounding mucosa and at capillaries. Time of exposure *(DBN):* 205 days. Total experimental period: 205 days. 100 X (Naturwissenschaften *56*, 639, 1969)

Fig. 5. Part of larger papilloma with loss of alkaline phosphatase activity; positive enzyme reaction (black) at blood vessels. Time of exposure *(DBN):* 260 days. Total experimental period: 260 days. 220 X (Z. Krebsforsch. *175,* 146–160, 1971)

Fig. 6. Well differentiated nonpapillary transitional cell carcinoma (grade II) showing complete loss of alkaline phosphatase activity; positive enzyme reaction (black) at small blood vessels within stroma. Time of exposure *(BBN):* 150 days. Total experimental period: 350 days. 190 X (Z. Krebsforsch. *84,* 143–160, 1975)

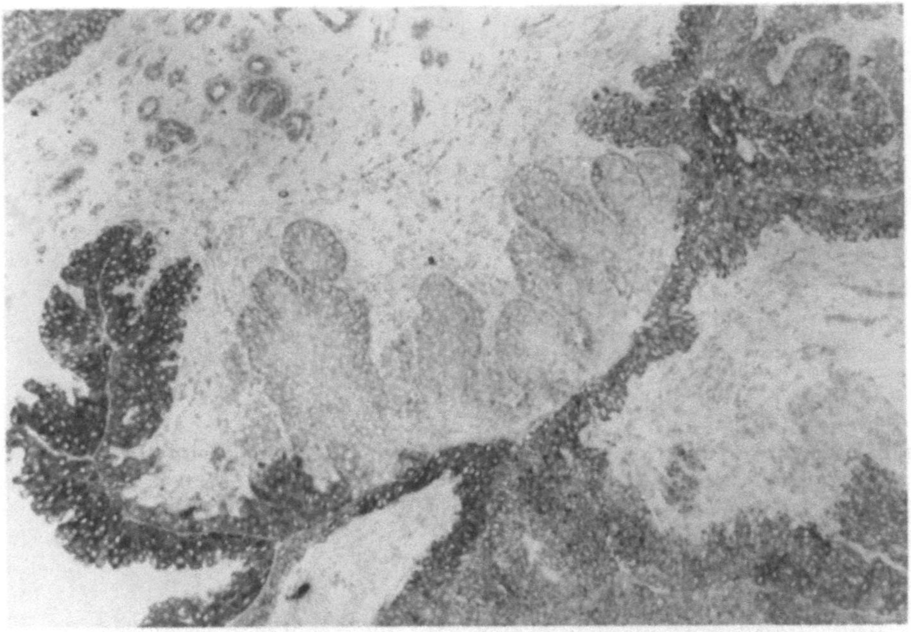

Fig. 8. Endophytic papillary hyperplasia exhibiting pronounced diminution of NADH-diaphorase activity. Time of exposure *(DBN)*: 290 days. Total experimental period: 290 days. 190 X (Z. Krebsforsch. *75*, 146–160, 1971)

phatase activity to be present with the same intensity in a papilloma as in the control urothelium. Papillomas with squamous cell metaplasia always showed a total loss of alkaline phosphatase activity in all parts. The capillaries and the smaller vessels of the stroma showed a very strong positive reaction.

Transitional cell carcinomas demonstrated basically the same enzyme-histochemical behavior as transitional cell papillomas (Table 6). Most were characterized by total loss of alkaline phosphatase activity in all parts (Fig. 6); in some cases enzyme activity was maintained in circumscribed areas. All squamous cell carcinomas revealed a total loss of enzyme activity throughout. There were no demonstrable differences in enzyme-histochemical behavior between well and poorly differentiated transitional cell carcinomas.

NADH-diaphorase: In papillomas the activity of NADH-diaphorase varied (Table 6). In some cases the activity was markedly decreased in all regions of the tumor, while in the adjacent parts it was comparable to that in the surrounding, apparently normal, urothelium (Fig. 10). Papillomas with squamous cell metaplasia showed an almost total loss of enzyme activity. Some papillomas, however, showed intact enzyme activity in all parts. Furthermore, certain areas of the tumor, or single cells, with increased activity were observed (Fig. 11).

Table 6. Enzyme-histochemical behavior of 53 BBN- and FANFT-induced papillomas and 31 carcinomas. Abbreviations: – = complete loss of enzyme activity in all regions of a tumor; focally + = positive enzyme reaction in small areas. + = positive enzyme reaction in all parts of a tumor; weak = diminished activity of NADH-diaphorase in all regions; focally weak = reduced activity in circumscribed areas (Z. Krebsforsch. *83*, 143–160, 1975)

Carcinogen	Papilloma						Carcinoma					
	Alkaline phosphatase			NADH-diaphorase			Alkaline phosphatase			NADH-diaphorase		
	–	Focally +	+	Weak	Focally weak	+	–	Focally +	+	Weak	Focally weak	+
BBN	26	6	1	15	16	2	14	8	1	8	13	2
FANFT	15	3	2	7	4	9	7	1	–	2	4	2
Total	41	9	3	22	20	11	21	9	1	10	17	4

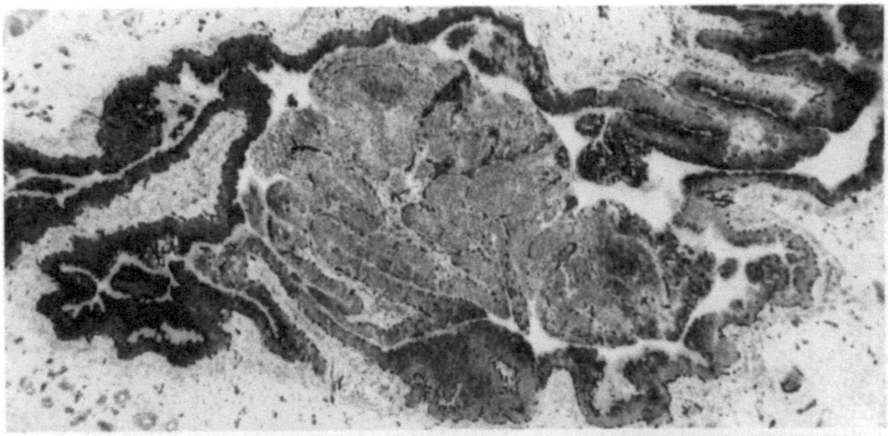

9

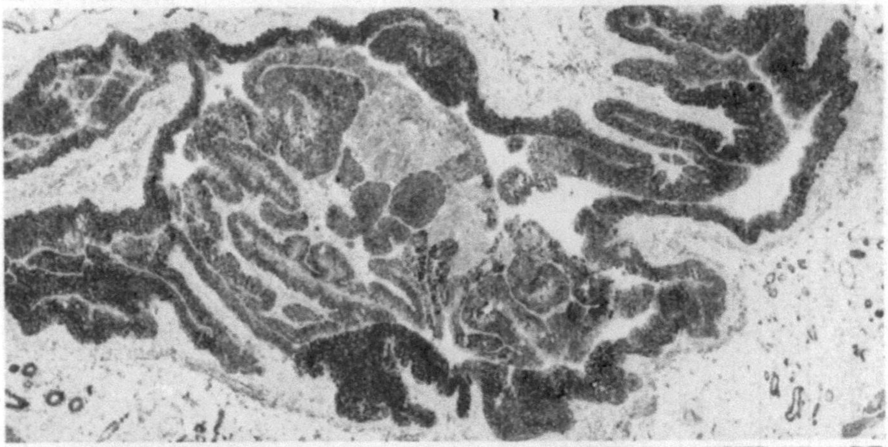

10

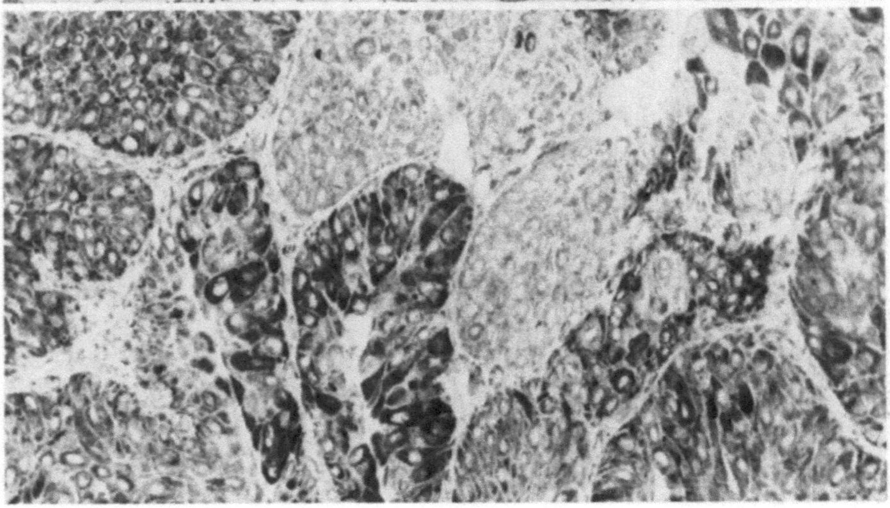

11

Figs. 9–11. Legends see page 165

In the majority of the transitional cell carcinomas the NADH-diaphorase activity was reduced – as in the papillomas – either in the whole tumor or in parts (Table 6; Fig. 12). Squamous cell carcinomas were always characterized by a complete loss of NADH-diaphorase activity throughout (Fig. 13).

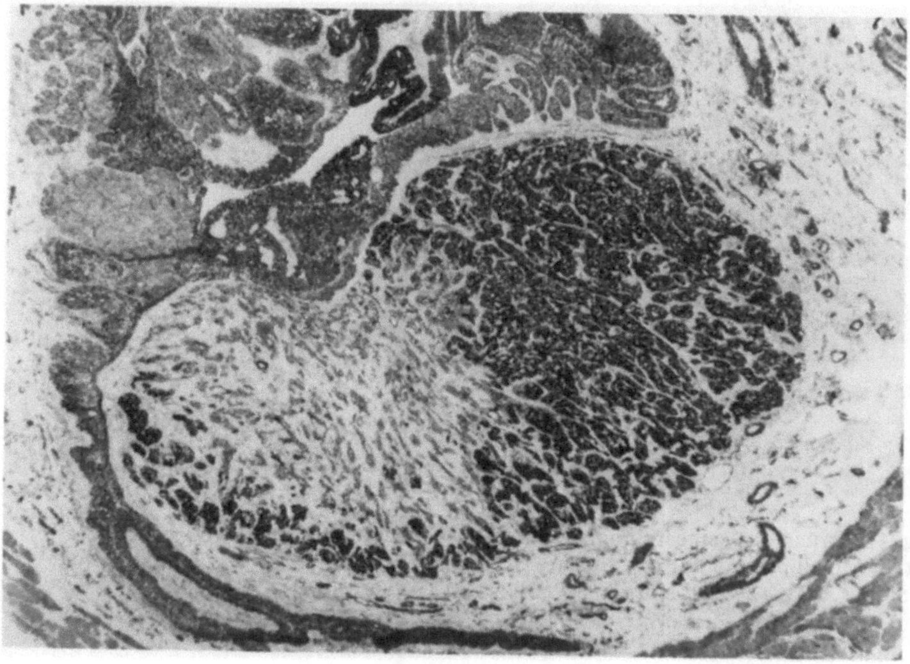

Fig. 12. Transitional cell carcinoma demonstrating reduced NADH-diaphorase activity in a large area. Time of exposure *(BBN):* 90 days; total experimental period: 270 days. 30 X (Z. Krebsforsch. *84,* 143–160, 1975)

Fig. 9. Papilloma characterized by almost complete loss of alkaline phosphatase activity; positive enzyme reaction (black) in most parts of surrounding urothelium. Time of exposure *(BBN):* 55 days. Total experimental period: 290 days. 30 X (Z. Krebsforsch. *84,* 143–160, 1975)

Fig. 10. Same papilloma as in Figure 9; NADH-diaphorase present in most parts, activity comparable to that in surrounding mucosa; decreased activity only in small limited areas (Z. Krebsforsch. *84,* 143–160, 1975)

Fig. 11. Part of papilloma in Figure 10. Besides areas with markedly decreased, some with markedly increased activity of NADH-diaphorase. 190 X (Z. Krebsforsch. *84,* 143–16o, 1975)

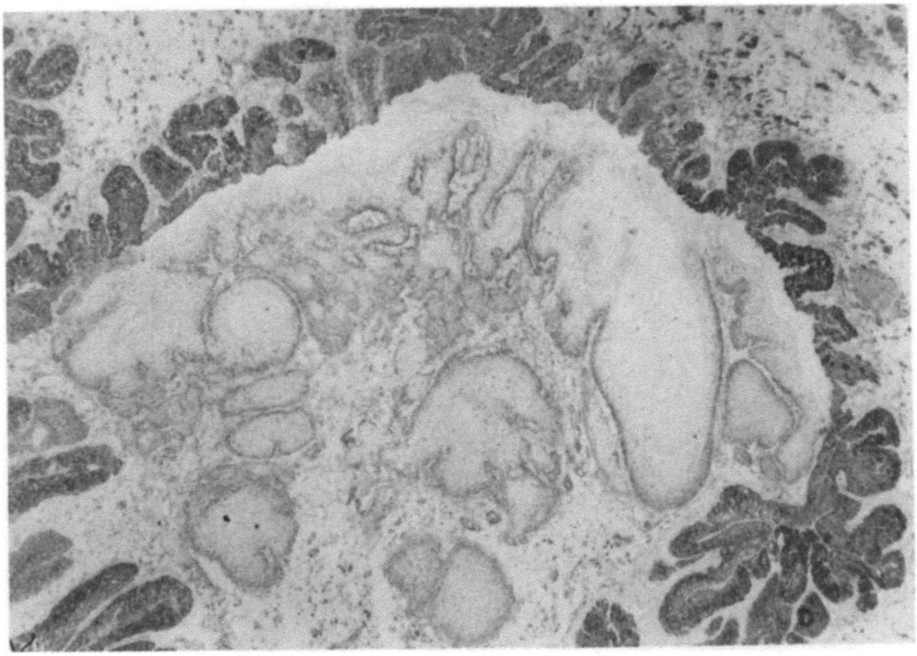

Fig. 13. Squamous cell carcinoma exhibiting strongly diminished NADH diaphorase activity in all parts. Time of exposure *(BBN):* 115 days. Total experimental period: 135 days. 30 X (Z. Krebsforsch. *84,* 143–160,1975)

γ) Activity of Lactate, Succinate and Glucose-6-Phosphatase Dehydrogenase in the Urothelium During Early Stages of Carcinogenesis and in Fully Developed Tumors

A reduction of lactate and glucose-6-phosphatase dehydrogenase activity occurred during the early phases of carcinogenesis in two-thirds of the urothelial regions that showed loss of alkaline phosphatase activity. This finding was demonstrable in all cases where the NADH-diaphorase activity was reduced. The lactate and glucose-6-phosphatase dehydrogenase activity was diminished in the papillomas and carcinomas at times in all parts and at times only focally, paralleling the behavior of NADH-diaphorase.

The activity of the succinate dehydrogenase was significantly increased in the foci deficient in alkaline phosphatase, where the activity of NADH-diaphorase was also reduced. Both enzymes also presented differing behavior in papillomas and carcinomas. The activity of succinate dehydrogenase was increased in foci exhibiting a decrease of NADH-diaphorase activity. The reaction precipitate of succinate dehydrogenase was particularly strong in papillomas with squamous cell metaplasia and in squamous cell carcinomas.

d) Discussion

Previous experimental studies of tumor development in the urinary bladder of different animal species have shown circumscribed hyperplasia of the urothelium to be the earliest carcinogenically induced lesion after application of several carcinogens (for reviews

Table 7. Occurrence of urothelial hyperplasias in the urinary bladder of various laboratory animals and in man

Species	Authors
Mouse	*Armstrong* and *Bonser,* 1944
	Sen Gupta, 1962
	Roe, 1964
	Bonser and *Clayson,* 1964
	Clayson et al., 1967a
	Clayson et al., 1967b
	Wood, 1969
	Betram and *Craig*, 1970
	Cooper et al., 1972
	Bertram and *Craig,* 1972
	Wood, 1970
	Akagi et al., 1973
Rat	*Sen Gupta*, 1962
	Santana , 1963
	Radomski et al., 1967
	Ito et al., 1969
	Ertürk et al., 1969
	Koss and *Lavin,* 1971
	Okajima et al., 1971
	Kunze et al., 1971
	Hashimoto et al., 1974
	Kunze et al., 1976
Hamster	*Mohr* et al., 1970
	Althoff et al., 1971
	So and *Wynder*, 1972
	Croft and *Bryan,* 1973
Dog	*Hueper* et al., 1938
	Bonser, 1958
	Jabara, 1963
Rabbit	*Wood,* 1968
Man	*Eisenberg* et al., 1960
	Temkin, 1963
	Austen and *Friedell,* 1965
	Allegra et al., 1972
	Koss et al., 1974

of the literature see *Clayson* et al., 1965; Table 7). A similar situation applies to the human bladder (Table 7). It would therefore seem consistent to consider hyperplasia an obligatory stage in the development of papillary tumors.

By means of enzyme histochemical methods we have been able to demonstrate circumscribed foci with loss of alkaline phosphatase activity, in an otherwise histologically and cytologically normal urothelium, as the earliest microscopically detectable change during carcinogenesis, i.e. prior to the appearance of hyperplasia. This finding was consistently obtainable with the application of BBN, DBN and FANFT (*Kunze* et al., 1969, 1971, 1975; *Kunze* and *Schauer,* 1971). *Stiller* and *Rauscher* (1971) reported identical results when they used the azo-dye method for histochemical assessment of alkaline phosphatase activity after subcutaneous administration of di-n-butylnitrosamine.

Recently *Highman* et al. (1975) described a reduced activity of alkaline phosphatase in hyperplastic epithelium and loss of activity in transitional cell carcinomas after administration of 2-acetylaminofluorene to mice. Loss of enzyme activity in fully developed tumors induced by BBN and DBN has been also confirmed by *Ito* et al. (1973). A lack of alkaline phosphatase activity in human bladder tumors has been described by *Mannheimer* and *Seligman* (1948), *Burghele* et al. (1965), and *Murata* et al. (1966).

Focal diminution of alkaline phosphatase activity in the bladder mucosa is not due to cytotoxic action of the carcinogen, nor is it a reversible effect; both conclusions are drawn from the absence of cell necrosis and from the irreversibility of the enzyme defect long after discontinuation of carcinogen. The reversible deficiency of alkaline phosphatase in hyperplasias induced by 4-ethylsulphonyl-naphthalene-1-sulfonamide in the mouse (*Levi* et al., 1971) can certainly be considered a toxic effect of the high dose of the carcinogen. The enzyme is thought to occur a long time after discontinuation of the carcinogen, i.e., a short time before the animals are sacrificed, as otherwise hyperplasias or tumors would have developed during the long period between withdrawal of the carcinogen and sacrifice, due to the high proliferative acitivy which is initiated immediately after onset of the enzyme defect (cf. Section III.2).

Tumor development in the human urinary bladder also has a considerable latency period; the tumors appear longer after cessation of exposure to carcinogens in the case of industrial workers. This fact is analogous to the results of animal experiments. The period of latency varies widely. *Temkin* (1963) gives an average latency period of 12.7 years (extreme values 1.2 years and 30 years). Other authors mention a much longer period (cf. *Temkin,* 1963). One assumes that very wide individual differences depend upon the length of exposure and the concentration of the carcinogen. The reason for the long latency period between transformation and manifestation, however, is still obscure.

Areas of urothelium showing a loss of alkaline phosphatase activity must be considered to be an initial stage of tumor development. Evidence of their preneoplastic state is based upon the following facts:

1. Morphological findings demonstrate a gradual transition of urothelial regions devoid of alkaline phosphatase activity into tumors passing through various stages of hyperplasia.
2. Enzyme-histochemically completely developed tumors (papillomas and carcinomas) exhibit extensive loss of alkaline phosphatase activity, as seen in hyperplasias and precursor areas.

3. Autoradiographic results (see Section III.2) show that there is always high proliferative activity in the enzyme-deficient foci, while the number of DNA-synthesizing cells is very low in the surrounding, apparently normal urothelium.

The occurrence of focal irreversible loss of alkaline phosphatase activity seems to characterize the initial stage of bladder tumor development in the rat. Loss of this enzyme can be observed after the action of carcinogens with different chemical structures, whose carcinogenicity may be based upon different modes of action.

The carcinogenic mechanisms of nitrosamines and FANFT are not known in detail. Both classes of compounds exert carcinogenicity only by gradual biotransformation. In the case of di-n-butyl-nitrosamine, a hydroxylation to n-butyl-(4-hydroxybutyl)-nitrosamine has been demonstrated. This intermediate, in turn, is oxidized to butyl-(3-carboxypropyl)-nitrosamine (*Okada* and *Suzuki,* 1972; *Hashimoto* et al., 1972, 1974; *Blattmann* and *Preussmann,* 1974). Further decomposition probably leads to the methylation of nucleic acids, proceeding via the formation of diazoalkanes and carbonium ions. It has also been suggested that decompositon comes about via mechanisms involving α-c- or ω-1-hydroxylation of di-n-butyl-nitrosamine and direct transfer to intact alkyl groups to nucleic acids (*Blattmann* and *Preussmann,* 1974). This is suggested by the presence of propylguanine and butylguanine in the urine of rats, in addition to methylguanine (*Krüger,* 1971).

The molecular basis of the carcinogenic action of FANFT is unknown. Available data suggest that the 5-nitro group of the furan ring plays a major role in the carcinogenic process, perhaps via formation of hydroxyl-amino furan as a reactive intermediate (*Ertürk* et al., 1971; *Cohen* et al., 1973).

The cause of the enzyme loss is not yet fully understood. One might conclude that loss of alkaline phosphatase activity results from an alteration in DNA and therefore gene expressivity; this is supported by the fact that the loss is irreversible and appears a long time after withdrawal of the carcinogen. A further point indicative of damage to genetic structure was the total loss of alkaline phosphatase activity; no gradual attenuation has been demonstrated. Nevertheless the relation between the alkylating action and the carcinogenicity of nitrosamines still remains a subject of controversy. The studies of *Ludlum* (1970) have shown that the base-pairing properties of 7-methylguanine do not differ from those of its parent compound. Further investigation will have to show whether the same is true for propyl- and butylguanine.

The histochemical behavior of NADH-diaphorase in the urothelium during carcinogenesis is even more difficult to interpret; its reaction pattern was very irregular. First, enzyme activity was attenuated in only about two-thirds of the preneoplastic foci of the urothelium showing a loss of alkaline phosphatase activity. Second, fully developed tumors frequently revealed decreased enzyme activity only in circumscribed areas. Third, NADH-diaphorase showed various grades of weakened activity and was only rarely completely absent. Furthermore, any statement regarding the significance of NADH-diaphorase activity is limited by the fact that it is not known – except in the case of lipoamiddehydrogenase (*Straub,* 1939; *Seidler,* 1973) – which enzymes are responsible for the histochemically demonstrable "diaphorase activity." For these reasons it could be assumed, for the time being, that NADH-diaphorase activity plays only a secondary role during carcinogenesis.

e) Summary

Focal loss of alkaline phosphatase activity was regularly demonstrable in histologically and cytologically apparently normal urothelium of the rat urinary bladder after oral application of BBN, DBN and FANFT. The enzyme loss occurred long before the appearance of tumors and must be considered the earliest microscopically detectable transformation stage in bladder carcinogenesis. Varying degrees of attenuation of NADH-diaphorase activity were observed in identical areas in two-thirds of the cases. The loss of alkaline phosphatase activity proved to be irreversible and was not of toxic origin, i.e., it developed long after discontinuation the carcinogen. The enzyme-negative areas of the urothelium are considered to be preneoplastic as papillomas and carcinomas develop from them via enzyme-deficient hyperplasias. In most cases papillomas and carcinomas also showed a loss of alkaline phosphatase activity as well as a variable reduction of NADH-diaphorase activity in circumscribed areas or, more rarely, in the entire tumor. The loss of alkaline phosphatase activity seems to be characteristic of the initial phase of tumor development in the urinary bladder in the rat, and is consistently reproducible after the application of chemically unrelated carcinogens. The cause for the enzyme defect is considered to be damage to DNA with a resultant change in gene expressivity.

2. Combined Enzyme-Histochemical and Autoradiographic Investigations

a) Introduction

We designed combined enzyme-histochemical and autoradiographic investigations with the aim of observing any changes in cellular proliferation in preneoplastic urothelium which showed in any way a loss of alkaline phosphatase activity. Of particular interest was the onset and the extent of proliferation in the enzyme-deficient areas compared with the surrounding mucosa, which exhibited preserved enzyme activity, and with the urothelium of control animals. We were also interested in clarifying the degree to which the cells in the various layers within the enzyme-deficient areas were involved in the proliferative process, and in determining any changes in the normal physiological regenerative process of the urothelium.

b) Material and Methods

The same animals were employed as in groups I–IV of the enzyme-histochemical investigations, with the exception of the controls (cf. Section III.1). The animals were given 6-^{3}H-thymidine (Radiochemical Centre, Amersham, England; specific activity 3 and 5 mCi/mmol) i.p. one hour before sacrifice, i.e. between 8.00 and 8.30 a.m. The rats in groups I and II received a dose of 0.3 mCi/100g, and the animals in group IV received 0.1 mCi/100 g. A group of 10 untreated female Sprague-Dawley rats served as controls (cf. Section II.3.). Each of these animals received a dose of 0.3 mCi 6-^{3}H-thymidine/100 g.

In order to determine the ^{3}H-thymidine labeling index over a fairly long radioactive exposure time, five female Wistar rats, who had been cancerized with BBN, received 0.1 mCi 6-^{3}H-thymidine/100 g i.p. every 6 h for a total of 54 h. Five female Wistar rats served as controls. They also received 0.1 mCi ^{3}H-thymidine/100 g every 6 h (cf. Section II.3.). The first injection was administered between 8.15 and 8.30 a.m.

Of the 70 rats in group III, 37 received ^{3}H-cytidine (Radiochemical Centre, Amersham, England; specific activity 27 Ci/mmol) i.p. for autoradiographic investigations of RNA-metabolism one hour before sacrifice, between 8.00 and 8.30 a.m. Each animal received a dose of 0.3 mCi/100 g. Four female Wistar rats served as controls.

The application of unlabeled precursors together with the tritiated thymidine or cytidine was not performed. We expected no essential effect upon the quantitative evaluation of the DNA synthesis. Comparison of the ^{3}H-cytidine incorporation was carried out only with the same animal, because of possible variations within the endogenic pool.

Cryostat serial and step sections were cut at 5 μm thickness; approximately half were subjected to the alkaline phosphatase reaction (cf. Section II.2.), while the rest were left untreated. All sections were covered with Kodak AR 10 stripping film.

After 14 days of exposure the autoradiograms were developed and fixed (time of developing: 12 min; the compositon of the developer solution: 7.2 g sodium sulfite, 3.2 ml 10% potassium bromide, 1.88 g amidol, 400 ml distilled water; length of fixation: 25–30 min; composition of fixation solution: 150 sodium thiosulfate, 15 g potassium metabisulfite, 500 ml distilled water). Then the sections were washed for 30 min with running water in the dark room and stained with Mayer's haemalaun. After 10 min of washing the sections were completely dried and embedded in Kaiser's glycerine gelatine.

The ^{3}H-thymidine labeling index (^{3}H-TdR index as %) was determined in nonhyperplastic sections of urothelium devoid of alkaline phosphatase activity, due to induction with BBN, DBN and FANFT. The index was calculated in all the cell layers taken as a whole, and compared with the surrounding apparently normal uorthelium. In addition, the ^{3}H-TdR index was determined separately in the basal cell layer and in the suprabasal cells of the defective areas and in the surrounding mucosa. The cell counts were carried out on two to five sections; 7000 to 8000 cells in the surrounding urothelium were counted in each animal. The ^{3}H-TdR index was determined in the same manner in nonhyperplastic and in slightly to moderately hyperplastic enzyme-defective areas after 54 h of continuous labeling.

In addition, the ^{3}H-TdR index was measured in areas of BBN- and FANFT-induced papillomas, which demonstrated a loss of alkaline phosphatase activity and simultaneously marked diminution of NADH-diaphorase activity. For comparison the index was calculated in the surrounding structures of the same papilloma, which showed normally high enzyme activity.

In order to determine the nuclear incorporation of ^{3}H-cytidine the number of silver granules overlying the nucleus was counted and the size of the nucleus measured with a planimeter (Leitz microscope Ortholux with drawing equipment). The density of silver grains was calculated from the quotient of the number of granules and the surface area of the nucleus. The counts were made in the enzyme-deficient areas and in the adjacent normal urothelium in 2–3 serial sections. The density of silver granules of the unaltered urothelium was equated with 100% and the enzyme-deficient areas compared with it. We have abstained from noting absolute numerical values, because the labeling differed in the individual sections and from one animal to the other. The density of silver granules in normal urothelium was calculated only in segments with three cell layers.

c) Results

α) ^{3}H-TdR Index of the Entire Urothelium in Enzyme-Deficient Areas after 1 Hour of Labeling

A marked increase of proliferative activity was determined consistently in the preneoplastic urothelial areas exhibiting a loss of alkaline phosphatase activity. The average ^{3}H-TdR index was 8.1% after application of BBN, 6.3% after DBN, and 6.1% after FANFT (Fig. 14; Tables 8 and 9). The value of the labeling index varied in the individual enzyme-deficient areas and was independent of the length of exposure and induction time. The ^{3}H-TdR index was sometimes higher after a shorter than after a longer

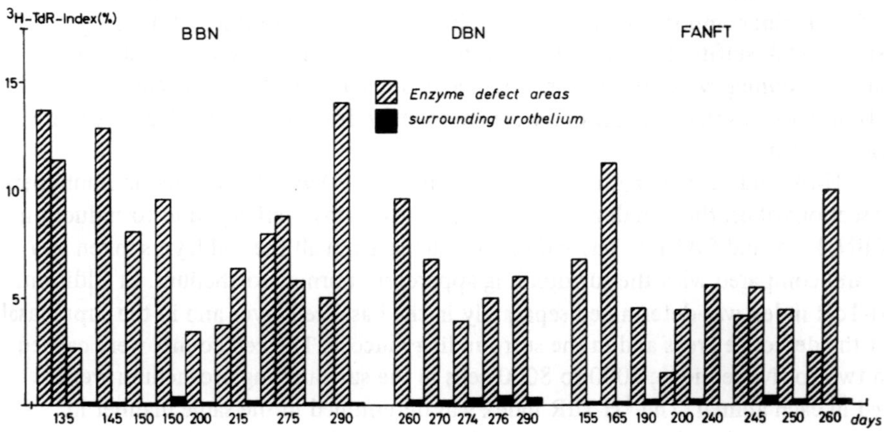

Fig. 14. ^{3}H-TdR index of non-hyperplastic urothelial areas devoid of alkaline phosphatase activity induced by *BBN, DBN* and *FANFT,* compared with surrounding urothelium showing positive enzyme reaction

total experimental time. Only rarely did we encounter enzyme-deficient areas without DNA-synthesizing cells. The comparative values for the surrounding enzyme-containing urothelium were: 0.188% for BBN, 0.36% for DBN, and 0.27% for FANFT. The ^{3}H-TdR index in the enzyme-active mucosa was only slightly changed compared with the urothelium of control animals, which had a labeling index of 0.26% (cf. Section II.3.). Compared with the surrounding mucosa with normal enzyme activity the ^{3}H-

TdR index in the enzyme-deficient areas demonstrated on average the following increase: 43-fold after BBN, 17-fold after DBN and 23-fold after FANFT.

β) ³H-TdR Index of the Basal and Suprabasal Cells in Enzyme-Deficient Areas after 1 hour of Labeling

When the labeled cells were counted separately in the various layers, the mean ^{3}H-TdR index in BBN-induced enzyme-deficient areas was 17.3% for the basal layer and 3.7% for the suprabasal cells (Table 8).

Table 8. ^{3}H-TdR index of the entire urothelium, i.e. of the basal and suprabasal cells in enzyme-deficient areas, induced by BBN after 1 h of labeling (Z. Krebsforsch. *84,* 143–160, 1975)

Experimental period (days)	Entire urothelium	Basal cells	Suprabasal cells
135	13.7	20.0	9.0
135	11.4	22.0	6.3
135	2.7	10.0	0.8
145	12.9	25.5	4.0
150	8.1	12.2	5.5
150	9.6	24.7	2.2
200	3.5	8.6	0.3
215	3.8	10.2	0.0
215	6.4	15.2	3.1
275	8.0	24.0	3.7
275	8.8	22.0	3.9
275	5.8	17.2	0.5
290	5.0	2.5	5.9
290	14.0	28.0	6.5
Average	8.1	17.3	3.7

Of all the labeled cells in the normal bladder mucosa, 19.1 ± 16.2% were located suprabasally. In the defective areas, however, 31.9% ± 13.0% of the DNA-synthesizing cells were found suprabasally ($p < 0.05$; Student's *t*-test).

In the urothelial areas with loss of alkaline phosphatase activity due to FANFT the mean ^{3}H-TdR index was 9.8% for the basal and 2.35% for the suprabasal cells; the surrounding enzyme-containing urothelium, by comparison, showed a mean value of 0.58% for the basal and 0.037% for the suprabasal cells (Table 9). Thus the FANFT-induced enzyme-deficient areas demonstrated a 17-fold increase in the labeling index in the basal cell layer and a 60-fold increase in the suprabasal cell layers compared with the surrounding urothelium.

Table 9. ^{3}H-TdR index in urothelial areas demonstrating a loss of alkaline phosphatase activity induced by FANFT, with comparative values for the surrounding normal enzyme active urothelium, referred to the entire urothelium as well as the basal and suprabasal cells. (Z. Krebsforsch. *84*, 143–160, 1975)

Experimental period (days)	Areas of urothelium devoid of alkaline phosphatase activity			Surrounding urothelium with preserved alkaline phosphatase activity		
	Total urothelium	Basal layer	Suprabasal layers	Total urothelium	Basal layer	Suprabasal layers
130	12.7	–	–	0.26	0.59	0.021
155	6.8	12.2	1.66	0.18	0.40	0.024
165	11.2	9.4	–	0.20	0.41	0.061
190	4.6	10.0	3.18	0.26	0.59	0.021
200	1.5	3.0	0.18	0.26	0.55	0.064
200	4.5	11.1	1.80	–	–	–
240	5.6	9.8	2.04	–	–	–
245	4.2	13.6	1.30	0.43	0.94	0.045
245	5.5	10.4	3.00			
250	4.5	7.8	1.00	0.30	0.64	0.000
260	2.5	6.1	1.10			
260	10.0	14.4	8.30	0.28	0.53	0.060
Average:	6.1	9.8	2.35	0.27	0.58	0.037

γ) ³H-TdR Index in Enzyme-Deficient Areas after 54 hours' Continuous Labeling

Nonhyperplastic enzyme-deficient areas induced with BBN demonstrated an average of 54.9% labeled cells after 54 h continuous labeling with 6-^{3}H-thymidine (individual values: 42.7%, 53.2% and 68.8%). Slight to moderate hyperplastic urothelial areas with loss of alkaline phosphatase activity exhibited an average ^{3}H-TdR index of 62.5% (individual values: 44.3%, 66.8%, 67.9% and 71.0%).

δ) ³H-TdR Index in Areas of Papillomas with Diminution of NADH-diaphorase Activity

The ^{3}H-TdR index in papillomas was not uniform, but showed marked differences from one region to another. Consistently high labeling was observed in areas of papillomas that showed a remarkable diminution of NADH diaphorase activity in addition to loss of alkaline phosphatase activity. In such areas of BBN-induced papillomas the ^{3}H-TdR index was 20.5%, as against 4.6% in the neighboring papilloma structures with preserved enzyme activity, and 0.25% in the surrounding apparently normal urothelium (Fig. 15). The papillomas induced with FANFT demonstrated in corresponding areas an average ^{3}H-TdR index of 13.7% (individual values: 10.1%, 13.2%,

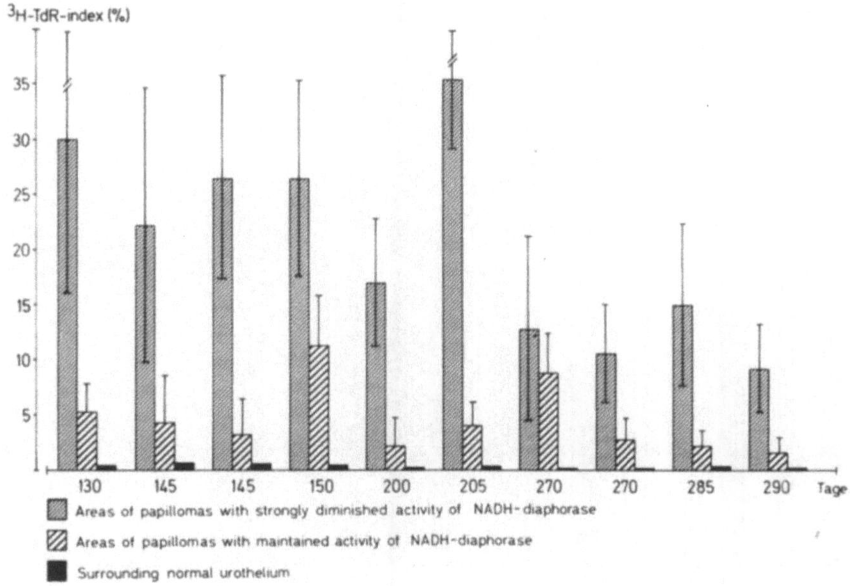

Fig. 15. ^{3}H-TdR index (means ± S.E.) in areas of *BBN*-induced papillomas with a marked reduction in NADH-diaphorase activity, compared with adjoining parts of the papillomas with positive enzyme reaction and the surrounding apparently normal urothelium. The differences are statistically highly significant (Student's *t*-test; $p < 0.001$). (Z. Krebsforsch. *84*, 143–160, 1975)

13.4% and 18.1%) compared with enzyme-containing papilloma areas, which showed an average labeling index of 4.9% (individual values: 3.5%, 4.2%, 5.4% and 6.6%).

ε) Incorporation of ^{3}H-Cytidine in Enzyme-Deficient Areas, Papillomas and Carcinomas

The incorporation of ^{3}H-cytidine was approximately equal in the nuclei of the basal, intermediate, and superficial cell layers within the normal mucosa. The density of silver granules overlying the basal cell nuclei was equated to 100%. The grain density of the intermediate nuclei by comparison varied between 91% and 106%, while that of the superficial nuclei was between 95% and 111%. No pronounced labeling of the nucleoli was observed. The nuclear incorporation of ^{3}H-cytidine varied within the individual alkaline phosphatase-deficient areas. Of the 33 enzyme-deficient areas tested, 18 showed an increased, three a decreased, and 12 an unchanged incorporation compared with the surrounding urothelium with preserved enzyme activity. The 10 areas exhibiting the most pronounced uptake of tritiated cytidine showed up to 2.5- to 4-fold increase in the density of silver grains compared with surrounding urothelium (Fig. 16); its labeling value was equated to 100%.

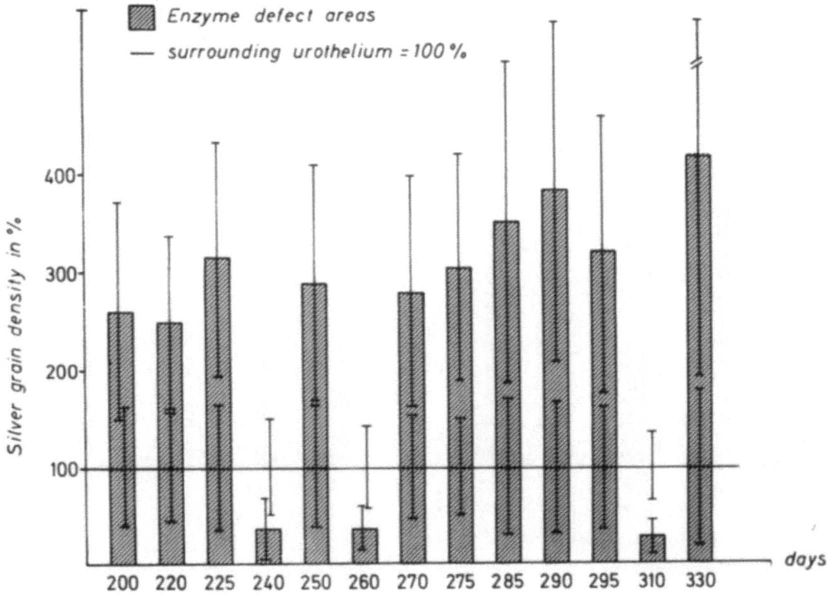

Fig. 16. Nuclear incorporation of ^{3}H-cytidine measured on basis of silver grain density within enzyme-deficient areas *(DBN)* and the surrounding normally enzyme-active urothelium. Grain density of neighboring bladder mucosa was equated to 100% and related enzyme-deficient areas compared with it. Differences were highly significant ($p < 0.001$; Z-test). (Z. Krebsforsch. 77, 236–248, 1971)

The standard deviations for each mean value revealed the expected wide range, corresponding to the large differences in labeling of the individual nuclei (Fig. 16). The increase in the grain concentration was highly significant in the evaluated enzyme-deficient areas in comparison to the unaltered bladder mucosa ($p < 0.001$; Z-test).

The nuclear incorporation of ^{3}H-cytidine in papillomas was not uniform. There were areas with a high number of granules over the nuclei as well as areas with a decreased or unchanged incorporation. Of the 27 papillomas observed, 13 showed an increase in ^{3}H-cytidine labeling within variously large areas, six showed a decrease and eight no change compared with the adjacent mucosa. Papillomas with squamous cell metaplasia more frequently showed an increased incorporation of ^{3}H-cytidine. Transitional cell carcinomas demonstrated variable incorporation rates in different areas, which were independent of the grade of cellular differentiation. They did not demonstrate any general increase in labeling compared with the papillomas.

d) Discussion

Combined enzyme-histochemical and autoradiographic investigations revealed a consistent increase in the ^{3}H-TdR index during the early phase of carcinogenesis in preneoplastic urothelial segments demonstrating a loss of alkaline phosphatase activity induced by the application of BBN, DBN and FANFT. Proliferation appears to begin simultaneously with the loss of alkaline phosphatase activity, since there was no occurrence of enzyme defects without labeled cells.

Precancerous areas defective in nucleoside-5'-triphosphatase activity in the rat liver induced by diethylnitrosamine only occasionally showed a slightly increased labeling index (*Schauer* and *Kunze,* 1968), compared with the immediate onset of proliferation in the enzyme-deficient areas of the bladder mucosa. An increase of up to 43-fold in the ^{3}H-TdR index after 1 h and a large percentage of labeled cells after 54 h of continuous labeling within the urothelial areas with loss of alkaline phosphatase activity indicate that the tumors develop very soon after the occurrence of the enzyme defect. The high labeling index within the preneoplastic urothelial segments at first seemed surprising, as the bladder mucosa is considered to be a tissue with a relatively low cell turnover. This finding is nevertheless quite understandable as the urothelium is capable of displaying a high proliferative potential after various stimuli (cf. Section II.3.).

Several authors believe that the carcinogenic effects are only possible within rapidly proliferating cells in hyperplastic urothelial areas following prior cellular necrosis (*Clayson* and *Pringle,* 1966; *Clayson* et al., 1967b). This opinion seemed quite unjustified on the basis of the present experimental series. Cellular necroses due to toxic effects were not demonstrable, and enzyme-deficient areas and hyperplasias that had developed from them were demonstrable long after the carcinogen had been discontinued, i.e., at a time when a possible toxic action was certainly no longer effective. The irreversible hyperplasias must therefore be regarded as an early stage in tumor development and not as its starting point.

With the onset of tumor development the physiological mode of regeneration was no longer maintained in the enzyme-deficient urothelial segments; not only the basal, but also the suprabasal cells were found to proliferate. The movement of the proliferative zone toward the suprabasal layers was much more pronounced in hyperplasias in which the majority of labeled cells were located in the suprabasal cell layers. This deviation from the physiological mode of regeneration is not, however, specific for carcinogenesis as such. Increased proliferative activity within the suprabasal cell layers has also been evidenced following various unspecific stimuli.

It was not possible to confirm the findings of American authors from in-vitro labeling experiments with human tumor material or in bladder tumors of rats induced by 2-N-acethylaminofluoren. They had found a close correlation between the degree of differentiation and the biological behavior of the tumors and the synthesis of nucleic acids (*Veenema* et al., 1963, 1965; *Battifora* et al., 1965; *Hainau* and *Dombernowsky,* 1974). In our experiments it was not uncommon to find a lower labeling index in transitional cell carcinomas than in papillomas. *Levi* et al. (1969) were also unable to confirm a simple relationship between the level of the labeling index and the degree of cell atypia in human urinary bladder tumors.

It is no easy task to interpret the autoradiographic findings concerning RNA metabolism, as there is no absolute correlation between the number of silver grains and the RNA synthesis. We might note at the outset that the uptake of ^{3}H-cytidine can be considered principally a measure for RNA metabolism, because incorporation into DNA is negligible. This also pertains to tissue with a high proliferative rate; findings in tumor cell populations and rapidly growing cell cultures have been reported, in which the incorporation of tritiated cytidine into DNA amounted to 5% (*Feinendegen* and *Bond,* 1964) and 13% (*Schaer* et al., 1969), respectively. In addition, the beta self absorption does not appear to have an essential influence upon the density of granules overlying the nuclei, because the mass of the cell nuclei was for the most part identical in the enzyme-deficient areas and in the surrounding urothelium under light microscopy.

Rat livers cancerized with diethylnitrosamine regularly demonstrated an increase of up to 2.5-fold increase in ^{3}H-cytidine incorporation compared with the surrounding enzyme-containing parenchyma in precancerous areas defective in nucleoside-5'-triphosphatase activity (*Schauer* and *Kunze,* 1968). By comparison, the urinary bladder demonstrated enzyme-deficient areas with increased, unchanged and even decreased incorporation. The increased labeling of the nucleoli in the enzyme-deficient areas of the liver was indicative primarily of new formation of ribosomal RNA; the nucleoli of the enzyme-negative urothelial cells did not demonstrate a pronounced density of silver granules typical for ribosomal RNA.

Changes in the ^{3}H-cytidine uptake in the urothelial segments with loss of alkaline phosphatase activity can be explained in a number of ways, of which the following seem to be most probable:

1. The increased incorporation of ^{3}H-cytidine correlates with an effective increase in RNA synthesis, which would be necessary for increased proliferative activity, i.e., for the synthesis of polymerases.

2. Assuming the existence of a small endogenic nucleotide pool originally, an increase in RNA synthesis would be simulated by filling up the pool with exogenous ^{3}H-cytidine. A diminution of the nucleotide pool has only been demonstrated in completely developed tumors, such as hepatomas (*Nodes* and *Reid,* 1963).

3. An alteration of the migration of nuclear RNA into the cytoplasm leads to an accumulation of tritiated cytidine in the cell nucleus. This, however, seems rather improbable from the findings of *Fingerhut* et al. (1969), who have demonstrated an undisturbed migration of RNA into the cytoplasm.

The variable incorporation of ^{3}H-cytidine in papillomas and carcinomas, like the level of the ^{3}H-TdR index, excludes any principally consistent relationship to the grade of cell differentiation. However, observations in experimentally induced tumors in rats and in human biopsy material have shown higher labeling in malignant than in benign tumors (*Veenema* et al., 1965; *Fingerhut* et al., 1969). Furthermore, it was not possible to confirm a predominantly extranuclear silver granule distribution in benign tumors in contrast to only intranuclear distribution of grains in malignant tumors (*Fingerhut* et al., 1969).

e) Summary

Combined enzyme-histochemical and autoradiographic investigations during carcinogenesis in the rat urinary bladder have led to the following conclusions:

1. Compared with the surrounding enzyme-containing urothelium, alkaline phosphatase-deficient areas demonstrated a 43-fold increase in the ^{3}H-TdR index after application of BBN, a 17-fold increase after administration of DBN and a 20-fold increase after FANFT.

2. The percentage of DNA-synthesizing cells after 54 h of labeling with ^{3}H-thymidine was on average 54.9% in nonhyperplastic enzyme-deficient areas and on average 62.5% in slightly to moderately hyperplastic urothelial segments demonstrating a loss of alkaline phosphatase activity.

3. The increased rate of proliferation of the suprabasal cells seen in the enzyme-deficient areas indicates a disturbance in the physiological mode of regeneration.

4. The histologically apparently normal urothelium of the cancerized urinary bladder with normal enzyme activity demonstrated only an insignificant change in the ^{3}H-TdR index compared with control animals.

5. Areas of papillomas with a marked reduction in NADH diaphorase activity showed a 4.5-fold (BBN) and a 3.1-fold (FANFT) higher ^{3}H-TdR index than the surrounding areas of the papilloma with retained enzyme activity.

6. The nuclear incorporation of ^{3}H-cytidine revealed a 2.5- to 4-fold increase in the majority of DBN-induced enzyme-deficient areas compared with the adjacent urothelium. The incorporation in papillomas and carcinomas showed considerable differences between the individual tumors and from area to area in the same tumor. No increase of incorporation occurred in carcinomas, in particular, as compared with papillomas. No clear-cut relationship was found to exist between degree of labeling and cellular differentiation in carcinomas.

3. Stages of Transformation in Papillomas

a) Introduction

It is known that carcinomas of the urinary bladder can develop either from a preexistent papilloma by malignant transformation or directly from a primary carcinoma-in-situ, the so-called intraurothelial carcinoma. *Zuckerkandl* (1919), *Stenius* (1922) and *Christeller* (1925) postulated the development of carcinomas from papillomas in man (for a review of the older literature see *Hückel,* 1934). *Stenius* coined the term "malignant papilloma," *Christeller* introduced the designation "atypical papillary fibroepithelioma," and *Zuckerkandl* (1910) spoke of a "latent carcinomatous nature" of papillomas. *Melicow* and coworkers were the first to note the direct development of a bladder carcinoma from a carcinoma-in-situ (*Melicow,* 1952; *Melicow* and *Hollowell,* 1952). To date it has not been definitely decided whether carcinomas arise predominantly from a papilloma or from carcinoma-in-situ. The aim of the present experiments was to clarify which of the two modes of origin predominates, and further, to find out any details regarding the proliferation kinetics of the urothelial cells during the malignant transformation of initially benign-seeming papillomas.

b) Material and Methods

Female Wistar rats (initially weighing between 150 g and 180 g) were given n-butyl-(4-hydroxybutyl)-nitrosamine (BBN) in their drinking water (20 mg/kg body weight/day). The 177 animals were divided into four main groups: group I received the carcinogen for 40 days, group II for 80 days, group III for 120 days and group IV for 150 days (time of exposure). Subsequently the carcinogen was discontinued. After a total experimental period (induction time) of 150, 200 and 250 days, respectively, 15 animals of each main group (with two exceptions; cf. Table 10) were killed by decapitation. All animals received a standardized compressed feed (Altromin).

For the purpose of autoradiographic studies each animal was injected with 6-^{3}H-thymidine (Radiochemical Centre, Amersham, England; specific activity 5 Ci/mmol) intraperitoneally one hour before sacrifice. The dose administered was 0.1 m Ci/100 g body weight, given between 8.15 and 9.00 a.m.

After fixation in 10% formaldehyde for 24 h, each urinary bladder was embedded in paraplast and then cut serially into 80 sections, each 5 μm thick. This number of sections proved to be quite sufficient to register carcinogenically induced preneoplastic and neoplastic lesions as well as to assess the different stages of tumor development. Thus it was possible to compare on a fairly exact basis the number of carcinogenic lesions of the individual animals in the different groups. The majority of the sections were stained with Mayer's haemalaun. PAS staining was performed occasionally. A smaller number of bladders were embedded in methacrylate and cut into 80 to 100 serial step sections approximately 1–2 μm thick. The semithin sections were stained with the Goldner trichrome stain.

Table 10. Distribution and number of preneoplastic and neoplastic lesions with and without transformation stages occurring in rats of the various groups after variously long exposure (BBN) and induction times

Time of induction (days)	Number of animals	Papillary hyperplasia	Papilloma	Papillary hyperplasia with atypia	Papilloma with focal atypia	Papilloma with ca in situ	Papilloma with focally invasive growth	Invasive carcinoma
				GROUP I (40 days BBN)				
150	15	31	21	10	19	14	1	—
200	15	25	11	5	24	6	3	1
250	13	12	9	7	20	6	5	3
				GROUP II (80 days BBN)				
150	15	53	61	19	39	11	3	1
200	15	71	25	24	46	18	2	—
250	15	18	6	13	44	25	28	2
				GROUP III (120 days BBN)				
150	15	66	62	12	51	11	1	—
200	15	33	18	20	79	52	24	1
250	14	13	9	13	56	33	24	4
				GROUP IV (150 days BBN)				
150	15	155	133	46	104	16	4	1
200	15	48	26	61	119	58	15	3
250	15	5	10	18	76	57	43	7

c) Results

The above experimental procedure, employing varying lengths of exposure and induction times, facilitated the investigation of various stages of development of papillomas and also of papillary and nonpapillary transitional cell carcinomas. Different stages were distinguishable on the basis of cytological and histological criteria. The following groups were delineated:

α) Preneoplastic and neoplastic lesions without significant cellular atypia (simple and papillary hyperplasias, papillomas).

β) Stages of development exhibiting focal atypia ⎤ within papillary
γ) Stages with carcinoma-in-situ ⎬ hyperplasias and
δ) Stages showing circumscribed infiltrative growth. ⎦ papillomas

ε) Transitional stages between α–δ.

ζ) Primary carcinoma-in-situ (intraurothelial carcinoma).

α) Preneoplastic and Neoplastic Lesions Without Atypia (Simple and Papillary Hyperplasias, Papillomas)

The first histologically detectable lesion of tumor development was evident in circumscribed simple hyperplasias of the urothelium generally consisting of layers of four to 10 cells. The urothelial cells within the hyperplastic regions were not distinguishable

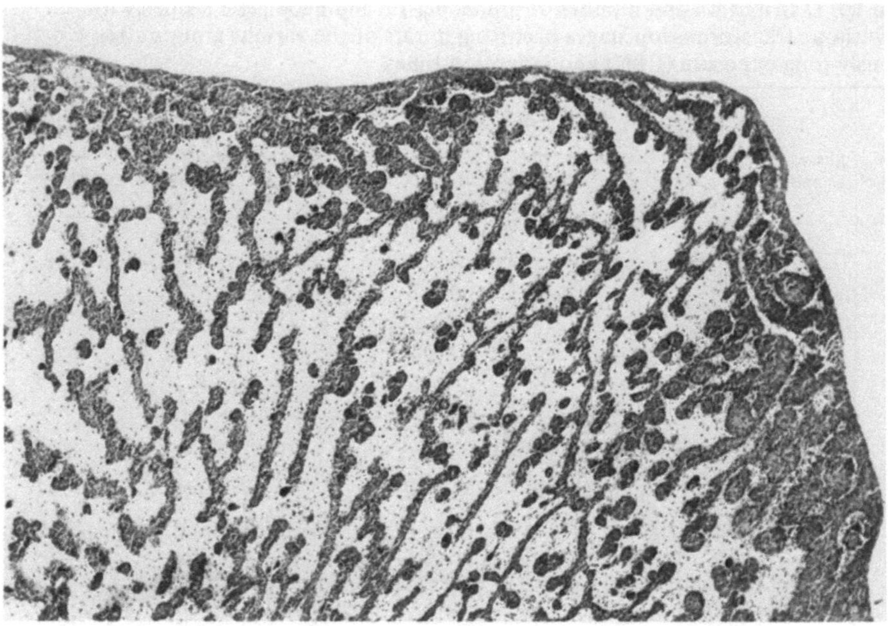

Fig. 17. Part of inverted papilloma consisting of small widely branched strands of neoplastic urothelial cells without cellular atypias. Time of exposure *(BBN)*: 150 days. Total experimental period: 250 days. 30 X. (Z. Krebsforsch. *87*, 139–160, 1975)

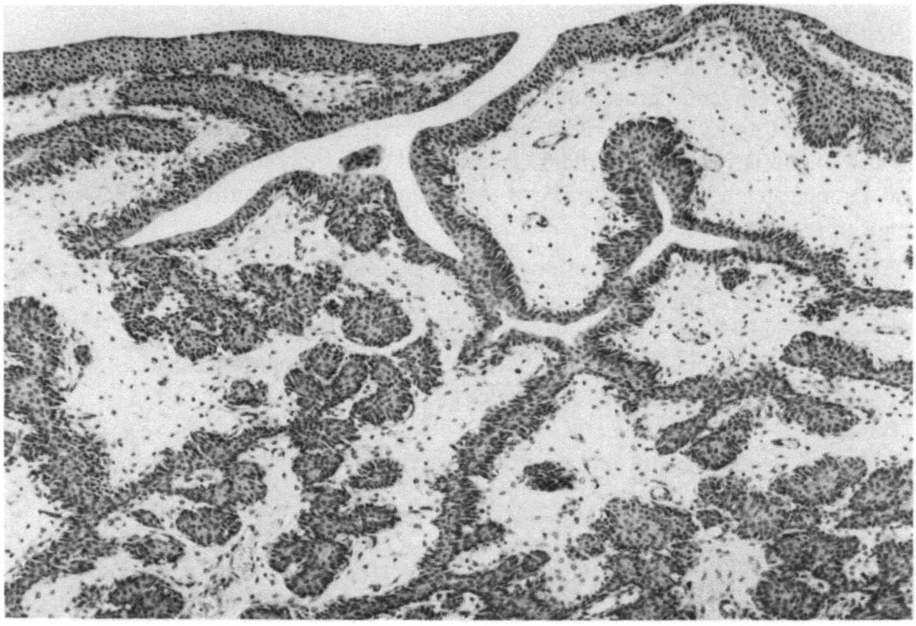

Fig. 18. Inverted papilloma showing indentations of the overlying urothelium into the stroma and pattern of bud-like branching cords of neoplastic urothelial cells. Time of exposure *(BBN)*: 120 days. Total experimental period: 250 days. 75 X (Z. Krebsforsch. *87*, 139–160, 1976)

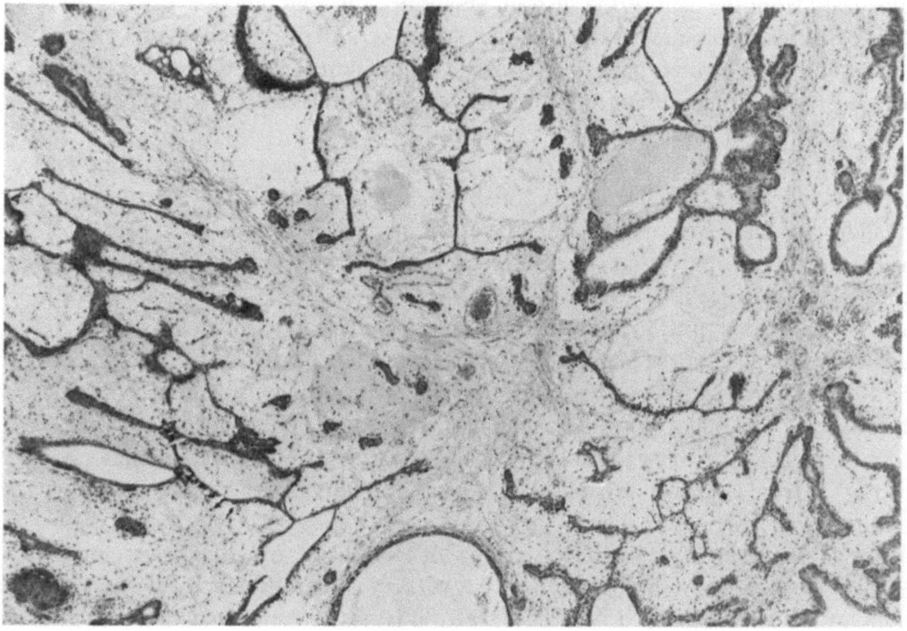

Fig. 19. Inverted papilloma with cyst formation. Marked edema of the intervening stroma. Time of exposure *(BBN)*: 150 days. Total experimental period: 250 days. 30 X. (Z. Krebsforsch. *87*, 139–170, 1976)

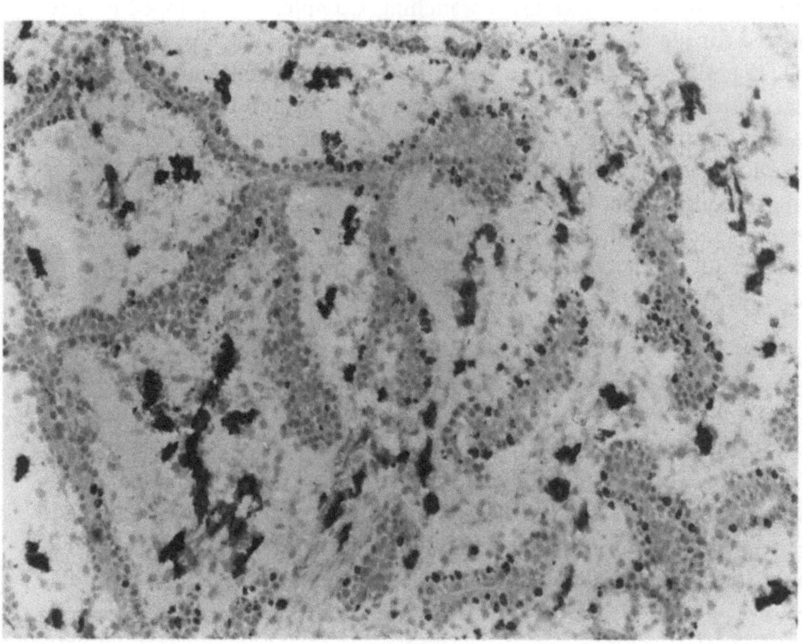

Fig. 20. Autoradiogram of an inverted papilloma. Numerous ^{3}H-thymidine-labeled cells basally (black) Positive alkaline phosphatase activity (black) at small blood vessels of the stroma. Time of exposure *(DBN)*: 150 days. Total experimental period: 360 days. 100 X. (Z. Krebsforsch. *87*, 139–160, 1976)

cytologically from the cells of the surrounding normal bladder mucosa. The urinary bladder of animals which received the carcinogen over a longer period of time in most cases demonstrated several foci of hyperplastic urothelium. These hyperplasias proved to be irreversible, being present long after withdrawal of the carcinogenic substance, i.e., they were not of toxic origin.

Papillary hyperplasia developed from simple hyperplasia. In its exophytic growth pattern it was formed of delicate stalks of stroma, which protruded into the lumen of the bladder and were covered by several layers of inconspicuous urothelial cells. In addition, papillary hyperplasias were observed in an endophytic growth pattern, though much less frequently (Fig. 8).

At a further stage, papillomas developed from papillary hyperplasias. These morphologically benign-seeming papillomas consisted of a tender core of highly branched, vascularized stroma, which was covered by several layers of inconspicuous neoplastic urothelial cells. The majority of the papillomas were connected to the wall of the bladder by means of a thin stalk of connective tissue. The papillary carcinomas grade I (*Koss,* 1975) were classified as papillomas because the tumors exhibited no cytological and histological criteria of malignancy.

Inverted papillomas were characterized by an endophytic growth pattern (Figs. 17–20). Histogenetically they developed first with an indentation of the bladder urothelium into the stroma (Fig. 18). Here all the cell layers of the urothelium were involved. At a further stage of development, secondary indentations developed from the primary indentations, which again built branches of their own, produced by a focal increased proliferative activity of the basal cells (Fig. 20). Often no further lumen could be discerned within the pattern of extensive branching. Completely developed inverted papillomas consisted for the most part of small strands of urothelial cells, which were widely branched (Fig. 17). As a rule, there was no recognizeable continuity with the overlying bladder urothelium. Occasionally pseudoglandular structures were observed within the strands of urothelial cells (Fig. 19). These were apparently the result of cellular necrosis, since necrotic cells were found in the lumina.

The papillomas frequently showed focal squamous metaplasia, but only rarely generalized squamous metaplasia. The benign-seeming papillomas did not reach any substantial size under the given experimental conditions. In general they developed atypical foci rather early.

β) Stages of Development Exhibiting Focal Atypia

After long exposure and induction times, an increase in papillary hyperplasias and papillomas was observed, which exhibited focally atypical cells (Figs. 21–23). Notable characteristics of these cells were a cytoplasmatic basophilia, prominent nucleoli, and enlargement of the cell nucleus, with an irregularly developed chromatin pattern. The atpyical areas were sharply delineated over and beside the apparently benign urothelial

---

Fig. 22. Papilloma showing atypical cells with marked cytoplasmatic basophilia *(right)* side by side with benign appearing papillomatous structures *(left).* Time of exposure *(BBN):* 80 days. Total experimental period: 150 days. 190 X. (Z. Krebsforsch. *87,* 139–160, 1976)

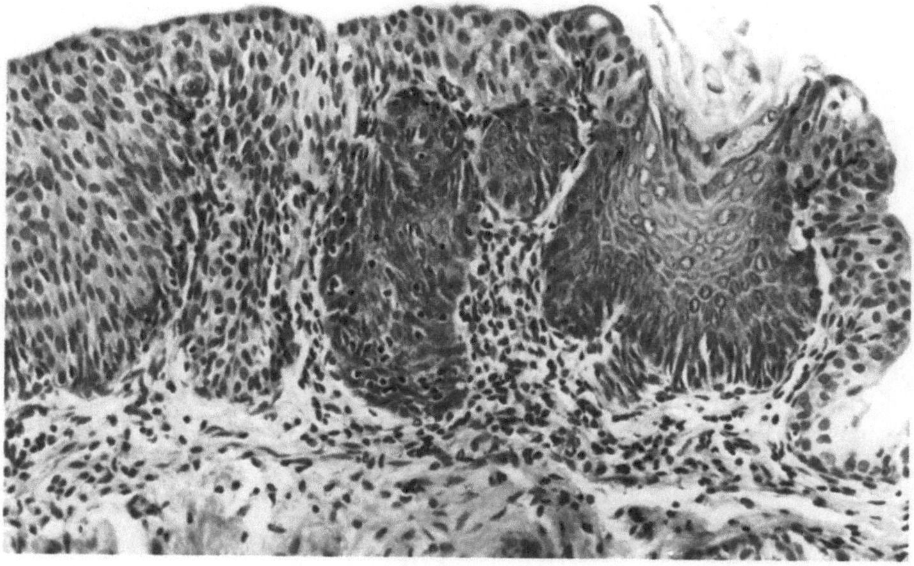

Fig. 21. Papillary hyperplasia exhibiting focally atypical cells with pronounced cytoplasmatic basophilia and squamous metaplasia *(right)*. Time of exposure *(BBN)*: 120 days. Total experimental period: 150 days. 190 X. (Z. Krebsforsch. *87*, 139–160, 1976)

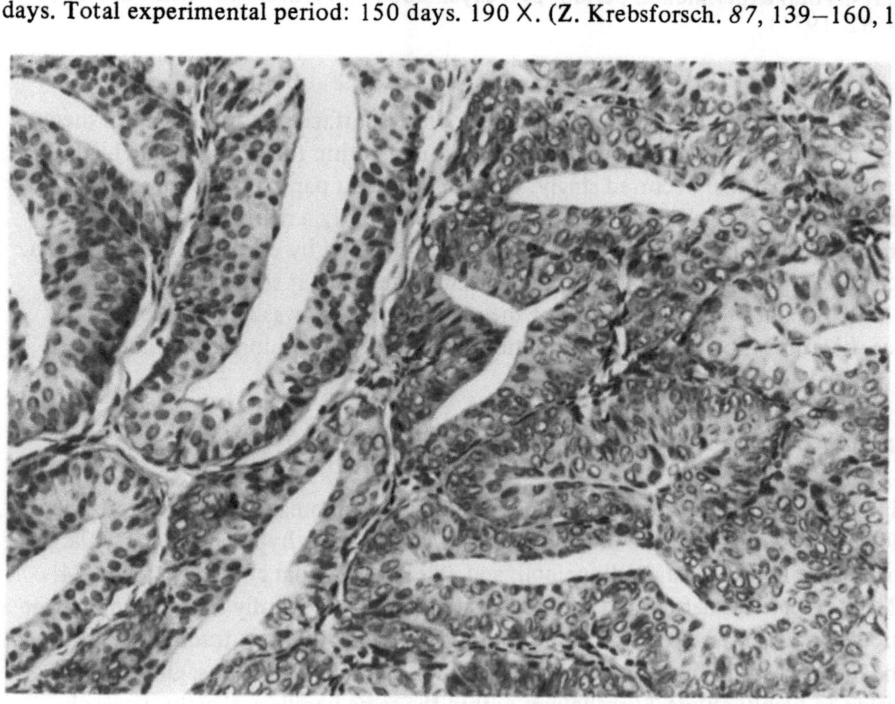

Fig. 22. Legend see page 184

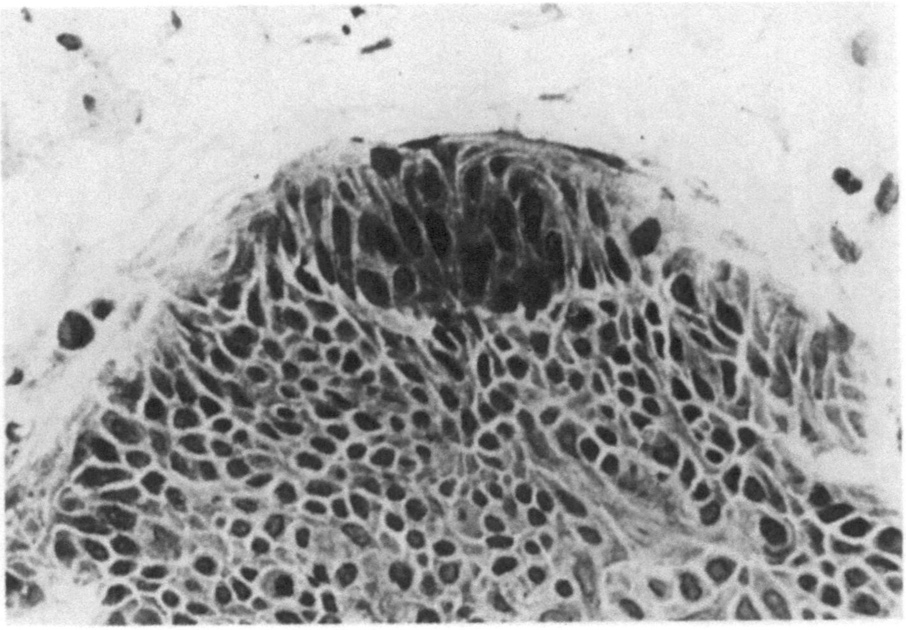

Fig. 23. Marked focal atypia within a papilloma showing enlargement and hyperchromasia of the nuclei and deep basophilia of the cytoplasm. Time of exposure *(BBN):* 290 days. Total experimental period. 290 days. 200 X. (Verh. Dtsch. Ges. Path. *55*, 577–582, 1971)

structures. Atypical foci lie either centrally or on the surface of a papilloma. In these cases exfoliated atpyical cells were frequently found within the lumen of the bladder. As a rule, atypical foci occurred singly. Only in the larger papillomas were several atypical foci observed close to each other. Very frequently a markedly developed squamous metaplasia was established, accompanied in part by excessive keratinization. If such areas were superficial, they exfoliated in large lamellar sheets, and in a few cases they filled up the entire lumen of the bladder. If there was no contact with the surface, keratinization with pearl formations was observed within the papilloma.

γ) Stages of Development with Carcinoma-in-situ

Carcinomas in situ within papillary hyperplasias and papillomas were characterized cytologically by a high degree of cellular atypia with nuclear hyperchromasia, enlarged and occasionally bizarre shaped nucleoli, and a deep basophilic cytoplasm (Figs. 24–26). Mitoses were numerous and frequently atypical. Histologically the most important feature was a preinvasive growth in the form of urothelial buds protruding toward the stroma or the surrounding apparently benign papillomatous structures. Occasionally a transition to highly atypical urothelium within the same papillary structure was observed (Fig. 24). This precancerous lesion within a papilloma or papillary hyperplasia

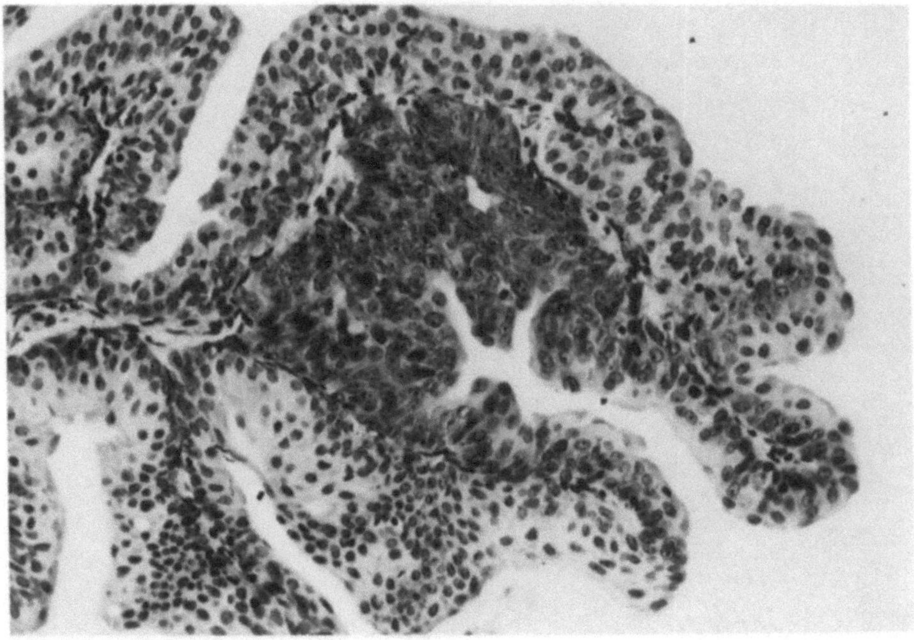

Fig. 24. Carcinoma in situ within a small papilloma. Transition of apparently benign papillary structures in highly atypical multilayered urothelium characterized by hyperchromasia of the nuclei and deep cytoplasmic basophilia. Time of exposure *(BBN):* 120 days. Total experimental period: 200 days. 190 X. (Z. Krebsforsch. *87,* 139–160, 1976)

we termed secondary carcinoma-in-situ, as against primary carcinoma-in-situ, which is located in the otherwise unchanged bladder mucosa. A frequently finding was squamous metaplasia with varying degrees of keratinization, similar to that within atypical foci. Carcinomas-in-situ occurred most frequently in papillomas; they were, however, also observed in papillary hyperplasias.

δ) Stages of Development Showing Circumscribed Infiltrative Growth

Papillomas that showed an infiltrative growth focally were considered manifestly malignant (Figs. 27 and 28). The term "malignantly transformed papilloma" seems meaningful, because the development of the carcinomatous growth took place within a preexistent papilloma. However, the invasive growth could have begun at a much earlier stage of carcinogenesis, for instance within a papillary hyperplasia. From a cytological standpoint it seems important to mention that the infiltrative growing cells quite often demonstrated a lesser degree of dysplasia and mitotic activity than the cells in a carcinoma-in-situ.

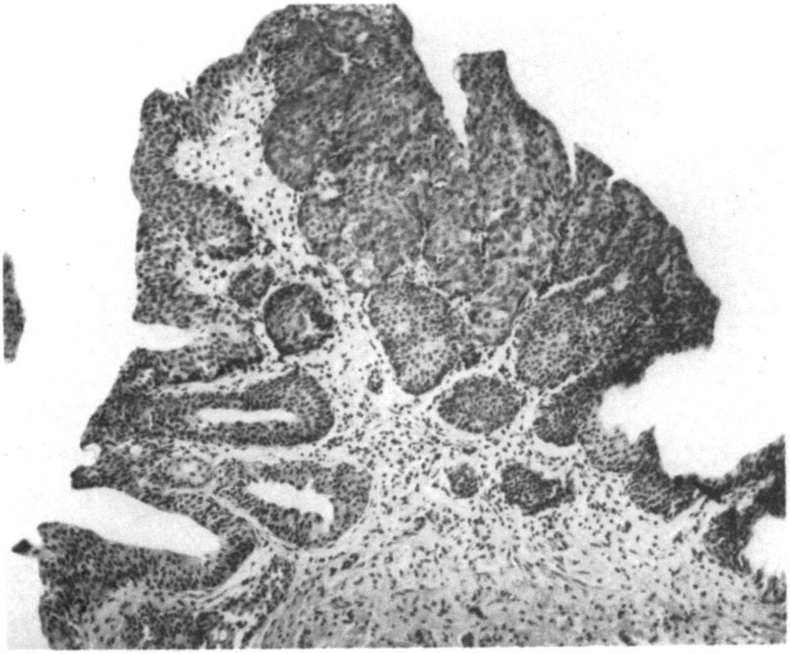

Fig. 25. Advanced carcinoma-in-situ within papilloma with urothelial buds growing toward stroma. Time of exposure *(BBN)*: 120 days. Total experimental period: 200 days. 75X

ε) Transitional Stages

Transitional stages of tumor development were observed, which do not clearly fit into the scheme defined above. Such transitions occurred throughout the carcinogenic process, e.g., between apparently benign papillomas and papillomas with focal atypia, as in the case of carcinoma-in-situ or of focally invasive growth. A tumor was designated a fully developed carcinoma if it was composed throughout of infiltratively growing cells and showed no apparently benign urothelial structures, as in the case of a malignantly transformed papilloma. The spectrum of BBN-induced tumors in the bladder of the rats covered all the types of carcinomas occurring in man, including the rare adenocarcinomas, squamous cell carcinomas and undifferentiated carcinomas (cf. Section III.5.).

ζ) Primary Carcinoma in situ (Intraurothelial Carcinoma)

The development of transitional cell carcinomas directly from a primary carcinoma in situ or intraurothelial carcinoma was observed infrequently. This precancerous lesion was characterized by the appearance of cells with marked nuclear and cytoplasmic abnormalities, these cells being part of the otherwise undisturbed mucosa of the urinary

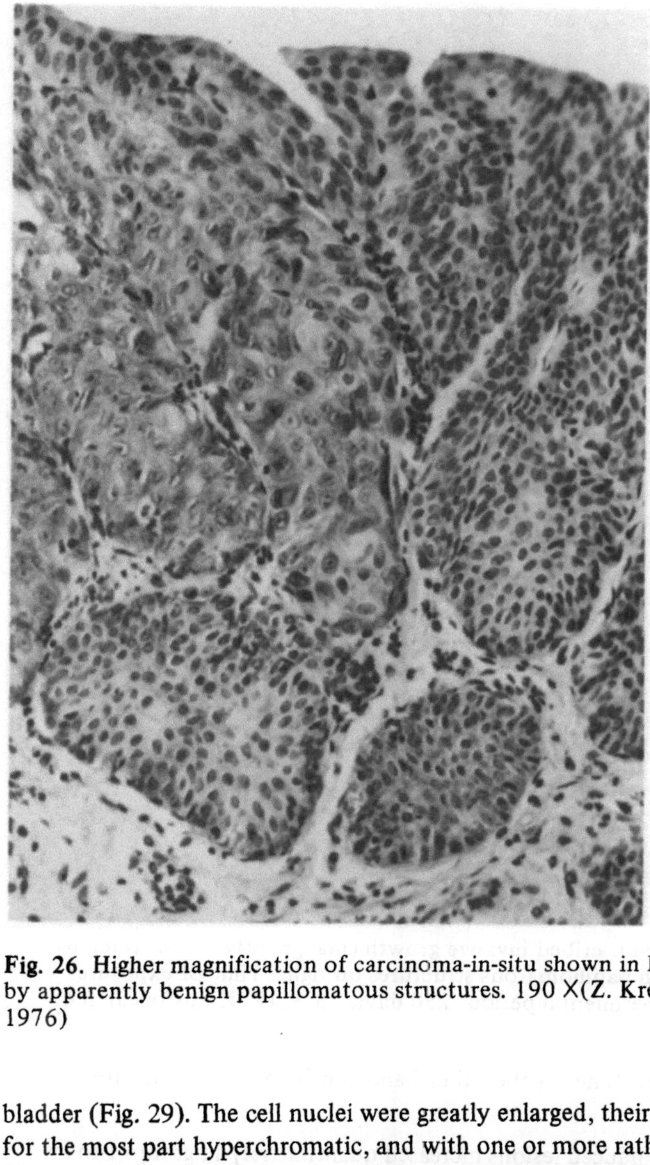

Fig. 26. Higher magnification of carcinoma-in-situ shown in Figure 25, surrounded by apparently benign papillomatous structures. 190 X(Z. Krebsforsch. *87*, 139–160, 1976)

bladder (Fig. 29). The cell nuclei were greatly enlarged, their shape and size irregular, for the most part hyperchromatic, and with one or more rather prominent nucleoli. The cytoplasm showed deep basophilia. Mitotic figures were common and occasionally atypical. At times the atypical cells demonstrated a decreased attachment to the underlying basement membrane, with the result that cells exfoliated into the lumen of the bladder, leaving small ulcerations. The primary carcinoma-in-situ was seen rather seldom; only 12 specimens were found in six animals among all the groups. On the other hand, carcinomas-in-situ within a papilloma or papillary hyperplasia (secondary carcinoma-in-situ) occurred rather frequently.

The distribution of the various preneoplastic and neoplastic lesions with and without transformation stages occurring in the rats of the various groups can be seen in Table 10. The following relationship between tumor development on the one hand

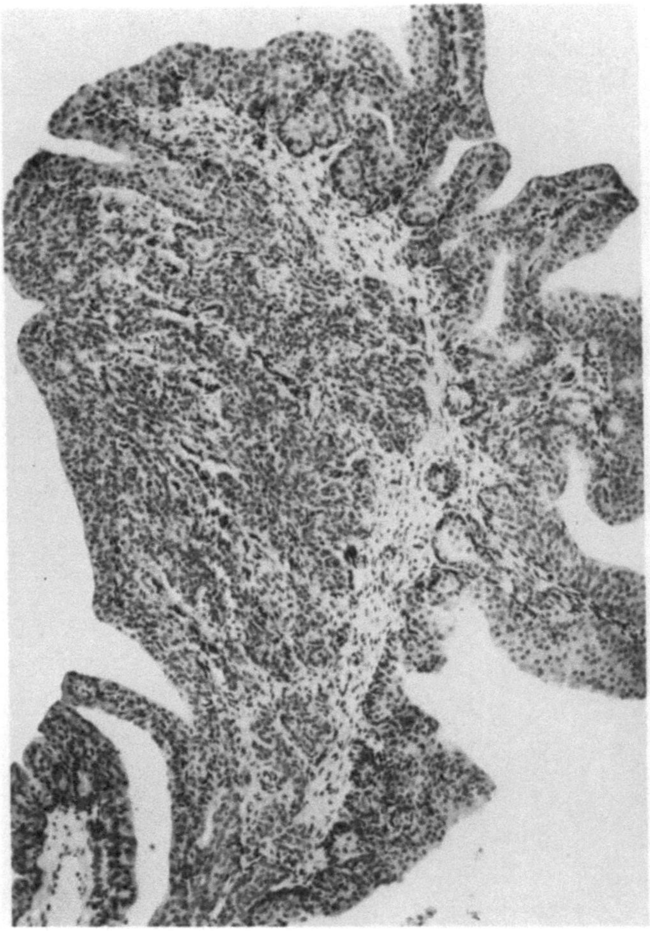

Fig. 27. Papilloma with circumscribed invasive growth (malignantly transformed papilloma). Apparently benign papillomatous structures on right. Time of exposure *(BBN):* 120 days. Total experimental period: 250 days. 75 X. (Z. Krebsforsch. *87,* 139–160, 1976)

and exposure and induction time on the other hand can be derived from this schedule:

1. All carcinogenically induced lesions increased quantitatively in groups I to IV with an increase in exposure time from 40 to 150 days. The highest incidence of lesions was found in the animals in group IV, which received BBN continuously for 150 days, i.e., up to the day they were killed. In the same group, after an induction time of 250 days, the number of changes was relatively low, because the bladders of these animals were usually completely filled by a few extensive tumors.

2. Proof for the multicentric theory of tumor development was found in the occurrence of multiple preneoplastic and neoplastic lesions in various places within the same bladder, each being independent of the others. The occurrence of various concomitantly existing stages of transformation supports the concept of a stepwise process of cancer development.

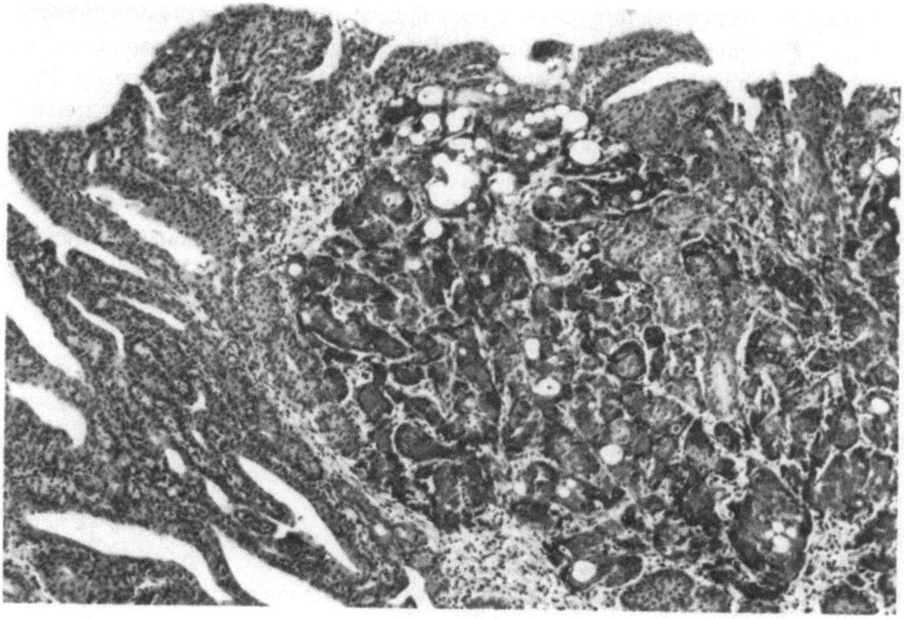

Fig. 28. Malignantly transformed papilloma with invasively growing atypical squamous cell epithelia. Time of exposure *(BBN)*: 80 days. Total experimental period: 250 days. 30 X. (Z. Krebsforsch. *87*, 139–160, 1976)

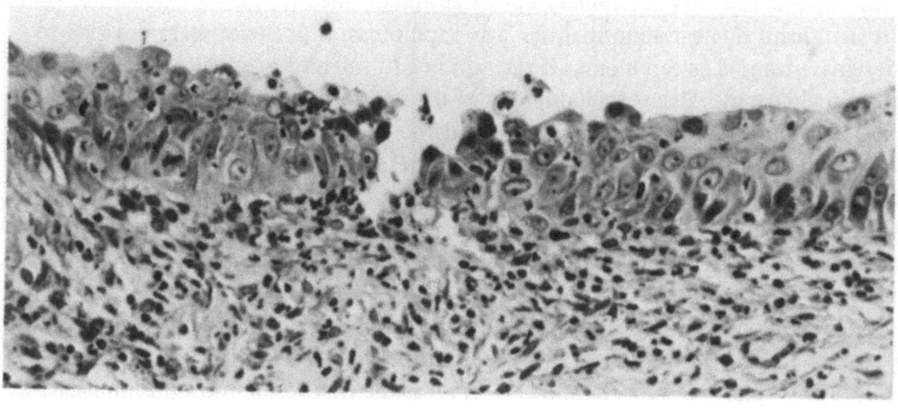

Fig. 29. Primary carcinoma in situ (intraurothelial carcinoma) with enlarged hyperchromatic nuclei and prominent nucleoli. In centre of lesion small area of ulceration with exfoliation of atypical cells in bladder lumen. Time of exposure *(BBN)*: 120 days. Total experimental period: 200 days. 190 X. (Z. Krebsforsch. *87*, 139–160, 1976)

3. There is a direct correlation between the length of exposure and the development of focal atypia, carcinoma-in-situ, and focally infiltrative growth within a papilloma. The number of such transformation stages was relatively low in animals receiving BBN for only 40 days, as in group I; however, in groups II, III, and IV the number of transformation stages increased in proportion to the duration of exposure. The same tendency was noted in the case of fully developed carcinomas.

4. The dependence of the development of the transformation stages upon the time of induction follows from the increase of papillomas with a carcinoma-in-situ or focally infiltrative growth and of carcinomas, when the induction time was prolonged from 150 to 250 days. The number of papillomas and papillary hyperplasias without atypia correspondingly decreased with an increase of the induction time.

5. Considering all groups as a whole, 74.4% of the papillomas showed various transformation stages; 44.3% of the papillomas exhibited focal atypias, 20.1% carcinomas-in-situ, and 10.0% focally infiltrative growth.

d) Discussion

The present experimental investigations have shown that the majority of papillary and nonpapillary transitional cell carcinomas of the urinary bladder developed by malignant transformation from preexistent papillomas or their precursors, the papillary hyperplasias. Urothelial tumors that showed no cellular atypia or increased proliferative activity at light-microscopic examination in serial sections of the entire tumor were designated "papillomas." We have also classified papillary carcinomas grade I according to the definition of *Koss* (1975) ("a papillary epithelial tumor lined by thickened urothelium without significant nuclear abnormalities") as papillomas. It does not seem justified to us to designate tumors as carcinomas if they do not fulfull any cytological or histological criterial of malignancy. This is probably one of the major reasons why the proportion of papillomas in our investigation is relatively high, compared with data on the incidence of papillomas in the human urinary bladder (*Pugh,* 1959: 3.2%; *Miller* et al., 1969: 2.0%). The papillomas of the rat bladder were as a rule very small. They occurred predominantly in animals of group I after a short exposure and induction time. It seems reasonable to believe that a large number of such small papillomas go undetected in humans.

Inverted papillomas were observed only rarely in our animal experiments, similar to its appearance in man (*Potts* and *Hirst,* 1963; *Trites,* 1969; *Assor* and *Taylor,* 1970; *Cummings,* 1974; *Koss,* 1975). *Paschkis* (1927) was the first to mention this unusual kind of papilloma in man, and provided a detailed description of it. It is characterized by its endophytic growth and should not be confused with the infiltrative growth of a well differentiated transitional cell carcinoma. Follow-up studies over up to 12 years in humans underscore the benign behavior of inverted papillomas (cf. *Koss,* 1975). Nevertheless, one must consider the possibility of malignant transformation analogous to exophytically growing papillomas. The present autoradiographic studies strongly suggest the conclusion that inverted papillomas are derived from the basal cells, and accordingly can be compared with the basal cell epithelioma of the skin and the adamantinomas and basal cell adenomas of the parotid gland.

Focal cellular abnormalities within papillomas and papillary hyperplasias developed more frequently after a longer exposure and induction time. Groups III and IV demonstrated more papillomas with transformation stages than did groups I and II. From these facts it can be concluded that the percentage of papillomas without atypia may be still smaller after longer exposure and/or after a higher total dose of BBN. Papillary urothelial tumors with focal cellular atypia and increased proliferative activity cannot be considered papillomas in the strict sense. In the present study we used the term papilloma nevertheless, i.e. papilloma with focal atypia, papilloma with carcinoma-in-situ, and papilloma with circumsribed invasive growth, to underscore the fact that the malignant growth developed in a primarily apparently benign urothelial tumor.

Histogenetically speaking, the transformation to malignant growth does not occur abruptly, but develops through different successive steps, each having its own distinct morphological and biological character. The various transformation stages within papillomas and papillary hyperplasias (focal atypia, carcinoma-in-situ, circumscribed invasive growth) were easily distinguished by light microscopy on the basis of their cytological properties and pattern of growth. The successive development of one stage out of another was evidenced by transitional stages and took place independently of any further carcinogen application after transformation was initiated. This conclusion was supported by the fact that the number of transformed papillomas increased in all test groups after the addition of the carcinogenic substance was stopped. The methods employed in these experiments did not allow us to determine how long any one stage of transformation would retain its biological distinctiveness. *Bettendorff* (1974) mentioned an average of 16.5 months for the malignant transformation of papillomas in man, the extreme values ranging from 1 to 48 months. Other authors, however, report a much longer time (*Deming,* 1950; *Mills,* 1964; *Lerman* et al., 1970; cf. *Koss,* 1975).

On the basis of the present experimental investigations, papillomas must be considered potentially highly malignant. Whether or not a papilloma in each case necessarily develops into a carcinoma could not be clarified by the methods employed in these experiments. The animal experiments confirmed the viewpoint of *Zuckerkandl* (1910); *Stenius* (1922), and *Christeller* (1925), that papillomas in man are capable of malignant transformation. Our results have proved as incorrect the opinion of *Kloos* and *Steffen* (1951) that bladder carcinoma must be viewed as nosologically distinct from papillomas.

The multicentric origin in the development of bladder tumors in the rat also applies to the human urinary bladder (*Lund* and *Lundwill,* 1955; *Pugh,* 1959; *Selberg,* 1961, 1964; *Pyrah* et al., 1964; *Zingg* and *Busser,* 1968; *Lerman* et al., 1970; cf. *Koss,* 1975). In animals the occurrence of a solitary neoplasm was a rarity, being found almost exclusively in group I. The number of preneoplastic and neoplastic lesions greatly increased with increasing doses of the carcinogenic substance applied and lengthening time of exposure. In rare cases the entire bladder was covered with innumerable very closely associated tumors, a finding which has been described in man as diffuse "papillomatosis."

In the present animal experiments, the malignant transformation of papillomas played the predominant role in the development of papillary and nonpapillary transitional cell carcinomas. It must be emphasized that primary carcinoma-in-situ occurred infrequently as an immediate precursor of carcinomas. The same results were achieved in earlier investigations with variously structured carcinogenic agents (*Kunze* et al., 1971, 1975) and by other authors (*Koss* and *Lavin,* 1971). However, it seems be possible that an increase in the daily dose of BBN would lead to an increase in primary carcinomata-in-situ. Inasmuch as the results of animal experiments are applicable to humans, of *Koss's* (1975) assumption that invasive nonpapillary carcinoma "most likely originates from nonpapillary carcinoma-in-situ" seems less likely to be true.

Since *Melicow* (1952) and *Melicow* and *Hollowell* (1952) first described primary carcinoma-in-situ, numerous reports have appeared about this early carcinogenic lesion in the bladder urothelium of man (*Eisenberg* et al., 1960; *Melamed* et al., 1960, 1964, 1966; *Simon* et al., 1962; *Austen* and *Friedell,* 1965; *Schade* and *Swinney,* 1968; *Utz* et al., 1970; *Yates-Bell,* 1971; *Cooper,* 1973; *Koss* et al., 1974; *Skinner* et al., 1974; *Thelmo* et al., 1974; *Koss,* 1975; *Seemayer* et al., 1975; *Farrow* et al., 1976). Very frequently carcinomas-in-situ were found in multiple foci in bladders where an invasive carcinoma had already developed. Quite often they were located in the immediate vicinity of the carcinoma. Approximately 60% of cases of carcinoma-in-situ in humans developed into an invasive carcinoma (cf. *Koss,* 1975). It appears to take a long time for a primary carcinoma-in-situ to develop into an infiltrative carcinoma. This is about all that can be said regarding this problem from the few investigations up to this time. *Melamed* et al. (1964) found it took an average of 26 to 33 months to develop, with extreme values ranging between 8 and 67 months. In isolated cases *Moloney* et al. (1974) found an invasive carcinoma even after 4 to 8 years. *Koss* et al. (1969) discovered invasive cancers after intervals of 18 to 77 months. The statistical relevance of such claims seems uncertain, inasmuch as statements regarding the time of development would have statistical relevance only if exactly the same lesion had been observed.

e) Summary

The present experimental investigations have shown that by far the largest proportion of papillary and nonpapillary transitional cell carcinomas of the urinary bladder developed by malignant transformation from preexistent papillomas or their precursors, the papillary hyperplasias. The transition into a focally malignant growth did not take place abruptly, but occurred in steps, passing through different successive stages of transformation, each with its own distinct morphological character. The first stage consisted of a focal, sharpely defined cellular atypia. In a further stage, carcinoma-in-situ developed out of the atypical foci and progressed in a last stage of transformation into a circumsribed infiltrative growth. The successive development of each stage occurred independently of any further carcinogen application after transformation was initiated at the molecular leve. The number of papillomas with transformation stages increased with lengthening exposure and induction time. Of the papillomas we saw, 74.4% had been transformed. This fact certainly underscores their high potential for malignancy. The development of transitional cell carcinomas from a primary carcinoma-in-situ (intraurothelial carcinoma) played a much less significant role.

4. Proliferation Kinetics of Transformation Stages within Papillomas

a) Introduction

Our morphological investigations have delineated transitional cell carcinomas as a tumor form which develops predominantly from papillomas via a stepwise malignant transformation. In order to gather more precise information about proliferation kinetics in the various transformation stages we carried out autoradiographic studies. We were particularly interested in knowing what relationship exists between the ^{3}H-TdR index and the cell cycle time on the one hand, and histological and cytological changes in the respective cell populations on the other. Furthermore, our interest was directed toward possible changes of the ^{3}H-TdR index that might occur in the transformation stages with variously long exposure and induction times.

b) Material and Methods

The 177 female Wistar rats were subdivided into four groups, as already mentioned (Section III.3.; cf. Table 10). One hour before sacrifice each animal received 0.1 m Ci/100 g of 6-^{3}H-thymidine (specific activity 5 Ci/mMol) by the intraperitoneal route between 8.15 and 9.00 a.m. Autoradiograms were prepared by coating histological sections with Kodak AR 10 stripping film. The time of exposure was 14 days. All sections were stained with Mayer's haemalaun.

The ^{3}H-TdR index was determined in atypical urothelial areas, carcinomas-in-situ within papillomas, and well differentiated nonpapillary transitional cell carcinomas. For comparison the ^{3}H-TdR index was calculated in the surrounding apparently benign papillomatous structures. In particular the ^{3}H-TdR index was determined from atypical areas within papillomas in 10 animals in group II (exposure time: 80 days) with an induction time of 150 and 250 days respectively, and in five animals group IV (exposure time 150 days) with an induction time of 250 days (cf. Table 10; Fig. 30). In carcinomas-in-situ within papillomas (secondary carcinoma-in-situ) the ^{3}H-TdR index was measured in 10 animals each in group III (exposure time: 120 days) with induction times of 150 and 250 days, in nine animals in group II (exposure time: 80 days) with an induction time of 200 days, and in five animals in group IV (exposure time: 150 days) with an induction time of 200 days (cf. Table 10; Fig. 31). The cells synthesizing DNA were counted within the entire area of an atypical focus or of a carcinoma-in-situ. The cell counts were performed in 2–10 sections. In well differentiated transitional cell carcinomas the ^{3}H-TdR index was measured within the entire tumor of 2–4 sections.

In a further experimental series BBN was added to the drinking water of 16 rats (20 mg/kg body weight/day) for 80 consecutive days. After discontinuation of the carcinogen and a total experimental period (induction time) of 250 days, 6-^{3}H-thymidine was administered by intraperitoneal injection every six hours for a total period of 54 h, the dose being 0.1 m Ci/100 g body weight. The percentage of cells synthesizing DNA in relation to the entire cell population was determined in atypical foci, carcinomas-in-situ, and well differentiated, nonpapillary transitional cell carcinomas (grade II).

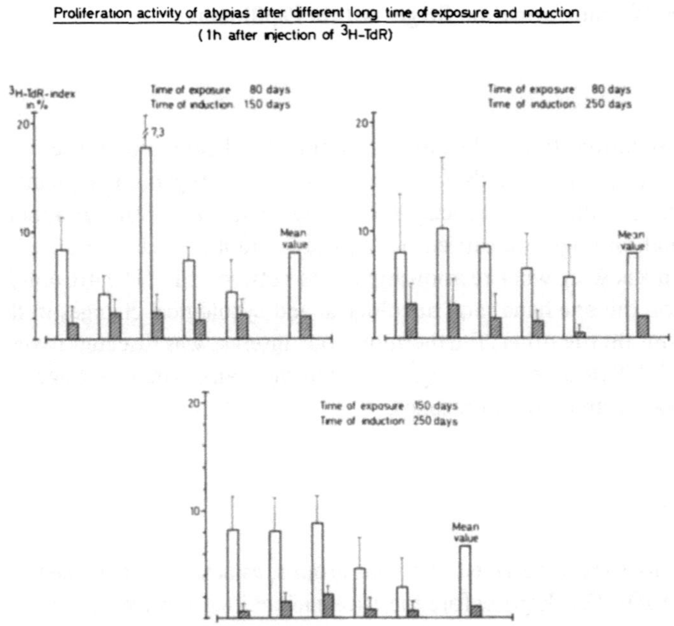

Fig. 30. ^{3}H-TdR index (% mean values ± S.E., using Student's *t*-test) of atypical areas within papillomas (white columns) and of surrounding apparently benign urothelial structures (hatched columns) after variously long exposure and induction times. (Z. Krebsforsch. *87*, 139–160, 1976)

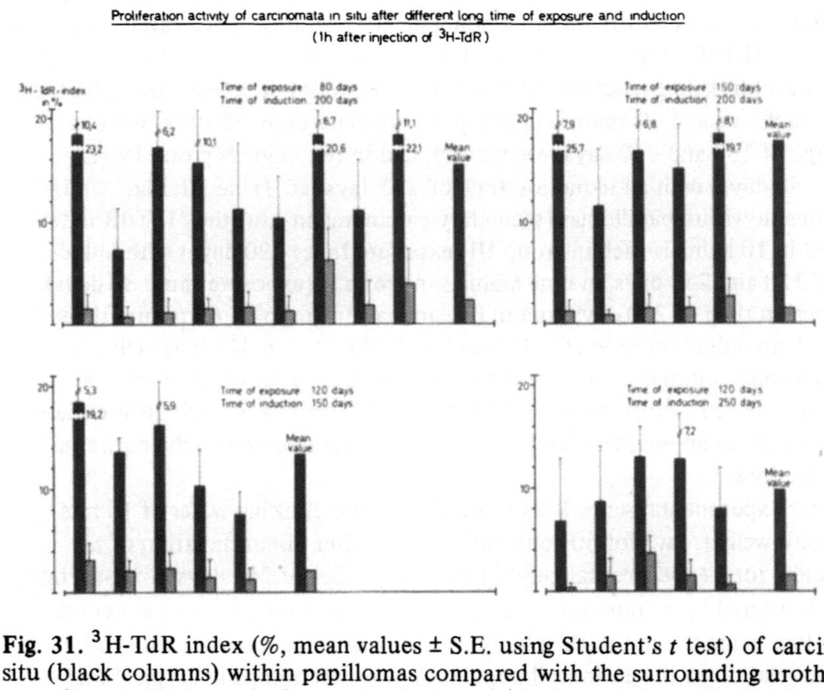

Fig. 31. ^{3}H-TdR index (%, mean values ± S.E. using Student's *t* test) of carcinomas in situ (black columns) within papillomas compared with the surrounding urothelial structures (hatched columns) after variously long time of exposure and induction. (Z. Krebsforsch. *87*, 139–160, 1976)

The duration of the cell cycle and its individual phases was determined by the percentage of labeled mitoses method (*Quastler* and *Sherman*, 1959) in atypical urothelial areas, carcinomas-in-situ within papillomas, and well differentiated nonpapillary transitional cell carcinomas (grade II). This method permits a direct measurement of the cell cycle and its phases, even with exponential growth. A total of 142 female Wistar rats (initial weight 180–220 g) were evaluated. The number of animals originally employed in the experiment was much larger. Each received 20 mg/kg/day BBN in its drinking water for an 80-day period. The total experimental time was 250 days. However, in many of the rats the evaluations could not carried out because the expected changes did not occur or were too slight. Before sacrifice, each rat received 0.1 m Ci/100 g of 6-^{3}H-thymidine (specific activity 3 Ci/mMol) intraperiteneally between 8.00 and 9.00 a.m. The radioactive testing time extended from one to 30 h, during which the animals were sacrificed at two-hour intervals. The urinary bladder of each animal was fixed for 24 h in 10% formaldehyde and cut into 60 to 80 sections 5 μm thick; autoradiograms were prepared from each one.

For setting up the curves for percentage of labeled mitoses the ratio of ^{3}H-labeled to nonlabeled mitoses was determined for the variously long radioactive testing periods. Only mitoses that contained at least five silver granules were considered labeled. At least 100 mitoses were counted from the late prophase to the early telophase. The incidence of labeled mitoses was plotted against time. The individual cycle phases were calculated as follows:

Mean cell cycle time (Tc): The difference in time between the two labeling peaks.

Mean DNA synthesis time (Ts): The difference between the intersection of the rising and falling parts of the curve at a labeling index of 50%.

Mean postsynthetic-premitotic phase and mitotic time ($TG_2 + M$): Difference between the time of injection and the point of reaching 50% labeling.

Mean postmitotic-presynthetic phase (TG_1): The difference between Ts and ($TG_2 + M$).

c) Results

α) ^{3}H-TdR Index after 1 hour of Radioactive Exposure

Atypical urothelial areas: The ^{3}H-TdR index, taking all the selected groups as a whole, averaged out to 7.6% in atypical urothelial areas within papillomas and to 1.8% in the surrounding apparently benign urothelial structures (Fig. 30). This meant a 4.3-fold increase ($P < 0.001$; Student's *t*-test). The degree of deviation from the mean, at times relatively large, corresponded to the wide differences in labeling values within the same atypical area. The length of the induction time did not substantially influence the proliferative activity (Fig. 30). This was confirmed by the fact that the ^{3}H-TdR index remained at average values of 8.0% and 7.8% for a total experimental time (induction time) of 150 and 250 days respectively. In both groups the exposure time was 80 days. Conversely, lengthening of the exposure time from 80 to 150 days, with a constant induction time of 250 days, caused no significant change in the ^{3}H-TdR index.

The mean mitotic index was 0.4% (n = 15) within atypical areas in all evaluated groups and 0.121% in the surrounding apparently benign urothelial structures. The increase of the mitotic index in focal atypias was 4.3-fold, which corresponded exactly to the rate of increase in the ^{3}H-TdR index.

Carcinomas-in-situ: An average ^{3}H-TdR index of 14.3% was determined in the carcinomas-in-situ within papillomas in all test groups; in the surrounding papillomatous structures a value of 1.9% was recorded (Fig. 31). The result here was a 7.5-fold increase, which was highly significant ($p < 0.001$; Student's *t*-test). Surrounding areas, which appeared benign by light microscopy, demonstrated approximately the same labeling index, irrespective of whether they bordered on atypia (1.8%) or carcinomas-in-situ (1.9%). Analogous to the result obtained from the atypical areas, there was no consistent relation between the exposure and induction time and the level of the ^{3}H-TdR index in the case of carcinomas-in-situ (Fig. 31). Thus there was no significant difference between the labeling index after an induction time of 150 and 250 days (13.4% and 9.9%) with a constant exposure time of 120 days. Nor did lengthening of the exposure time from 80 to 150 days with a constant induction time of 200 days lead to any significant change in the ^{3}H-TdR index (15.5% and 17.8%).

The mean mitotic index amounted to 0.77% (n = 21) in carcinomas-in-situ among the various test groups. An index of 0.124% was determined for the surrounding apparently benign urothelial structures. The 5.4-fold increase in the mitotic index was somewhat smaller than the increase in the ^{3}H-TdR index.

An average ^{3}H-TdR index of 8.2% was counted in well differentiated invasive nonpapillary transitional cell carcinomas (grade II; Table 11). The labeling index varied widely from carcinoma to carcinoma, as extreme values of 1.47% and 20.5% show. As a rule, the number of labeled cells was also very different within the same tumor from one area to another. The mean mitotic index amounted to 0.67% (Table 11).

Table 11. ^{3}H-TdR index (%; mean values ± S.E.) and mitotic rate (%; mean values ± S.E.) of well differentiated nonpapillary transitional cell carcinomas (grade II)

No. of animal	^{3}H-TdR index	Mitotic rate
1	3.09 ± 3.81	0.16 ± 0.43
2	1.83 ± 2.35	0.08 ± 0.28
3	8.67 ± 3.52	0.33 ± 0.66
4	13.93 ± 5.41	1.11 ± 0.76
5	13.54 ± 5.95	1.29 ± 0.85
6	20.50 ± 7.06	1.48 ± 0.97
7	8.93 ± 4.20	0.95 –
8	1.47 ± 5.15	0.01 –
9	2.93 ± 2.06	0.35 ± 0.56
10	7.01 ± 4.03	0.93 ± 0.85
Average	8.19	0.67

β) ^{3}H-TdR Index after 54 hours' Continuous Labeling

Average ^{3}H-TdR indices of 42.5% and 66.5%, respectively, were determined in atypical areas and carcinomas-in-situ within papillomas after 54 h of continuous labeling with ^{3}H-thymidine (Table 12). The differences in labeling between atypia and carcinoma-in-situ were highly significant ($p < 0.001$; Student's *t*-test).

γ) The Cell Cycle

The curves for percentage of labeled mitoses were almost identical in atypical urothelial areas and carcinomas-in-situ within papillomas and in well differentiated nonpapillary transitional cell carcinomas (Fig. 32). The three cell populations tested consistently exhibited a mean cell cycle time (Tc) of 16–18 h and a mean DNA-synthesis time of 8 h. The mean premitotic-postsynthetic phase together with the duration of mitosis (TG_2 + M) was between 2 and 3 h. The resulting mean time for the postmitotic-presynthetic phase (TG_1) would then be 6–7 h.

Table 12. ^{3}H-TdR index (%; mean values ± S.E.) of atypical urothelial areas and carcinomas-in-situ within papillomas after 54 h continuous labeling

No. of animal	Atypia	Carcinoma-in-situ
1	56.7 ± 12.2	72.6 ± 13.6
2	51.2 ± 16.4	59.7 ± 8.2
3	36.2 ± 10.7	64.9 ± 11.3
4	38.3 ± 12.5	57.2 ± 12.7
5	53.7 ± 14.6	68.6 ± 15.9
6	43.0 ± 11.0	76.9 ± 7.9
7	34.2 ± 11.9	50.2 ± 12.9
8	47.8 ± 14.2	80.4 ± 7.9
Average	45.2	66.5

d) Discussion

During the malignant transformation of papillomas it was possible to recognize a stepwise increased proliferative activity (*Kunze* et al., 1976). Atypical urothelial areas within papillomas had a ^{3}H-TdR index of 7.6%, carcinomas-in-situ one of 14.3%. This means 4.3-fold and 7.5-fold higher values than that in the surrounding papillomatous regions. The increase in proliferation activity was correspondingly much higher when compared with the urothelium of control bladders, in which we found an ^{3}H-TdR index of 0.26% (*Kunze* et al., 1975). The surrounding apparently benign urothelial structures had approximately the same ^{3}H-thymidine labeling index whether they bordered on atypical foci (1.8%) or carcinomas-in-situ (1.9). This fact underscores their biological equivalence, particularly regarding their potential for proliferation.

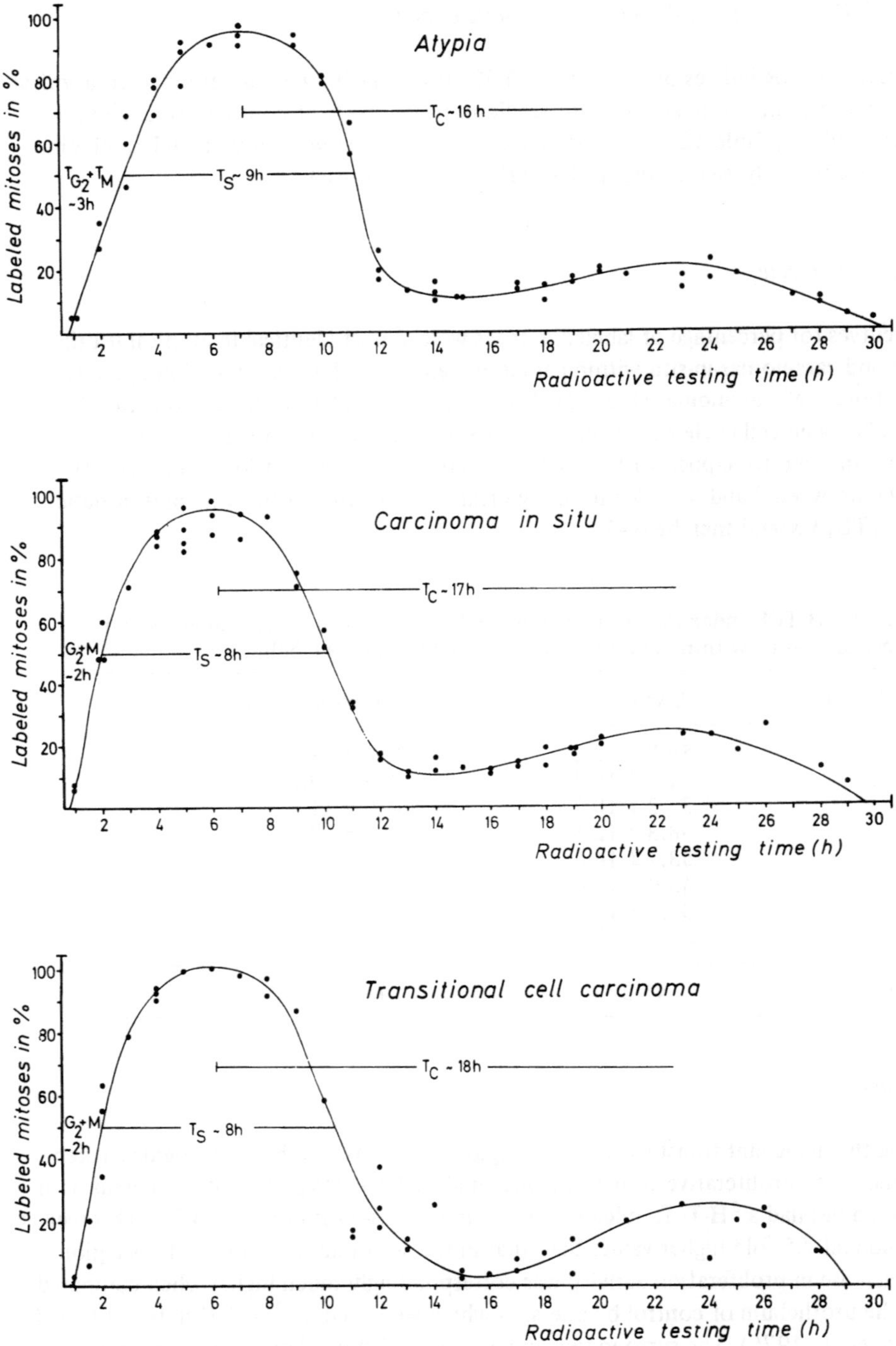

Fig. 32. Time of cell cycle and of individual phases of atypias, carcinomas-in-situ and well differentiated nonpapillary transitional cell carcinomas (percent labeled mitoses method). *Tc* = median cell cycle time. *Ts* = median DNA synthesis time; TG_2 + M = median postsynthetic-premitotic phase and mitotic time)

A likely explanation for the increase of the ^{3}H-TdR index is an enlargement of the proliferating pool or the p-compartment; shortening of the cell cycle time could not be proved. An increase in the fraction of proliferating cells would depend upon cells of the G_0 phase or "resting period," i.e., of the "q-compartments," which otherwise do not form a part of the proliferating pool, entering the cell cycle during carcinogenesis. The size of the p-compartment in the various transformation stages can best be estimated by approximation from the high ^{3}H-TdR index of 45.2% in the atypia or 66.5% in the carcinomas-in-situ, compared with the index of 1.22% in normal urothelium after 54 h of continuous labeling (cf. Section II.3.).

The time of the cell cycles and their individual phases averaged out to almost identical values in the cell populations of atypical foci, carcinomas-in-situ and well differentiated nonpapillary transitional cell carcinomas. Of course, cells or cell clones might have a cycle or phases deviant from the ascertained mean values. It would seem, however, that the determined duration of the cycles and the individual phases corresponds largely to the existent conditions, particularly since the atypias, carcinomas-in-situ and well differentiated transitional cell carcinomas were found to consist of a relatively homogeneous cell population under light microscopy. The situation was different in less differentiated transitional cell carcinomas, which exhibited as a rule a very heterogeneous cell population.

There are a number of possible explanations for the low level of the second labeling peak:

1. Some of the cells leave the p-compartment for the q-compartment after the first division and exclude themselves from further division for one or more cycles.
2. The cell cycle duration of some of the cells has such a prolonged G_1 phase that a second division extends beyond the 30 h of autoradiographic testing.
3. Some of the cells are lost after the first division due to necrosis. This cell loss factor cannot satisfactorily explain the low second peak; there were no extensive necroses in the cell populations tested as they were in most cases taken from completely developed tumors.
4. False-negativ findings in evaluation of labeled and nonlabeled mitoses result in a low percentage of labeled mitoses if the number of silver granules is reduced by prior division.

It seems particularly important to compare the cell cycle duration of the transformation stages and transitional cell carcinomas with that of papillomas without atypia and the normal bladder mucosa. Unfortunately there have been no investigations dealing with the cell cycle of the normal urothelium and papillomas. This is because the determination of the cell cycle with the percentage of labeled mitoses method is hardly practicable, because the normal bladder mucosa and papillomas exhibit a very low mitotic activity (cf. Section II.3.). Using the double-labeling method with ^{3}H- and ^{14}C-thymidine would permit measurement only of the DNA synthesis time, and not of the duration of the other cell-cycle phases. Furthermore it is questionable to determine the cell cycle time merely on the basis of the labeling and mitotic indices and the DNA synthesis time (*Leblond* et al., 1955; *Regele* and *Lunglmayer,* 1969; *Schreiber* et al., 1969), because it is not known whether all the cells participate in the proliferation. To be sure, one must assume that a large number of the normal urothelial cells remain in the q-compartment or even in the G_0 phase, as the bladder mucosa is tissue of the slow-proliferative type. A calculated cycle duration of the actually proliferating cells would thus be much too long.

After a comparison with investigations of other models of carcinogenesis one would be more likely to expect neoplastic cells to exhibit a shorter cycle time than cells of corresponding normal tissue (for a review of the literature see *Bresciani,* 1968). *Dörmer* et al. (1964) found a shortening of the cell cycle duration during carcinogenesis of the skin in the mouse: the normal epidermis exhibits a cycle time of 150 h, hyperplasia of 56 h and squamous cell carcinoma of 32 h. *Reiskin* and *Mendelsohn* (1964), inducing carcinomas in the cheek of the hamster, computed a cycle duration of 142 h for the basal cells of the normal mucosa, 42 h for hyperplasias and 20.7 h for carcinomas. *Bresciani* (1968) examining the breast of the mouse, ascertained a cell cycle time of 64 h in the normal "alveoli," 41 h in hyperplastic nodes, and 33 h in completely developed tumors. A shortening of the entire cycle duration was brought about by a shortening of all individual phases. Frequently there was a shortening of the post-mitotic-presynthetic TG_1 phase only, as in the case of fully developed tumors (for a review of the literature see *Lennartz,* 1969). A shortening of the cycle time does not appear to be essential for carcinogenesis, as it was once thought to be (review of literature: *Baserga,* 1964); a lengthed cycle has moreover been reported during tumor development. *Post* and coworkers (*Post* et al., 1963; *Post* and *Hoffmann,* 1964) were able to determine a cycle duration of 31 h in hepatomas induced with 3-methyl-4-dimethylaminoazobenzol; the cycle of normal hepatocytes of 4-week-old rats was just 21.5 h.

The great variability in labeling of well differentiated invasive nonpapillary transitional cell carcinomas (grade II), with indices of 1.5–20%, showed definitely that no clear-cut relation exists between the degree of differentiation and the synthesis of nucleic acids, as many authors assumed from their in-vitro labeling experiments with human tumor material (*Veenema* et al., 1965, 1971; *Battifiora* et al., 1965; *Hainau* and *Dombernowsky,* 1974). This underscores basically the results of *Levi* et al. (1969), who stated that no simple correlation exists between the labeling index and the histological grade in human bladder tumors of varying differentiation.

e) Summary

Autoradiographic investigations of the proliferation kinetics of transformation stages in bladder papillomas and well differentiated nonpapillary transitional cell carcinomas (grade II) yielded essentially the following results:

1. The ^{3}H-TdR index was 4.2 times higher in atypical urothelial areas (7.6%) and 7.5 times higher in carcinomas-in-situ (14.3%) than in the surrounding papillomatous structures which appeared benign under light microscrope. The length of exposure and induction times exercised no significant influence on the degree of proliferative activity.

2. The papillomatous structures without atypia demonstrated a rather constant ^{3}H-TdR index, whether they bordered on atypical foci (1.8%) or carcinomas-in-situ (1.9%).

3. The percentage of proliferating cells within the entire population after 54 h of continuous labeling was 54.2% in atypical urothelial areas and 66.5% in carcinomas-i-situ within papillomas. Normal bladder mucosa exhibited a mere 1.22% of DNA-synthesizing cells.

4. The mean cell cycle time (Tc), determined with the percentage of labeled mitoses method, was consistently 16–18 h in atypical urothelial areas and carcinomas-in-situ within papillomas and well differentiated nonpapillary transitional cell carcinomas. The mean DNA-synthesis time (Ts) took 8 h, the mean postsynthetic-premitotic phase and mitosis (TG_2 + M) 2.3 h.

5. It seems conceivable that the cause of the increased proliferative activity in the transformation stages in papillomas was due to an enlargement of the p-compartment, because the cell cycles and the individual phases were approximately equal in duration in the cell populations tested.

5. Morphology, Classification, and Histogenesis of Carcinomas

a) Introduction

The following investigations were carried out to clarify whether the various histological types of carcinomas occurring in the human bladder, their growth forms, and their biological behavior were reproducible with n-butyl-n-(4-hydroxybutyl)-nitrosamine in rats. The value of such an experimental model lies in the degree of conformity between induced tumors and human tumors; if this were high, it would permit conclusions to be drawn from animal experiments and applied to human pathology.

b) Material and Methods

The evaluation of the carcinoma findings included the 177 female Wistar rats (4 subgroups) which received BBN orally in the drinking water for variously long exposure and induction times, as already mentioned in Section III.3. Most of the bladders were fixed in 10% formaldehyde for 24 h, embedded in paraplast, and then cut into 80 serial and step sections of 5 μm thickness. As a rule the sections were stained with Mayer's haemalaun. PAS staining was used occasionally. A smaller number of bladders were embedded in methacrylate and cut into 80 to 100 serial sections of approximately 1–2 μm thickness. The semithin sections were stained with the Goldner trichrome stain.

c) Results

α) Macroscopic Findings

The largest number of fully developed invasive carcinomas and papillomas with circumscribed invasive growth (malignantly transformed papillomas) was observed in the animals subjected to the longest induction time of 250 days (time of exposure: 80 or 120 days, respectively). The same finding was seen in the rats that received the highest total dose of carcinogen [time of exposure: 150 days; time of induction: 200 or 250 days (cf. Table 10)]. The size of the tumors increased in proportion to the length of

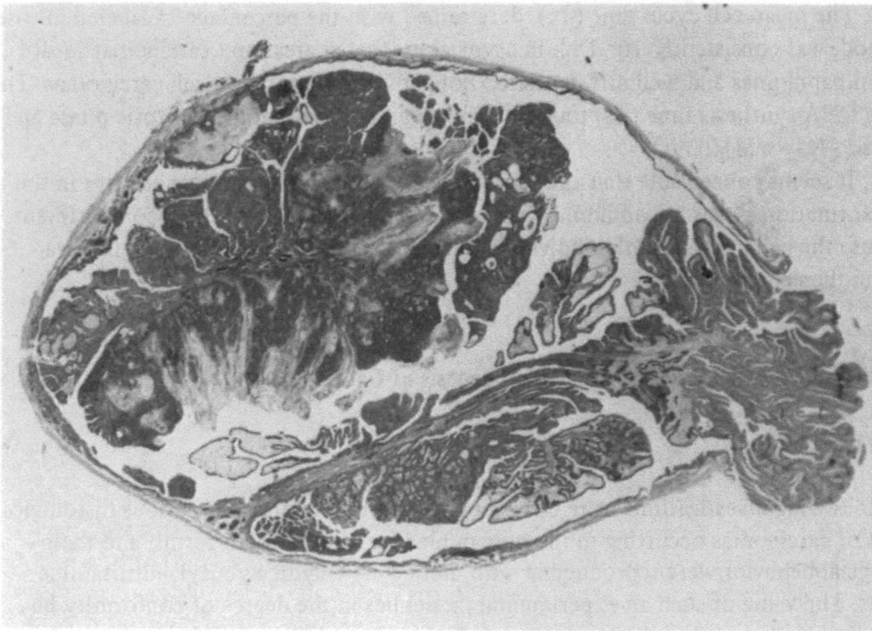

Fig. 33. Enormously enlarged urinary bladder filled up with papillary tumors induced by *BBN*

the induction time as well as to the total dose of the carinogen. The completely developed carcinomas exhibited predominantly an exophytic growth pattern and were generally attached to the bladder wall by a broad base. Quite frequently the entire bladder was filled with the extending tumor mass (Fig. 33). The largest bladder measured was 2.5 × 1.5 × 1 cm. Animals with advanced carcinomas usually showed hematuria. Only in isolated cases did we find hydronephrosis or a hydroureter. No tumors of the ureter were demonstrable. In two animals we found metastases in the lung. No primary tumors were found other than in the bladder.

β) Microscopic Findings

We have designated fully developed carcinomas only such tumors as were composed throughout of invasively growing cells and showed no papillomatous structures. However, in the statistical evaluation we included malignantly transformed papillomas exhibiting an invasive growth focally. Our classification of bladder carcinomas is based on those of *Dukes* and *Masina* (1949), Institute of Urology, London (1955), *Mostofi* (1973), and *Koss* (1975):

αα) Transitional cell carcinoma
Nonpapillary (solid) type
Papillary type
Variants with squamous and glandular metaplasia.
ββ) Squamous cell carcinoma
γγ) Adenocarcinoma
δδ) Undifferentiated carcinoma.

Table 13 lists the frequency of each tumor type occurring in our experimental series:

Table 13. Frequency (%) of various histological type of carcinomas induced with n-butyl-n-(4-hydroxybutyl)-nitrosamine (n = 176). The classification includes fully developed invasive carcinomas and malignantly transformed papillomas (papillomas with focally invasive growth).

Type of Carcinoma	Frequency (%)
Transitional cell carcinoma	88.8
Squamous cell carcinoma	5.1
Mixed type (transitional and squamous cell carcinomas)	2.8
Adenocarcinoma	2.2
Undifferentiated carcinoma	1.1

αα) Transitional cell carcinoma
Nonpapillary (solid) type)

When we began our investigations we distinguished between well and poorly differentiated transitional cell carcinomas in accordance with the Institute of Urology, London (1955). The well differentiated type corresponds broadly to grade I–II, the poorly differentiated to grade III by the definition of *Mostofi* (1973) and *Koss* (1975), as used first by *Broders* (1922).

The well differentiated nonpapillary transitional cell carcinoma (grade II) was characterized by invasively growing cancer cells arranged in broad strands, sheets or nests (Fig. 34a). The amount of interspersed stroma varied widely. As a rule it was barely developed; however, sometimes it occurred abundantly, demonstrating only scattered small clusters of carcinoma cells. The neoplastic urothelial cells appeared uniform and contained a round to oval nucleus, which showed minimal to moderate enlargement. One prominent nucleolus was generally present; in rare instances several were seen. The nuclear-cytoplasmic ratio was largely unchanged, the mitotic activity low to moderate. Pseudoglandular structures appeared occasionally in the tumors and consisted of irregulary shaped gland-like structures of varying size (Fig. 35). At times

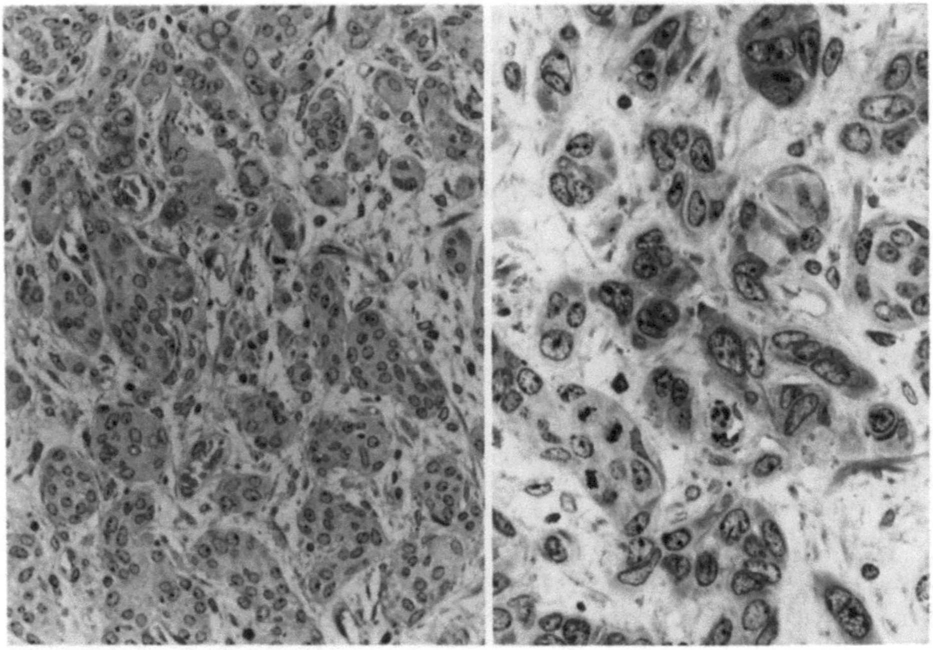

Fig. 34a and b. a Well differentiated nonpapillary transitional cell carcinoma (grade II) with moderate stroma development (methacrylate embedding; Goldner trichrome strain). Time of exposure *(BBN)*: 120 days. Total experimental period: 200 days. 190 X. **b** Poorly differentiated nonpapillary transitional cell carcinoma (grade III) showing marked polymorphism of the nuclei and increased mitotic activity (methacrylate embedding; Goldner trichrome stain. Time of exposure *(BBN)*: 120 days. Total experimental period: 250 days. 240 X. (Z. Krebsforsch. *88*,273–289, 1977)

the pseudoglandular structures were cystically dilated and bordered by a layer of highly flattened neoplastic urothelial cells reminiscent of endothelium. Frequently exfoliated and necrotic cells were seen in the lumina.

The poorly differentiated transitional cell carcinoma (grade III) displayed marked disorganization in tissue and cell structure in comparison with the well differentiated type (Fig. 34b). Yet derivation of the cancer cells from the urothelium was still recognizable. The cells of this tumor type were characterized by enlarged and irregularly shaped, polymorphic nuclei, an irregular chromatin pattern, and greatly enlarged and sometimes bizarrely formed nucleoli. The nuclear-cytoplasmic ratio shifted in favor of the nucleus. Many atypical mitoses were present.

Fig. 36a and b. a Partial view of a papillary transitional cell carcinoma with moderate nuclear atypism (grade II; hematoxylin). Time of exposure *(BBN)*: 150 days. Total experimental period: 250 days. 190 X. **b** Clear-cell variant of a papillary transitional cell carcinoma exhibiting markedly distended and pale cytoplasm of the neoplastic urothelial cells. Time of exposure *(BBN)*: 150 days. Total experimental period: 150 days. 480 X. (Z. Krebsforsch. *88*, 273–289, 1977)

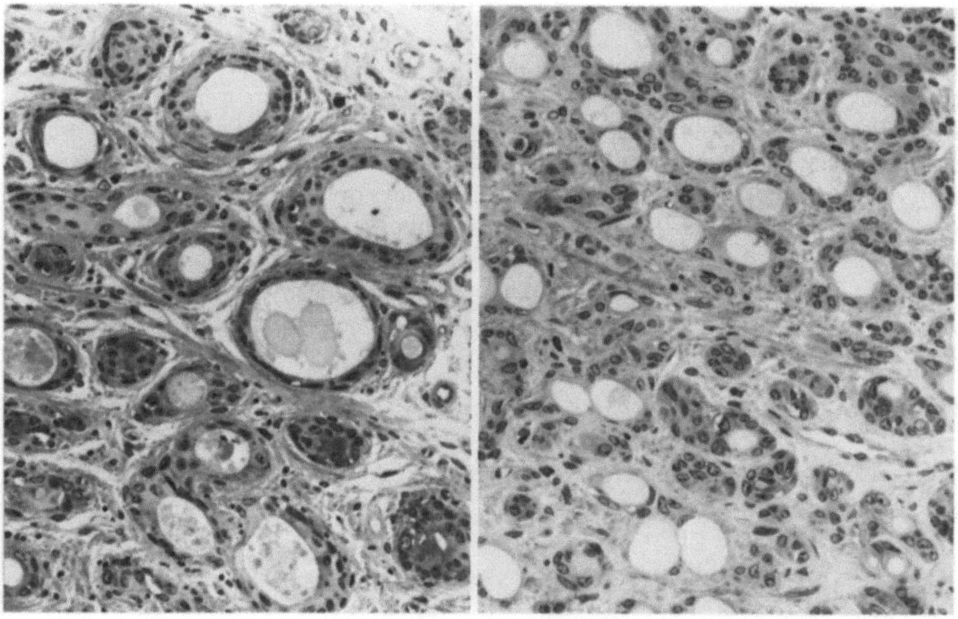

Fig. 35a and b. Well differentiated nonpapillary transitional cell carcinoma with pseudoglandular structures (methacrylate embedding; Goldner trichrome stain). Time of exposure *(BBN)*: 120 days. Total experimental period: 200 (**a**) and 250 (**b**) days. 190 ×. (Z. Krebsforsch. *88*, 273–289, 1977)

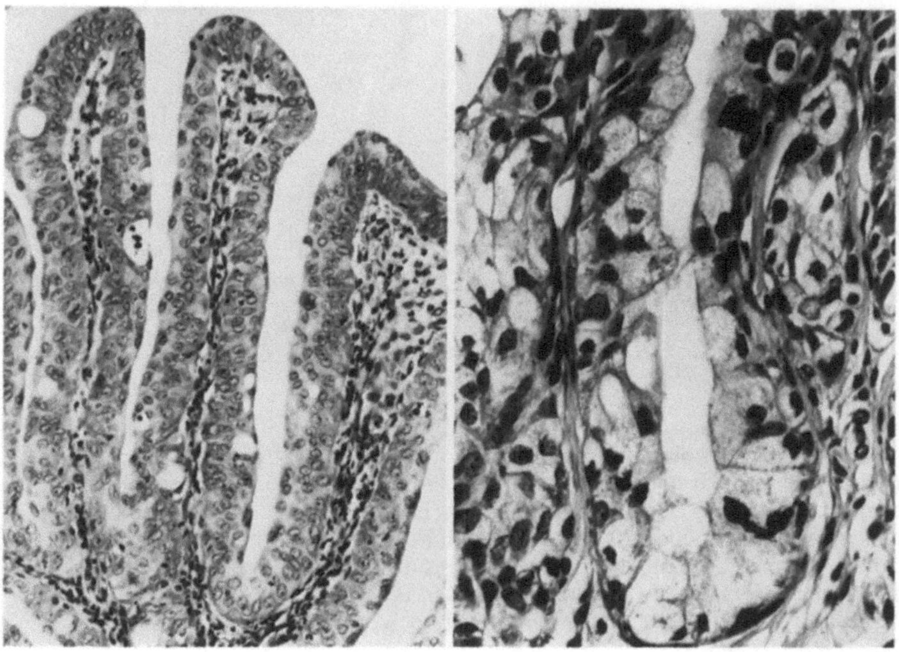

Fig. 36a and b. Legend see page 206

Papillary type

The papillary type of transitional cell carcinoma was composed of papillary fronds covered by a varying number of cell layers (Fig. 36). As a rule there were between two and eight layers. The vast majority of papillary carcinomas showed cells with only minimal to moderate atypism (grade II). Invasive growth occurred seldom. Where no invasive growth was present the only distinguishing features over and against a papilloma were the atypism of the nuclei and the increased mitotic activity. At times a clear cell variant was observed whose cells showed an extremely distended and pale cytoplasm (Fig. 36b). Besides carcinomas formed of either solid or papillary elements throughout, mixed types occurred containing both elements.

Variants with squamous and glandular metaplasia

Nonpapillary transitional cell carcinomas quite often showed focal squamous metaplasia, at times with extreme keratinization. Circumsribed areas of columnar meta-

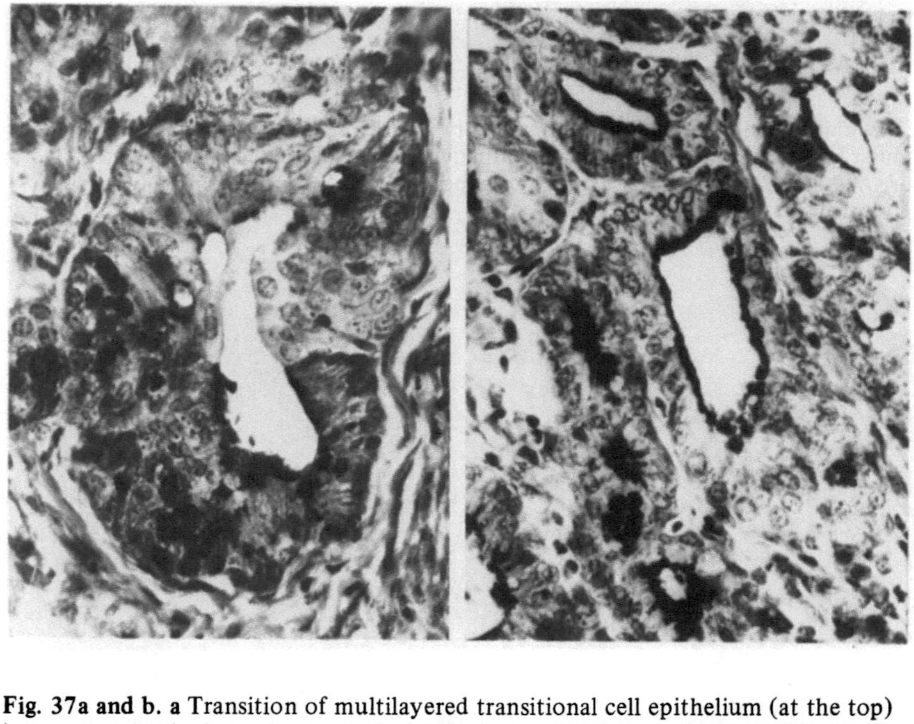

Fig. 37a and b. a Transition of multilayered transitional cell epithelium (at the top) into mucus-producing columnar cells (at the bottom). Mucus substances (black) distributed in fine granular deposits throughout cytoplasm or in form of large globules. Incipient extrusion into the lumen (PAS stain). Time of exposure *(BBN):* 80 days. Total experimental period: 250 days. 480 X. **b** Focal glandular metaplasia within a nonpapillary transitional cell carcinoma. Mucus substances (black) localized predominantly in the apical parts of the cytoplasm and in the lumen (PAS stain). Time of exposure *(BBN):* 80 days. Total experimental period: 250 days. 480 X. (Z. Krebsforsch. *88,* 273–289, 1977)

plasia with glandular structures were seen far less frequently (Fig. 37). The glands were generally lined with a single layer of mucus-producing columnar cells with a basally displaced nucleus. Sometimes the epithelium was also multilayered. In PAS staining the mucous substances were seen to have a diffuse though fine granular distribution within the entire cytoplasm.

Sometimes the mucus was predominantly located in the apical parts of the cytoplasm prior to extrusion into the lumen. Not infrequently the lining cells were packed with mucus and appeared severely distended and pale (Fig. 38). At times areas of pseudoglandular structures demonstrated a direct transition of transitional epithelium into mucus-producing columnar cells (Fig. 37a). More rarely, areas of neoplastic urothelial cells, squamous cell formations, and glandular strucutres were seen all next to each other in the same tumor (Fig. 38).

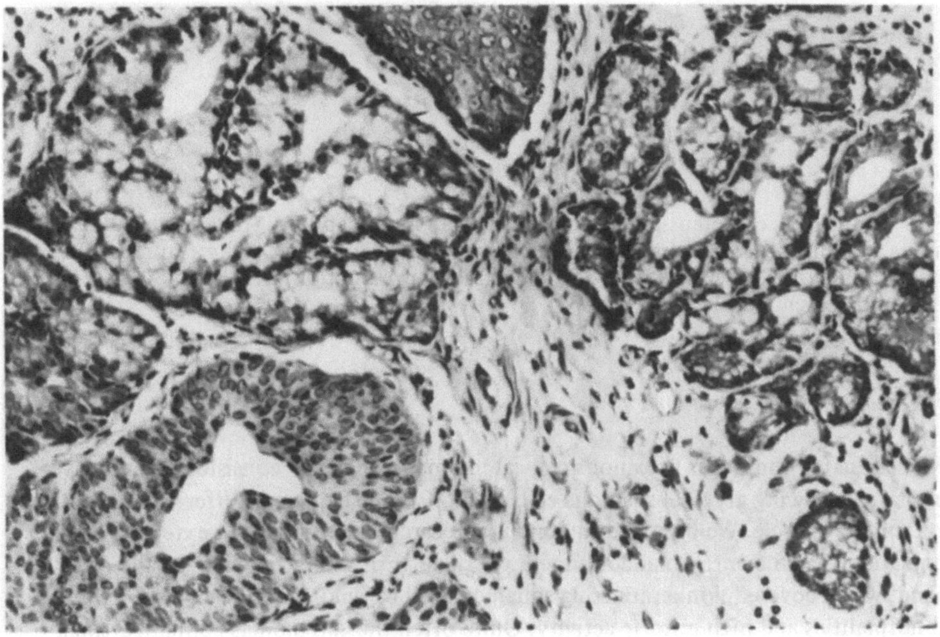

Fig. 38. Close association of neoplastic urothelial cell groups (lower left), squamous epithelia (upper middle) and glandular, mucus-producing structures (upper left and right; hematoxylin). Time of exposure *(BBN):* 120 days. Total experimental period: 200 days. 190 X. (Z. Krebsforsch. *88,* 273–289, 1977)

Infrequently, clusters of mucus-producing cells were found in nonpapillary transitional cell carcinomas without the formation of glandular structures or columnar cell metaplasia (Fig. 39). The distribution of the mucus varied: in some cells fine granular deposits were noted only within the Golgi area, while in others the entire cytoplasm showed a massive storage of fine and coarse granular mucus. Typical signet ring cells were not observed.

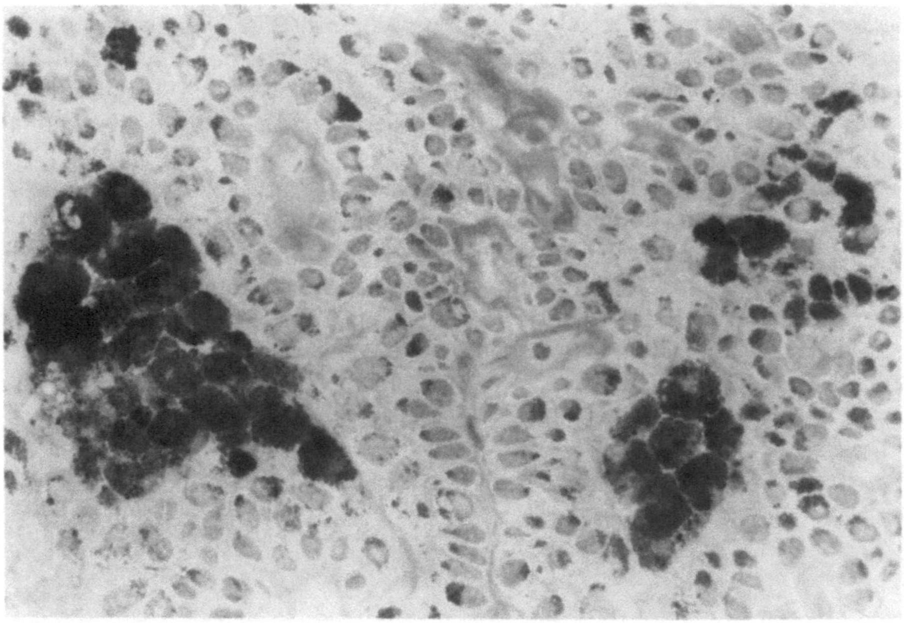

Fig. 39. Clusters of mucus-producing cells within a nonpapillary transitional cell carcinoma without development of glandular structures or columnar cell metaplasia (PAS stain). Time of exposure *(BBN)*: 350 days. Time of induction: 150 days. 500 X. Z. (Z. Krebsforsch. *88*, 273–289, 1977)

ββ) Squamous cell carcinoma

We designated tumors as squamous cell carcinomas when they consisted exclusively of invasively growing atypical sqamous cells (Fig. 40). The degree of differentiation was extremely variable. We observed squamous cell carcinomas with such extensive keratinization that the entire bladder lumen was filled with a keratin mass. On the other hand, we discovered nonkeratinizing squamous cell carcinomas with marked cellular abnormalities and high mitotic activity. Quite often the carcinomas contained small necrotic areas, which upon resorption produced a pseudoglandular appearance (Fig. 40b).

γγ) Adenocarcinoma

Adenocarcinomas consisted of irregularly shaped, sometimes cystically dilated glands, which were lined with one or more layers of cuboidal or columnar cells (Fig. 41a). The cellular atypism and the mitotic activity were moderate. No highly differentiated mucus-producing adenocarcinomas or colloid carcinomas were observed. Not to be confused or identified with invasive adenocarcinomas are the tumor-like forms of proliferative cystitis cystica and cystitis glandularis (Fig. 41b). The glandular structures of

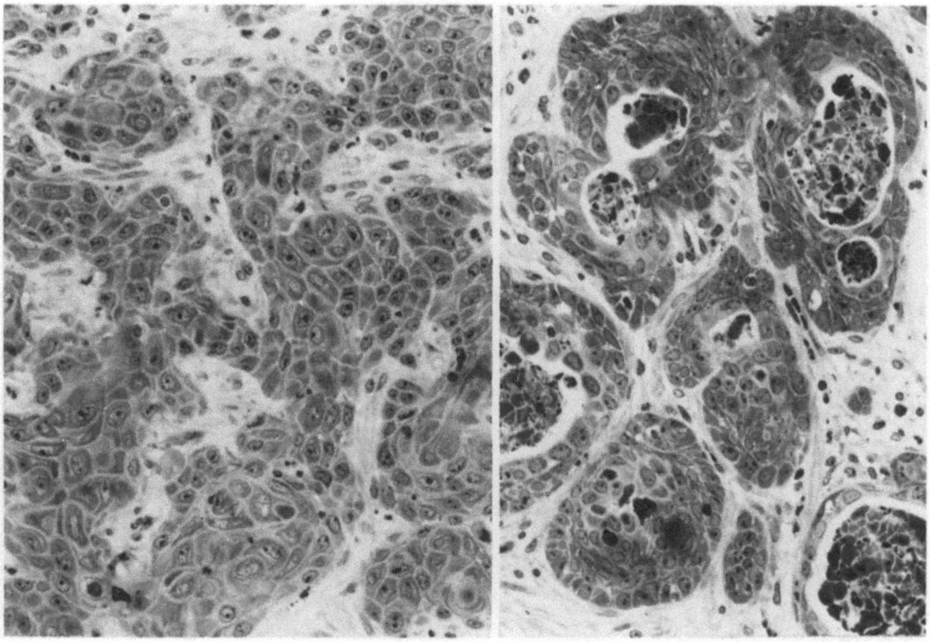

Fig. 40a and b. Squamous cell carcinoma. Note central necrotic areas with incipient development of pseudoglandular structures **b** (methacrylate embedding; Goldner trichrome stain). Time of exposure *(BBN)*: 150 **a** and 120 **b** days. Total experimental period: 250 days. 190 X. (Z. Krebsforsch. *88*, 273–289, 1977)

cystitis cystica and glandularis showed no cellular atypism and no essential mitotic activity in the present experimental series, which distinguishes them from carcinomas. Furthermore, we did not find transition of von Brunn's nests, cystitis cystica and cystitis glandularis into invasive adenocarcinomas. However, these proliferative lesions of the urothelium were observed rather infrequently in the present experimental series.

δδ) Undifferentiated carcinoma

We were able to distinguish a small-cell, a giant-cell and a spindle-cell variant of undifferentiated bladder carcinomas. The small-cell carcinoma (Fig. 42a) was composed of relatively uniform cells with a small round to oval nucleus, a dense chromatin structure and only a small rim of cytoplasm. Certain similarities with the oat-cell carcinoma of the lung were thus apparent. It was not possible to recognize an origin of the small cancer cells from the urothelium.

In one case we found a giant-cell carcinoma, which consisted of highly polymorphic cells with bizarrely formed and hyperchromatic nuclei (Fig. 42b). Frequently multinucleated giant cells occurred. There was a large number of predominantly atypical mitoses. The stroma was made up of loosely packed and edematous connective tissue.

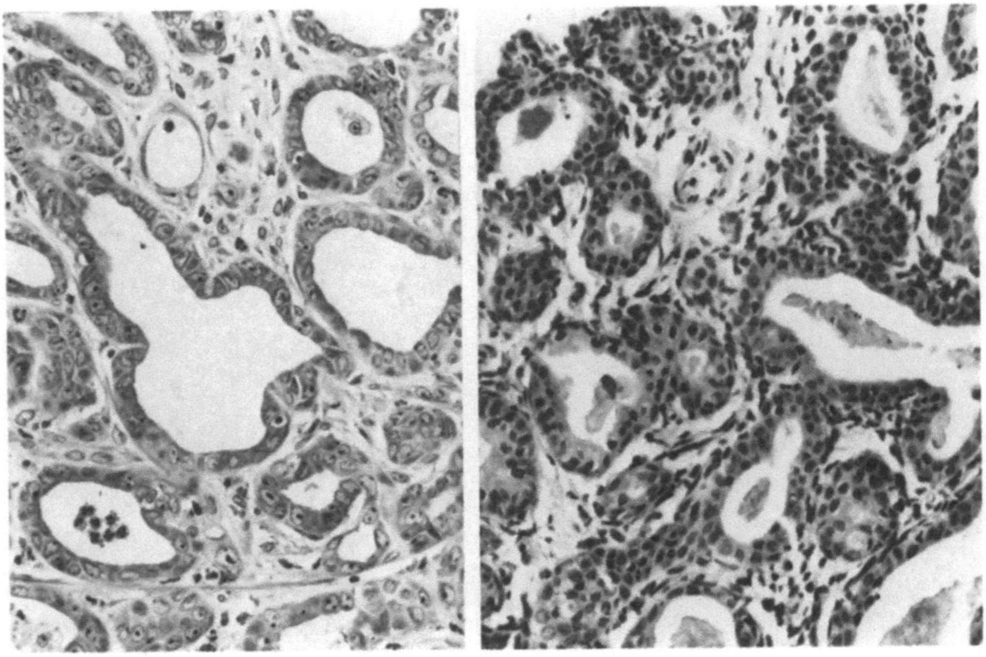

Fig. 41a and b. a Non-mucus producing adenocarcinoma with abundant stroma development (methacrylate embedding; Goldner trichrome stain). Time of exposure *(BBN):* 120 days. Total experimental period: 250 days. 190 X. **b** Pronounced cystitis cystica with tumorlike proliferating urothelial cells without cellular atypism. Part of the bladder lumen in the left upper corner (hematoxylin). Time of exposure *(BBN):* 80 days. Time of induction: 250 days. 180 X. (Z. Krebsforsch. *88,*, 273–289, 1977)

The histological features of the giant-cell carcinomas closely resembled the embryonal rhabdomyosarcoma (botryoid sarcoma). However, cytoplasmic cross-striations were not demonstrable. In addition in this case, a transition of nonpapillary transitional cell carcinoma into the giant-cell carcinoma was present; this surely indicates an epithelial origin of the tumor.

Undifferentiated spindle-cell carcinomas were made up of spindly, elongated cells, often arranged in parallel or whorled bundles. This histological pattern was very much like that of sarcomas, but we regularly observed the transition of squamous or transitional cell carcinomas into spindle-cell carcinomas. Mixed tumor types occurred, frequently consisting of well differentiated and undifferentiated forms (Figs. 43–45).

Fig. 43. Mixed type of well differentiated nonpapillary transitional cell carcinoma and undifferentiated carcinoma (hematoxylin). Time of exposure *(BBN):* 150 days. Total experimental period: 250 days. 190 X. (Z. Krebsforsch. *88,* 273–289, 1977)

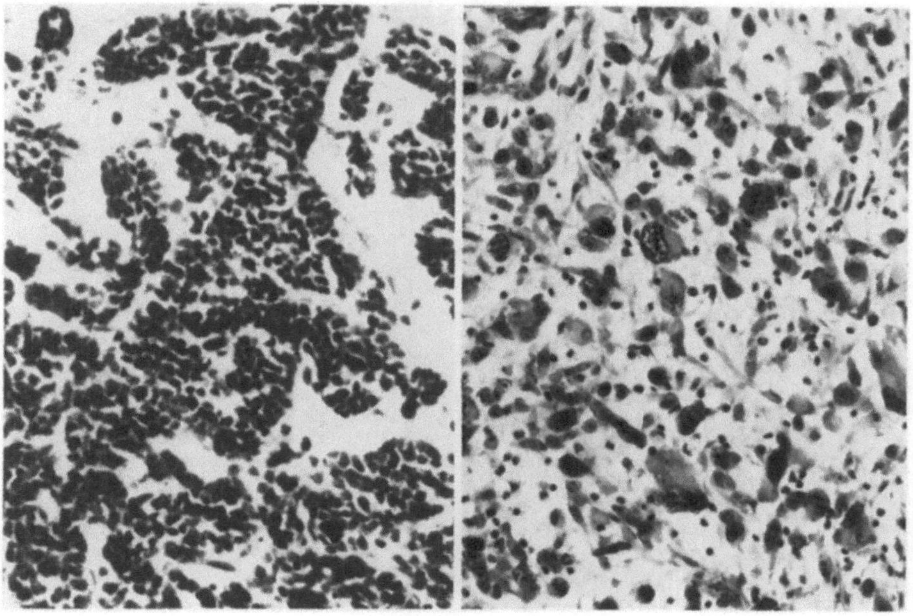

Fig. 42a and b. Undifferentiated carcinoma. Small **a** and giant cell type **b** (hematoxylin). Time of exposure *(BBN):* 150 **a** and 80 **b** days. Total experimental period: 250 days. 150 X **a** and 190 X **b**. (Z. Krebsforsch. *88*, 273–289, 1977)

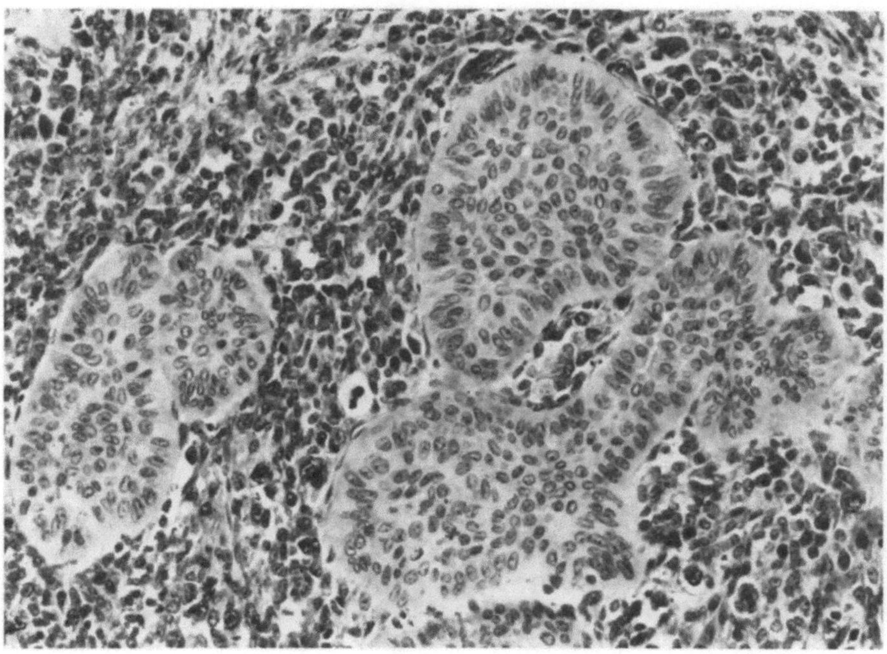

Fig. 43. Legend see page 212

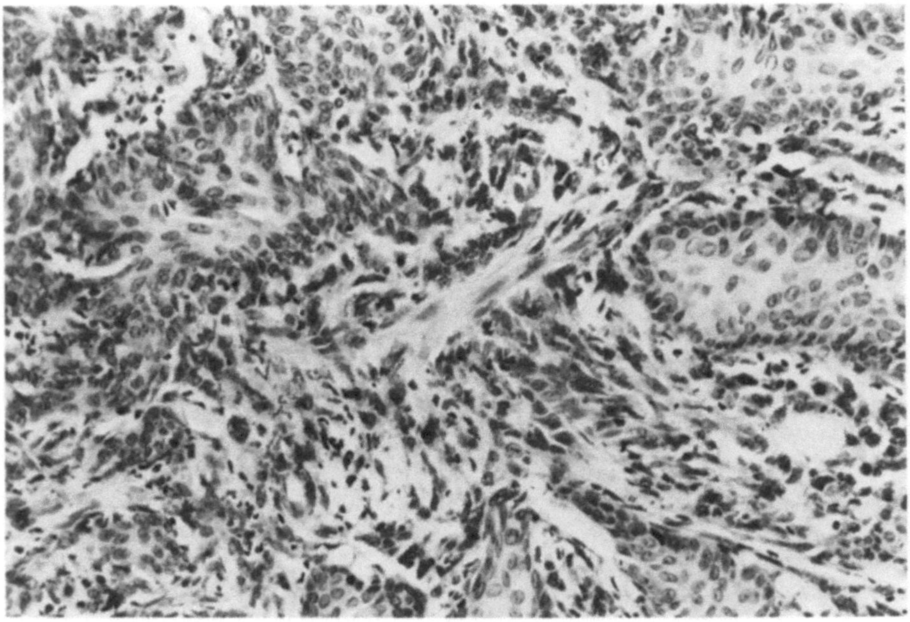

Fig. 44. Nonpapillary transitional cell carcinoma with an undifferentiated spindle-cell component. Time of exposure *(BBN)*: 150 days. Total experimental period: 200 days. 180 X

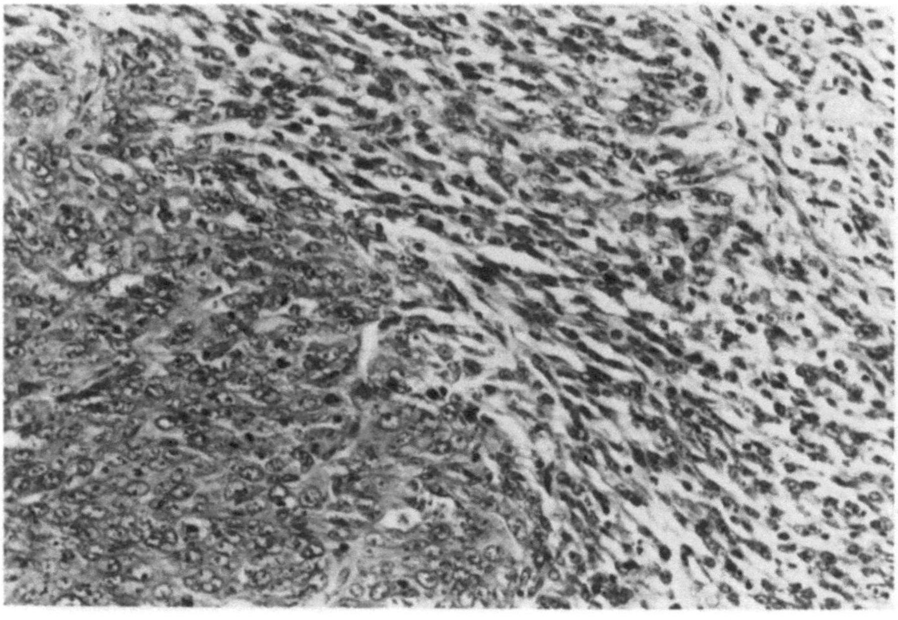

Fig. 45. Transition of a squamous cell carcinoma in a spindle-cell component. Time of exposure *(BBN)*: 80 days. Total experimental period: 250 days. 190 X

d) Discussion

The experiments have shown that all the usually occurring types of carcinomas in the human bladder were reproducible in rats with n-butyl-n-(4-hydroxybutyl)-nitrosamine (*Kunze* and *Schauer,* 1977). In addition, we might note that the relative frequency of each type of carcinoma, its form of growth, and, apparently, its biological behavior were for the most part quite similar in humans and rats. These findings are true for the carcinomas caused by occupational carcinogens such as β-naphthylamine, benzidine or 4-aminodiphenyl (for a review of the literature see *Temkin,* 1963), as well as for tumors whose etiology is still unknown.

Transitional cell carcinomas were by far the most frequently occurring type of carcinoma in rats (88.8%). This is quite consistent with the findings in the human bladder. The papillary type, as against the nonpapillary, rarely exhibited invasive growth. Delineation of these forms over and against papillomas was often only possible on the basis of cellular atypism and the increased proliferative activity. From this point of view it is understandable that in man the prognosis of papillary transitional cell carcinomas is essentially better than that of the nonpapillary type.

Squamous cell carcinomas were found in the animal experiments with a frequency of 5.1%. Statistics relating to squamous cell carcinoma in the human bladder give an incidence of 1.6–11.4% (Table 14). In the case of bilharziasis the situation is quite different; 40–60% of the tumors encountered are squamous cell carcinomas (*Goebel,* 1905; *Ferguson,* 1911; *Dimette* et al., 1956; *Hashem,* 1961; *Gilman* and *Prates,* 1962 *Aboul Nasr* et al., 1962).

Adenocarcinomas made up 2.2% of the carcinomas in the animal experiments. In the human bladder they occur with an incidence of 0.2–2.0% (Table 15), being more frequently encountered in the exstrophic bladder (for reviews of the literature see *Goyanna* et al., 1951; *Wattenberg* et al., 1956). Besides, carcinomas of urachal origin are almost exclusively adenocarcinomas (*Wheeler* and *Hill,* 1954; *Mostofi* et al., 1955;

Table 14. Incidence (%) of squamous cell carcinomas in the urinary bladder of man

Incidence (%)	Authors
1.6	*Pugh,* 1959
1.6	*Miller* et al., 1969
2.9	*Schauer* et al., 1971
3.4	*Ludvig* and *Zinnbauer,* 1971
3.9	*Hollands,* 1952
4.3	*Dunham* et al., 1968
5.0	*Maruchi* et al., 1974
5.0	*Selberg,* 1964
6.2	*Urlesberger,* 1965
6.7	*Francis,* 1961
7.8	*Kretschmer* et al., 1934
8.5	*Guira,* 1971
9.0	*Cox* et al., 1969
11.4	*Melicow,* 1955

Table 15. Incidence (%) of adenocarcinomas in the urinary bladder of man

Incidence (%)	Authors
0.2	*Miller* et al., 1969
0.4	*Culver* et al., 1942
0.4	*Pugh*, 1959
0.5	*Peacock* and *Corbett*, 1930
0.5	*Melicow*, 1955
0.6	*Howard* and *Bergmann*, 1948
0.6	*Sandrey*, 1967
0.8	*Thomas* et al., 1971
0.9	*Urlesberger*, 1965
1.0	*Dean* et al., 1954
1.0	*Francis*, 1961
1.1	*Dunham* et al., 1968
1.5	*Dean* and *Ash*, 1950
1.8	*Guira*, 1971
2.0	*Cox* et al., 1969
2.0	*Ludvig* and *Zinnbauer*, 1971
2.0	*Maruchi* et al., 1974

Thomas et al., 1971). Highly differentiated mucus-producing adenocarcinoma of the exstrophic bladder of urachal origin did not occur in animal experiments. Signet ring cell carcinomas, which rarely develop in humans (*Mostofi* et al., 1955; *Saphir*, 1955; *Rosas-Uribe* and *Luna*, 1969; *Naeim* et al., 1972), were not among the induced tumors. Clusters of mucus-producing cells occurred rather infrequently in nonpapillary transitional cell carcinomas of the rat; however, when they did, the typical appearance of signet ring cells was missing. An analogous finding has been reported in man (*Hamperl* and *Hellweg*, 1957; *Feyrter*, 1956; *Fischer*, 1958; *Forster* and *Levine*, 1963). It is conceivable that signet ring cell carcinomas develop at some later date in such areas.

Only 1.1% of the carcinomas in the rat were of the undifferentiated type. In humans undifferentiated carcinomas are just as infrequent.

Epithelial tumors were the only type induced experimentally, one difference in the tumor spectrum between humans and rats. In the human urinary bladder 95–97% of the tumors encountered are of epithelial origin, and approximately 3–5% are either benign or malignant tumors of nonepithelial origin. The incidence of sarcomas was 0.25–0.6% (*Thompson* and *Coppridge*, 1959; *Francis*, 1961; *Dunham* et al., 1968). Rhabdomyosarcomas (*Kretschmer*, 1947; *Young-Blood* et al., 1952; *Mostofi* and *Morse*, 1952; *Flocks* and *Culp*, 1955; *Maletta* and *Horton*, 1959; *Legier*, 1961; *Hellstrom* and *Fischer*, 1961; *Batsakis*, 1963) and leiomyosarcomas (*Silbar* and *Silbar*, 1955; *Bohne* et al., 1962; *Brown*, 1965) have been frequently observed, and rarely fibrosarcomas (*Thompson* and *Coppridge*, 1959), osteogenic sarcomas (*Powers* et al., 1956; *Pang Shu-Chao*, 1958; *Nicolai* and *Spjut*, 1959) and primary malignant lymphomas (*Borski*, 1960; *Pontius* et al., 1963; *Santino* et al., 1970).

The existence of carcinosarcomas has been much disputed, although it has been reported in isolated cases in humans (*Saphir* and *Vass*, 1938; *Du Bose Dent*, 1961; *Brinton* et al., 1970). The animal experiments presented evidence that does not support existence of genuine carcinosarcomas. The sarcoma-like portions of the transitional and squamous cell carcinomas revealed their origin from the epithelial part of the tumor, and as such must be considered as an undifferentiated epithelial component.

The histogenesis of adenocarcinoma and squamous cell carcinomas presents a problem, as the bladder normally contains neither columnar nor squamous epithelium (for reviews of the literature see *Coppridge* et al., 1951; *Mostofi* et al., 1955; *Shaw* et al., 1958; *Allen* and *Henderson,* 1965). Three possible explanations have been proposed:

1. The anatomical hypothesis which claims that adenocarcinomas develop from normally occurring glandular tissue of the trigone can be discarded; every attempt to demonstrate glandlike tissue in the trigone to date has failed. Even if the supposed glandular tissue described by *Albarran* (1892) did exist in the trigone, it would be very difficult to explain the development of adenocarcinomas outside of the tirgone. For the same reason it seems rather improbable that adenocarcinomas of the bladder develop from prostatic glands located in the trigone (for a review of the literature see *Begg,* 1931).

2. An embryological hypothesis claims that adenocarcinomas start from residual tissue of the cloaca. This hypothesis seems quite plausible at first, because both the rectum and the largest part of the bladder originate from the cloaca, which is potentially capable of differentiating into glandular and transitional cell epithelium. However, residual cloacal tissue in the bladder has not been demonstrated, which makes it seem that this hypothesis is untrue after all.

3. A metaplastic theory postulates the transformation of transitional epithelium into columnar and glandular epithelium; this would then provide the basis for the development of adenocarcinomas after a malignant transformation was induced. This theory is accepted by the majority of authors as the most probable (*Patch* and *Rhea,* 1935; *Mostofi,* 1954; *Wheeler* and *Hill,* 1954; *Melicow,* 1955; *Mostofi* et al., 1955; *Johnson,* 1957; *Shaw* et al., 1958; *Gordon,* 1963; *Allen* and *Henderson,* 1965; *Ward,* 1971). The most important facts in favor of this hypothesis are that adenocarcinomas in man develop almost exclusively in the exstrophic bladder (*Graham,* 1942; *Abeshouse,* 1943; *Goyanna* et al., 1951; *Wattenberg* et al., 1956) or in the urachus (*Begg,* 1931; *Wheeler* and *Hill,* 1954; *Mostofi* et al., 1955; *Fischer,* 1958; *Thomas* et al., 1971) although the urachus (*Begg,* 1931) and the exstrophic bladder (*Enderlen,* 1904; *Formiggini,* 1920; *Graham,* 1942) are both primarily lined with transitional epithelium and possess neither embryonic remnants nor glandular tissue.

The metaplastic theory was substantiated in our experiments. They showed quite clearly that glandular structures developed histogenetically in two successive steps. In a first stage pseudoglandular structures were formed in areas of solid transitional cell or squamous cell carcinomas by focal necrosis and ensuing resorption of the necrotic material, with resulting development of "lumina." In a second stage, the cells bordering the lumina were transformed into columnar epithelium, with concomitant development of true glands. In the experiments it was possible at times to observe this transition directly. Foci of glandular metaplasia can also be found in transitional cell carcinoma of the human urinary bladder (*Ash,* 1940; *Dukes* and *Masina,* 1949; *Pugh,* 1959; *Dukes,* 1959; *Mills,* 1964; *Sandrey,* 1967; *Mostofi,* 1968; *Ward,* 1971). Paneth or argentaffin cells were not observed in the experimentally induced metaplasias. *Gordon* (1963) has reported the occurrence of paneth and argentaffin cells in human bladder carcinomas. This would then explain the frequently combined appearance of transitional cell carcinomas and adenocarcinomas.

In this context the much discussed question arises as to whether adenocarcinomas develop from von Brunn's nests, cystitis cystica or cystitis glandularis which were first described by *von Brunn* (1893), *Lubarsch* (1893), and *Aschoff* (1894) and later confirmed by *Bayer* (1904) as well as *Störck* and *Zuckerkandl* (1907). Opinions differ widely whether to regard these lesions as premalignant (*Patch* and *Rhea,* 1935; *Patch,* 1948; *Wheeler* and *Hill,* 1954; *Mostofi* et al., 1955; *Shaw* et al., 1958; *Kitteredge* and *Brannam,* 1959; *Pugh,* 1959; *Grieve,* 1965; *Schade* and *Swinney,* 1969; *Parker,* 1970). There is now general agreement that the afore-mentioned changes are primarily a proliverative rather than a true neoplastic process (*Koss,* 1975); furthermore, that the proliferative lesions should generally be considered as a predisposing factor in subsequent carcinoma development. *Mostofi* (1976) considers von Brunn's nests, cystitis cystica and cystitis glandularis as premalignant lesions. His conclusion stems from cytological abnormalities observed within proliferative changes as well as from transitions to an invasive carcinoma. It remains, however, the task of prospective studies to determine just how often von Brunn's nests remain as such or do indeed develop into carcinoma.

It was not possible to clarify the problem of the biological significance of von Brunn's nests entirely in these experiments. The number of such proliferative changes in the animals was relatively small, but nevertheless they could be followed step by step up to tumorlike structures. However, we found no proof for the transition into an invasive adenocarcinoma. *Giani* (1907) came to the same conclusion after he induced cystitis cystica and cystitis glandularis in rabbits by implanting foreign bodies. Their relatively infrequent occurrence in the experiments points to their insignificance in the development of carcinomas in the bladder, as compared with the malignant transformation of papillomas and with the origin of carcinoma-in-situ (*Kunze* et al., 1976).

The particular biological potential of squamous metaplasia and leukoplakia of the bladder in the development of bladder carcinoma is widely contested. *Rabson* (1936) found no convincing reason to see a connection between leukoplakia and the development of carcinomas. Most authors now consider leukoplakia as a precursor of squamous cell carcinoma (*Koss,* 1975; *Mostofi,* 1976). Our experiments offered no basis for postulating the direct development of squamous cell carcinomas from squamous cell metaplasia of the urothelium. Our findings would seem to support more readily the conclusion that squamous cell carcinomas developed from focal squamous metaplasia within completely developed transitional cell carcinomas. This possibility is probably relevant also to the situation in man – if one excludes the development of squamous cell carcinomas in Bilharziasis – because transitional cell carcinomas demonstrate not infrequently squamous metaplasia (*Ash,* 1940; *Dukes* and *Massina,* 1949; *Dean* et al., 1954; *Pugh,* 1959; *Mostofi,* 1968; *Miller* et al., 1969).

In summary, one can say that n-butyl-n-(4-hydroxybutyl)-nitrosamine must be considered an excellent selective carcinogen, as it can induce the entire spectrum of bladder carcinomas that occur "spontaneously" in humans. Similar findings have recently been reported by *Fukushima* et al. (1976). It is of particular significance for the application of the findings in animal experiments to humans to note that it was also possible to induce inverted papillomas, primary carcinomas-in-situ (*Kunze* et al., 1976), and proliferative lesions such as von Brunn's nests, cystitis cystica and cystitis glandularis. For this reason this experimental model seems particularly suited to advance our knowledge of carcinogenesis in the human urinary bladder.

e) Summary

The spectrum of carcinomas induced with BBN in the urinary bladder of rats embraces all the types known to occur in man. The various tumor types occurred with the same frequency as in man and exhibited the same growth patterns. Variously differentiated papillary and nonpapillary transitional cell carcinomas comprised 88.8% of all carcinomas registered. A further 5.1% were squamous cell carcinomas, 2.8% carcinomas of mixed squamous and transitional cell differentiation, 2.2% adenocarcinomas, and 1.1% undifferentiated carcinomas.

Histogenetically, adenocarcinomas were found to originate from glandular metaplasia, and squamous cell carcinomas from squamous metaplasia within completely developed transitional cell carcinomas. In addition, it was possible to induce proliferative lesions such as von Brunn's nests, cystitis cystica and cystitis glandularis. However, we found no clues to substantiate the development of adenocarcinomas from these proliferative lesions, or for that matter squamous cell carcinomas from squamous metaplasia of the otherwise unchanged urothelium. The present experimental model seems particularly suited to the search for further information regarding the development of tumors in the human bladder.

IV. General Conclusions

Our experimental investigations of the tumor development in the urinary bladder of rats after application of various carcinogens (Di-N-butylnitrosamine, N-butyl-N-(4-hydroxybutyl)-nitrosamine, N-[4-(5-nitro-2-furyl)-2-thiazolyl] formamide) revealed that transitional cell carcinomas develop mainly through successive stages of transformation.

The first stage was demonstrable only by means of enzyme-histochemical methods and consisted of a focal irreversible loss of alkaline phosphatase activity in histologically and cytologically normal urothelium. The enzyme loss occurred long before the appearance of tumors and represents the earliest light-microscopically detectable transformation stage in bladder carcinogenesis. The loss of alkaline phosphatase activity seems to be characteristic of the initial phase of tumor development in the urinary bladder of rats, and is consistently reproducible after the application of chemically unrelated carcinogens. The enzyme-negative areas of the urothelium must be considered preneoplastic. This conclusion follows particularly from the finding that papillomas develop from such areas via enzyme-deficient hyperplasias after marked proliferative activity of the urothelial cells that are devoid of alkaline phosphatase activity. Papillomas and carcinomas also showed a loss of alkaline phosphatase activity in most cases.

By far the largest proportion of carcinomas developed by way of malignant transformation of preexisting papillomas or their precursors, the papillary hyperplasias. The transition into focally malignant growth did not take place abruptly, but occurred stepwise through different successive stages of transformation, each of which had its own distinctive morphological character. The first stage consisted of a focal, sharply defined cellular atypia. In a further stage carcinomas-in-situ developed from the atypical foci, followed by a circumscript infiltrative growth as the last stage. The successive development of each stage occurred independently of any further carcinogen application after transformation was initiated at the molecular level. The number of papillomas with transformation stages increased with a lengthening of the exposure and induction time. How long each stage retained its biological behavior could not be clarified under the experimental conditions used. As 74.4% of the papillomas had been transformed, papillomas must be considered potentially highly malignant. It remains for further investigations to find out whether papillomas necessarily transform into carcinomas. The various transformation stages within papillomas were distinguishable from the surrounding papillomatous structures without atypia not only on the basis of their cytological and histological characteristics, but also by a stepwise increased proliferation activity. The length of exposure and induction time exercised no significant influence on the degree of proliferative activity. The development of transitional cell carcinomas from papillomas occurred in the vast majority of cases, whereas they seldom developed directly from a primary carcinoma-in-situ (so-called intraurothelial carcinoma).

The spectrum of carcinomas induced in the urinary bladder of rats included all types known to occur in man. Even rare tumors, such as inverted papillomas, adenocarcinomas, squamous cell carcinomas and undifferentiated carcinomas, were observed. The various tumor types occurred with the same frequency as in man and exhibited the same growth pattern. Histogenetically, adenocarcinomas were found to originate from glandular metaplasia and squamous carcinomas from squamous metaplasia within completely developed transitional cell carcinomas.

The experiments showed that the changes commonly found in the human urinary bladder during carcinogenesis could be reproduced very successfully in experimental animals by application of DBN, BBN and FANFT. This aspect of our results makes the experimental models employed particularly suited for the collection of facts relevant to the tumor development in the human urinary bladder.

References

Abeshouse, B.S.: Exstrophy of the bladder, complicated by adenocarcinoma of the bladder and renal calculi. J. Urol. *49,* 259–289 (1943)

Aboul Nasr, A.L., Gazayerli, M.E., Fawzi, R.M.: Epidemiology and patholoy of cancer of the bladder in Egypt. Acta Un. int. Cancr. *18,* 528–537 (1962)

Akagi, G., Akagi, A., Kimura, M., Otsuka, H.: Comparison of bladder tumors induced in rats and mice with N-butyl-N-(4-hydroxybutyl)-nitrosamine. Gann *64,* 331–336 (1973)

Albarran, J.: Les tumeurs de la vessie. Paris: Steinheil 1892

Allegra, S.R., Broderick, P.A., Covese, N.L.: Cytologic and histogenetic observations in well differentiated transitional cell carcinoma of bladder. J. Urol. *107,* 777–782 (1972)

Allen, T.D., Henderson, B.W.: Adenocarcinoma of the bladder. J. Urol. *93,*50–56 (1965)

Althoff, J., Krüger, F.W., Mohr, U., Schmähl, D.: Dibutylnitrosamine carcinogenesis in Syrian golden and Chinese hamsters. Proc. Soc. Exp. Biol. *136*, 168–173 (1971)

Amon, H., Petry, G.: Fermenthistochemische Untersuchungen am Übergangsepithel verschiedener Säugetiere. Experientia *18*, 442–444 (1962)

Armstrong, E.C., Bonser, G.M.: Epithelial tumours of the urinary bladder in mice induced by 2-acetylaminofluorene. J. Path. Bact. *56*, 507–512 (1944)

Aschoff, L.: Ein Beitrag zur normalen und pathologischen Anatomie der Schleimhaut der Harnwege und ihrer drüsigen Anhänge. Virchows Arch. path. Anat. *138*, 119–161 (1894)

Ash, J.E.: Epithelial tumors of the bladder. J. Urol. *44*, 135–145 (1940)

Assor, D., Taylor, J.N.: Inverted papilloma of the bladder. J. Urol. *104*, 715–717 (1970)

Austen, G., Friedell, G.H.: Observations on local growth patterns of the bladder cancer. J. Urol. *93*, 224–229 (1965)

Baserga, R.: The relationship of the cell cycle to tumor growth and control of cell division: a review. Canc. Res. *25*, 581–592 (1965)

Batsakis, J.G.: Urogenital rhabdomyosarcoma: histogenesis and classification. J. Urol. *90*, 180–186 (1963)

Battifora, H.A., Eisenstein, R., Sky-Peck, H.H., McDonald, H.J.: Electron microscopy and tritiated thymidine in gradation of malignancy of human bladder carcinomas. J. Urol. *93*, 217–223 (1965)

Bayer, R.: Ein schleimbildendes Cystadenom der Harnblase. Virchows Arch. path. Anat. *196*, 350–370 (1904)

Begg, C.: The colloid adenocarcinomata of the bladder vault arising from the epithelium of the urachal canal: with a critical survey of the tumours of the urachus. Br. J. Surg. *18*, 422–466 (1931)

Beltzow, A.: Zur Regeneration des Epithels der Harnblase. Virchows Arch. path. Anat. *97*, 279–288 (1884)

Bern, H.A.: The distribution of alkaline phosphatase in the genital tract of male mammals. Anat. Rec. *104*, 361–369 (1949)

Bertram, J.S., Craig, A.W.: Induction of bladder tumors in mice with dibutylnitrosamine. Br. J. Cancer *24*, 352–359 (1970)

Bertram, J.S., Craig, A.W.: Specific induction of bladder cancer in mice by butyl-(4-hydroxybutyl)-nitrosamine and the effects of hormonal modifications on the sex difference in response. Eur. J. Cancer *8*, 587–594 (1972)

Bettendorf, M.: 630 Biopsien von Harnblasentumoren aus pathologisch-anatomischer Sicht unter besonderer Berücksichtigung der Dignität von Harnblasenpapillomen. Urologe A *13*, 56–58 (1974)

Blattmann, L., Preussmann, R.: Biotransformation von carcinogenen Dialkylnitrosaminen. Weitere Urinmetaboliten von Di-n-butyl- und Di-n-pentyl-nitrosamin. Z. Krebsforsch. *81*, 75–78 (1974)

Bohne, A.W., Osborn, R.W., Hettle, P.J.: Regeneration of the urinary bladder in the dog, following total cystectomy. Surg. Gynec. Obstet. *100*, 259–264 (1955)

Bohne, A.W., Urwiller, R.D., Pantos, T.G.: Leiomyosarcoma of the urinary bladder, with review of the literature. Henry Ford Hosp. Med. Bull. *10*, 445–448 (1962)

Bonser, G.M.: Epithelial tumours of the bladder in dogs induced by pure β-naphthylamine. J. Path. Bact. *55*, 1–6 (1958)

Bonser, G.M., Clayson, D.B.: A sulphonamide derivative which induces urinary tract epithelial hyperplasia and carcinomas of the bladder epithelium in the mouse. Br. J. Urol. *36*, 26–34 (1964)

Borski, A.A.: Lymphosarcoma of the bladder. J. Urol. *84*, 551 (1960)

Bourne, G.: The distribution of alkaline phosphatase in various tissues. J. exp. Physiol. *32*, 1–19 (1943)

Bresciani, F.: Cell proliferation in cancer. Eur. J. Cancer *4*, 343 (1968)

Brinton, J.A., Ito, Y., Olsen, B.S.: Carcinosarcoma of the urinary bladder. Cancer *25,* 1183–1186 (1970)
Broders, A.C.: Epithelioma of the genito-urinary organs. Ann. Surg. *75,* 574–604 (1922)
Brown, H.E.: Leiomyosarcoma of the bladder: follow up report of two cases with 4 and 10 years' survival. J. Urol. *94,* 247–251 (1965)
Brunn, A. von: Über drüsenähnliche Bildungen in der Schleimhaut des Nierenbeckens, des Ureters und der Harnblase beim Menschen. Arch. mikroskop. Anat. *41,* 294–303 (1893)
Bucher, O., Délèze, J.: Recherches complémentaires sur les cellules binuclées (foie et épithélium de transition). Anat. Anz. *102,* 1–20 (1955)
Burckhardt: Das Epithel der ableitenden Harnwege. Virchows Arch. path. Anat. *17,* 94–134 (1859)
Burghele, T., Mares, V., Vlad, C., Vulcan, R.: Contribution à l'étude histochimique des tumeurs de la vessie. Urol. Int. *20,* 42–60 (1965)
Campobasso, O., Berrino, F.: Early effects of cyclophosphamide on mouse bladder epithelium. Path. Microbiol. *38,*144–157 (1972)
Christeller, E.: Pathologie und pathologische Anatomie der Geschwülste der Harnblase. Z. Urol. *19,* 103–117 (1925)
Clayson, D.B., Cooper, E.H.: Cancer of the urinary tract. Advanc. Cancer Res. *13,* 271–381 (1970)
Clayson, D.B., Pringle, J.A.S.: The influence of a foreign body on the induction of tumours in the bladder epithelium of the mouse. Br. J. Cancer *20,* 564–568 (1966)
Clayson, D.B., Lawson, T.A., Santana, S., Bonser, G.M.: Correlation between the chemical induction of hyperplasia and of malignancy in the bladder epithelium. Br. J. Cancer *19,*297–310 (1965)
Clayson, D.B., Lawson, T.A., Pringle, J.A.S.: The carcinogenic action of 2-aminodiphenyleneoxide and 4-aminodiphenyl on the bladder and liver of the $C_{57} \times$ FJ mouse. Br. J. Cancer *21,*755–762 (1967a)
Clayson, D.B., Pringle, J.A.S., Bonser, G.M.: 4-Ethylsulphonylnaphthalene-1-sulphonamide: a new chemical for the study of bladder cancer in mouse. Biochem. Pharmacol. *16,* 619–626 (1972b)
Cohen, S.M., Alter, A., Bryan, G.T.: Distribution of radioactivity and metabolism of formic acid 2-[4-(5-nitro-2-furyl)-2-^{14}C-2-thiazolyl] hydrazide following oral administration to rats and mice. Cancer Res. *33,* 2802–2809 (1973)
Connally, J.G., Morales, A., Minaker, L., Raeburn, H.: The origin of regenerating bladder mucosa after partial mucosal stripping. Invest. Urol. *8,* 481–487 (1971)
Cooper, E.H., Cowen, D.M., Knowles, J.C.: The recovery of mouse bladder epithelium after injury by 4-ethylsulphonylnaphthalen-1-sulphonamid. J. Path. *108,* 151–156 (1972)
Cooper, P.H.: Severe atypia of transitional epithelium and carcinoma of the urinary bladder. Cancer *31,*, 1055–1060 (1973)
Coppridge, W.M., Roberts, L.C., Culp, D.A.: Glandular tumors of the bladder. J. Urol. *65,* 540–549 (1951)
Cox, C.E., Cass, A.S., Boyce, W.H.: Bladder cancer: a 26-year review. J. Urol. *101,* 550–558 (1969)
Cox, R.P., Gilbert, P., Griffin, M.J.: Alkaline inorganic pyrophosphatase activity of mammalian-cell alkaline phosphatase. Biochem. J. *105,* 155 (1967)
Croft, W.A., Bryan, G.T.: Production of urinary bladder carcinomas in male hamsters by N[4-(5-nitro-2-furyl)-2-thiazolyl]formamide, N-[4-(5-nitro-2-furyl)-2-thiazolyl]-acetamide, or formic acid 2-[4-(5-nitro-2-furyl)-2-thiazolyl]hydrazide. J. Nat. Cancer Inst. *51,*941–949 (1973)
Culver, H., Baker, W.J., Lakin, H.S.: Adenocarcinoma of the urinary bladder: three instructive cases. Trans. Am. Assoc. Genito-Urin. Surg. *35,* 247–265 (1942)
Cummings, R.: Inverted papilloma of the bladder. J. Path. *112,* 225–227 (1974)

Danini, E.S.: Zur Frage über den Bau des Übergangsepithels. Z. Anat. *74*, 297–317 (1924)

Dean, A.L., Ash, J.E.: Study of the bladder tumors in the registry of the American Urological Association. J. Urol. *63*, 618–621 (1950)

Dean, A.L., Mostofi, F.K., Thomson, R.V., Clark, M.L.: A restudy of the first fourteen hundred tumors in the bladder tumor registry, Armed Forces Institute of Pathology. J. Urol. *71*, 571–590 (1954)

Deming, C.L.: The biological behaviour of transitional cell papilloma of the bladder. J. Urol. *63*, 815–820 (1950)

Dimette, R.M., Sproat, H.F., Sayegh, E.S.: Classification of carcinoma of the urinary bladder associated with schistosomiasis and metaplasia. J. Urol. *75*,680–686 (1956)

Dörmer, P., Tulinius, H., Oehlert, W.: Untersuchungen über die Generationszeit, DNS-Synthesezeit und Mitosedauer von Zellen der hyperplastischen Epidermis und des Plattenepithelcarcinomas der Maus nach Methylcholantrenpinselung. Z. Krebsforsch. *66*, 11–28 (1964)

Dogiel, A.S.: Zur Frage über das Epithel der Harnblase. Arch. mikrosk. Anat. *35*, 389–406 (1890)

Druckrey, H., Preussmann, R., Ivankovic, S., Schmidt, C.H., Mendel, H.D., Stahl, K.W.: Selektive Erzeugung von Blasenkrebs an Ratten durch Dibutyl- und N-Butyl-N-butanol (4)-nitrosamin. Z. Krebsforsch. *66*, 280–290 (1964)

Druckrey, H., Preussmann, R., Schmähl, D., Müller, M.: Erzeugung von Blasenkrebs an Ratten mit N, N-Dibutylnitrosamin. Naturwissenschaften *49*,19 (1962)

Du Bose Dent, E.: Carcinosarcoma ("collision tumour") of the urinary bladder. J. Urol. *85*, 104–108 (1961)

Dukes, C.E.: Tumours of the bladder (D.M. Wallace, ed.) Edinburgh, London: Livingstone 1959

Dukes, C.E., Masina, F.: Classification of epithelial tumours of the bladder. Br. J. Urol. *21*, 273–295 (1949)

Dunham, L.J., Rabson, A.S., Stewart, H.L., Frank, A.S., Young, J.L.: Rates, interview and pathology study of cancer of the urinary bladder in New Orleans, Louisiana. J. Nat. Cancer Inst. *41*, 683–687 (1968)

Eaton, R.H., Moss, D.W.: Action of purified alkaline phosphatases from human liver and small intestine on nucleosidphosphates. Biochem. J. *104*, 65p (1967)

Eisenberg, R.B., Roth, R.B., Schweinsberg, M.H.: Bladder tumors and associated proliferative mucosal lesions. J. Urol. *84*, 544–550 (1960)

Enderlen, E.: Zur Histologie der Schleimhaut der ektophierten Blase. Verh. Dtsch. path. Ges. *7*, 167–170 (1904)

Ertürk, E., Price, J.M., Morris, J.E., Cohen, S., Leith, R.S., Esch, A.M. von, Crovetti, A.J.: The production of carcinoma of the urinary bladder in rats by feeding N-[4-(5-nitro-2-furyl)-2-thiazolyl]formamide. Cancer Res. *27*, 1998–2002 (1967)

Ertürk, E., Cohen, S.M., Price, J.M., Bryan, G.T.: Pathogenesis, histology and transplantability of urinary bladder carcinoma induced in albino rats by oral administration of N-[4-(5-nitro-2-furyl)-2-thiazolyl]formamide. Cancer Res. *29*, 2219–2228 (1969)

Ertürk, E., Morris, J.E., Cohen, S.M., Esch, A.M. von, Crovetti, A.J., Price, J.M., Bryan, G.T.: Comparative carcinogenicity of formic acid 2-[4-(5-nitro-2-furyl)-2-thiazolyl] hydrazide and related chemicals in the rat. J. nat. Cancer Inst. *47*, 437–445 (1971)

Farrow, G.M., Utz, D.C., Rife, C.C.: Morphological and clinical observations of patients with early bladder cancer treated with total cystectomy. Cancer Res. *36*, 2495–2501 (1976)

Feinendegen, L.E., Bond, V.P.: Zur Ribonucleinsäure-Synthese im Chromatin und im Nucleolus der menschlichen Krebszelle HELA-S_3 in Kultur. Atomkernenergie *V9*, 283–292 (1964)

Ferguson, A.R.: Associated bilharziasis and primary malignant disease of the urinary bladder, with observations in a series of forty cases. J. Path. Bact. *16*, 76–94 (1911)

Feyrter, F.: Zur Pathologie des Polysaccharidstoffwechsels im Epithel. I. Im Epithel der menschlichen Harnblase. Virchows Arch. path. Anat. *328,* 378–390 (1956)
Fingerhut, B., Veenema, R.J., Graf, S., Butler, M.: Observations on RNA in prostate and bladder neoplasms. J. Urol. *101,* 608–614 (1969)
Fischer, E.R.: Transitional cell carcinoma of the urachal apex. Cancer *11,* 245–249 (1958)
Fleroff, N.: Studien über den Bau und die funktionelle Struktur des Harnblasenepithels der Nagetiere. Z. Zellforsch. mikrosk. Anat. *24,* 360–392 (1936)
Flocks, R.H., Culp, D.A.: Polypoid fibromyxosarcoma of the urinary bladder in a child. J. Urol. *73,* 299–306 (1955)
Formiggini, B.: Contributo allo studio istologico della mucosa vesicele extro fica. Riv. med. *36,* 252–254 (1920)
Forster, E.A., Levine, A.J.: Mucin production in metastatic carcinomas. Cancer *16,* 506–509 (1963)
Francis, R.R.: Carcinoma of the bladder. J. Urol. *85,* 552–555 (1961)
Fukushima, S., Hirose, M., Tsuda, H., Shirai, T., Hirao, K., Arai, M., Ito, N.: Histological classification of urinary bladder cancers in rats induced by N-butyl-N-(4-hydroxy-butyl)-nitrosamine. Gann *67,* 81–90 (1976)
Gauer, J.P.: Kerngrößenuntersuchungen am Übergangsepithel. Ein Beitrag zum Studium der Amitose. Mitt. naturforsch. Ges. Bern N.F. *6,* 85–114 (1949)
Giani, R.: Neuer experimenteller Beitrag zur Entstehung der Cystitis cystica. Beitr. path. Anat. *42,* 1–22 (1907)
Gilman, J., Prates, M.D.: Histological types and histogenesis of bladder cancer in the Portuguese East African with special reference to bilharzial cystitis. Acta Univ. Int. Eur. *18,* 560–574 (1962)
Goebel, C.: Über die bei Bilharziakrankheit vorkommenden Blasentumoren mit besonderer Berücksichtigung des Carcinoms. Z. Krebsforsch. *3,* 369–513 (1905)
Göldi, K.: Histochemische Reaktionen in der normalen Harnblasenschleimhaut. Z. mikrosk.-anat. Forsch. *58,* 265–288 (1952)
Gössner, W., Friedrich-Freska, H.: Histochemische Untersuchungen über die Glucose-6-Phosphatase in der Rattenleber während der Kanzerisierung durch Nitrosamine. Z. Naturforsch. *19b,* 862–683 (1964)
Gomori, G.: The distribution of phosphatase in normal organs and tissues. J. Cell. Comp. Physiol. *17,* 71–80 (1941)
Gordon, A.: Intestinal metaplasia of the urinary tract epithelium. J. Path. Bact. *85,* 441–444 (1963)
Goyanna, R., Emmett, J.L., McDonald, J.R.: Exstrophy of the bladder complicated by adenocarcinoma. J. Urol. *65,* 391–400 (1951)
Graham, N.H.: Ectopia vesicae complicated by adenocarcinoma: with review of literature. Br. J. Surg. *30,* 23–32 (1942)
Grieve, J.: Contrasting cases of cystitis cystica. Br. J. Urol. *37,* 157–159 (1965)
Guira, A.C.: Bladder carcinoma in rubber workers. J. Urol. *106,* 548–552 (1971)
Hainau, B., Dombernowsky, P.: Histology and cell proliferation in human bladder tumors. Cancer *33,* 115–126 (1974)
Hamperl, H., Hellweg, G.: On mucoepidermoid tumors of different sites. Cancer *10,* 1187–1192 (1957)
Hashem, M.: The aetiology and pathogenesis of the bilharzial bladder cancer. J. Egypt. med. Assoc. *44,* 857–966 (1961)
Hashimoto, Y., Suzuki, E., Okada, M.: Induction of urinary bladder tumors in ACI/N rats by butyl (3-carboxyl-propyl)nitrosamine, a major urinary metabolite of butyl-(4-hydroxybutyl)nitrosamine. Gann *63,* 637–638 (1972)
Hashimoto, Y., Suzuki, K., Okada, M.: Induction of urinary bladder tumors by intravesicular instillation of butyl-(4-hydroxybutyl)-nitrosamine and its principal urinary metabolite, butyl(3-carboxylpropyl)nitrosamine in rats. Gann *65,* 69–73 (1974)

Hellstrom, H.R., Fischer, E.R.: Embryonal rhabdomyosarcoma of the bladder in the aged. J. Urol. *86,* 336–339 (1961)
Hess, R., Scarpelli, D.G., Pearse, A.G.E.: The cytochemical localisation of oxidative enzymes. II. Pyridine nucleotide-linked dehydrogenases. J. biophys. biochem. Cytol. *4,* 753–760 (1958)
Hicks, R.M.: The fine structure of the transitional epithelium of rat ureter. J. Cell Biol. *26,* 25–48 (1965)
Hicks, R.M.: The permeability of rat transitional epithelium. Keratinization and the barrier to water. J. Cell Biol. *28,* 21–31 (1966a)
Hicks, R.M.: The function of the Golgi complex in transitional epithelium. Synthesis of the thick cell membrane. J. Cell Biol. *30,* 623–643 (1966b)
Highman, B., Frith, C.H., Littlefield, N.A.: Alkaline phosphatase activity in hyperplastic and neoplastic urinary bladder epithelium of mice fed 2-acetylaminofluorence. J. Nat. Cancer Inst. *54,* 257–261 (1975)
Hoffmann-Ostenhof, O.: Enzymologie. Berlin, Göttingen, Heidelberg: Springer 1954
Hollands, F.G.: Malignant disease of the urinary bladder. Ann. Roy. Coll. Surg. Engl. *11,* 265–286 (1952)
Howard, A.H., Bergman, R.T.: Mucous adenocarcinoma of the urinary bladder. J. Urol. *59,* 455–460 (1948)
Hückel, R.: Die Gewächse der ableitenden Harnwege (Nierenbecken, Harnleiter und Blase.) In: Handbuch der speziellen Pathologischen Anatomie und Histologie. Berlin: Springer 1934
Hueper, W.C., Wiley, F.H., Wolfe, H.D.: Experimental production of bladder tumours in dogs by administration of β-naphthylamine. J. Industr. Hyg. *20,* 46–84 (1938)
Institute of Urology, London: The classification of tumours of the bladder. London: The University 1955 (Broadsheet no. 1)
Ito, N., Hiasa, Y., Okajima, E., Kitamura, H.: Histogenesis of urinary bladder tumors induced by N-butyl-N-(4-hydroxybutyl)nitrosamine in rats. Gann *60,* 401–410 (1969)
Ito, N.: Experimental studies on tumors of the urinary system of rats induced by chemical carcinogens. Acta path. Jap. *23,* 87–109 (1973)
Ito, N., Matayoshi, K., Arai, M., Yoshioka, Y., Kamamoto, Y., Makiura, S., Sugihara, S.: Effect of various factors on induction of urinary bladder tumors in animals by N-butyl-N-(4-hydroxybutyl)nitrosamine. Gann *64,* 151–159 (1973)
Jabara, A.: A comparison of the pathologcial effects of 2-acetylaminofluorene, 4-acetylaminobiphenyl and 2-acetylaminobiphenyl in the dog. Cancer Res. *23,* 921–927 (1963)
Johnson, F.R.: Some proliferative and metaplastic changes in transitional epithelium Br. J. Urol. *29,* 112–120 (1957)
Johnson, F.M.: Development of differences of alkaline phosphatase zymograms for Drosophila melanogaster and D-ananassae. Nature *212,* 843–844 (1966)
Kabat, E.A., Furth, J.: A histochemical study of the distribution of alkaline phosphatase in various normal and neoplastic tissues. Am. J. Path. *17,* 303–317 (1941)
Kagawa, S.: Enzyme histochemistry of bone induction by urinary bladder epithelium. J. Histochem. Cytochem. *13,* 255–264 (1965)
Kitteredge, W.E., Brannan, W.: Cystitis glandularis. J. Urol. *81,* 419–430 (1959)
Kloos, K., Steffen, J.: Histologische und cytologische Untersuchungen an Fibroepitheliomen der Harnblase. Z. Krebsforsch. *57,* 577–613 (1951)
Koss, L.G.: A light and electron microscopic study of the effects of an single dose of cyclophosphamide on various organs in the rat. I. The urinary bladder. Lab. Invest. *16,* 44–65 (1967)
Koss, L.G.: The asymmetric unit membrane of the epithelium of the urinary bladder of the rat. An electron microscopic study of a mechanism of epithelial maturation and function. Lab. Invest. *21,* 154–168 (1969)

Koss, L.G.: Tumors of the urinary bladder. Armed Forces Institute of Pathology, Fascicle 11 (1975)
Koss, L.G., Lavin, P.: Studies of experimental bladder carcinoma. I. Induction of tumors with diet low in vitamin B_6 containing N-2-fluorenylacetamide after single dose of cyclophosphamide. J. Nat. Cancer Inst. *46,* 585–595 (1971)
Koss, L.G., Melamed, M.R., Kelly, R.E.: Further cytologic and histologic studies of bladder lesions in workers exposed to paraamino-diphenyl. Progress report. J. Nat. Cancer Inst. *43,* 233–243 (1969)
Koss, L.G., Tiamson, E.M., Robbins, M.A.: Mapping cancerous and precancerous bladder changes. Y.A.M.A. *27,* 281–286 (1974)
Kretschmer, H.L.: Rhabdomyosarcoma of the bladder; report of a case and review of the literature. Arch. Path. *44,* 350–355 (1947)
Kretschmer, H.L., Barringer, B.S., Braasch, W.F., Dean, A.L., Ferguson, R.S., Keyes, E.L., Smith, C.C.: Cancer of the bladder. J. Urol. *31,* 423–472 (1934)
Krüger, F.W.: Metabolismus von Nitrosaminen in vivo. I. Über die β-Oxidation aliphatischer Di-n-alkylnitrosamine: Die Bildung von 7-Methylguanin neben 7-Propyl- bzw. 7-Butylguanin nach Applikation von Di-n-propyl- oder Di-n-butylnitrosamin. Z. Krebsforsch. *76,* 145–154 (1971)
Krüger, F.W.: New aspects in metabolism of carcinogenic nitrosamines. In: Topics in Chemical Carcinogenesis. W. Nakahara, S., Takayama, T. Sugimura, S. Odashima (eds.). Tokyo: University of Tokyo Press 1972
Kunze, E., Schauer, A.: Enzymhistochemische und autoradiographische Untersuchungen an Dibutylnitrosamin-induzierten Harnblasenpapillomen der Ratte. Z. Krebsforsch. *74,* 146–160 (1971)
Kunze, E., Schauer, A.: Morphology, classification and histogenesis of N-butyl-N-(4-hydroxybutyl)-nitrosamine-induced carcinomas in the urinary bladder of rats. Z. Krebsforsch. *88,* 273–289 (1977)
Kunze, E., Schauer, A., Calvör, R.: Zur Histochemie von Harnblasenpapillomen der Ratte, induziert durch Dibutylnitrosamin. Naturwissenschaften *56,* 639 (1969)
Kunze, E., Schauer, A., Krüssmann, G.: Focal loss of alkaline phosphatase and increase of proliferation in preneoplastic areas of the rat urothelium after administration of N-butyl-N-(4-hydroxybutyl)-nitrosamine and N[4-(5-nitro-2-furyl)-2-thiazolyl] formamide. Z. Krebsforsch. *84,* 143–160 (1975)
Kunze, E., Schauer, A., Schatt, S.: Morphologie und Proliferationskinetik der Entwicklungsstadien von Harnblasentumoren der Ratte. Verh. Dtsch. Ges. Path. *58,* 508 (1974)
Kunze, E., Schauer, A., Schatt, S.: Stages of transformation in the development of N-butyl-N-(4-hydroxybutyl)-nitrosamine-induced transitional cell carcinomas in the urinary bladder of rats. Z. Krebsforsch. *87,* 139–160 (1976)
Kunze, E., Schauer, A., Spielmann, J.: Autoradiographische Untersuchungen über den RNS-Stoffwechsel während der Entwicklung von Dibutylnitrosamin-induzierten Harnblasentumoren der Ratte. Z. Krebsforsch. *77,* 236–248 (1971)
Leblond, C.P., Vulpe, M., Bertalanfey, F.D.: Mitotic activity of epithelium of urinary bladder in albino rat. J. Urol. *73,* 311–313 (1955)
Leeson, R.: Histology, histochemistry and electron microscopy of the transitional epithelium of the rat urinary bladder in response to induced physiological changes. Acta Anat. *48,* 297–315 (1962)
Legier, J.F.: Botryoid sarcoma and rhabdomyosarcoma of the bladder: review of the literature and report of 3 cases. J. Urol. *86,* 583–590 (1961)
Lendorf, A.: Beiträge zur Histologie der Harnblasenschleimhaut. Anat. Hefte *17,* 55–179 (1901)
Lennartz, K.J.: Proliferationskinetik von Tumorzellen. In: Fortschritte in Krebsforschung: Molekularbiologie, Wachstum, Klinik. Stuttgart, New York: Schattauer 1969
Lerman, R.I., Huttler, R.V.P., Whitmore, W.F.: Papilloma of the urinary bladder. Cancer *25,* 333–342 (1970)

Levi, P.E., Cooper, E.H., Anderson, C.K., Path, M.C., Williams, R.E.: Analysis of DNA content, nuclear size and cell proliferation of transitional cell carcinoma in man. Cancer *21,* 1074–1085 (1969a)

Levi, P.E., Cowan, D.M., Cooper, E.H.: Induction of cell proliferation in the mouse bladder by 4-ethylsulphonylnaphthalene-1-sulphonamide. Cell Tissue Kinet. *2,* 249–262 (1969b)

Levi, P.E., Knowles, J.C., Cowen, D.M., Wood, M., Cooper, E.H.: Disorganization of mouse bladder epithelium induced by 2-acetyl-aminofluorene and 4-ethylsulphonyl-naphthalene-1-sulphonamide. J. Nat. Cancer Inst. *46,* 337–352 (1971)

Lezava, A.: Experimentell-histologische Untersuchungen über das Übergansepithel. Z. Anat. *103,* 844–884 (1934)

Locher, G.W., Cooper, E.H.: Repair of rat urinary bladder epithelium following injury by cyclophosphamide. Invest. Urol. *8,* 116–123 (1970)

Lubarsch, O.: Über Cysten der ableitenden Harnwege. Arch. mikrosk. Anat. *41,* 303–323 (1893)

Ludlum, D.B.: The properties of 7-methylguanine-containing templates for ribonucleic acid polymerase. J. Biol. Chem. *245,* 477–482 (1970)

Ludvig, W., Zinnbauer, B.: Die urologisch-chirurgische Therapie des Blasenkarzinoms. Wien. Klin. Wochenschr. *83,* 524–525 (1971)

Lund, F., Lundwall, F.: Papillomas of the urinary bladder. Acta Path. Scand. Suppl. *105,* 118–134 (1955)

Lunglmayer, G., Breitenecker, G., Pecherstorfer, M.: Die Bedeutung proliferativer und metaplastischer Urothelveränderungen für die Karzinomentwicklung in der Harnblase. Urol. Int. *27,* 24–36 (1972)

Maletta, T., Horton, B.: Botryoidal sarcoma of the bladder in children: a case report. J. Urol. *82,* 490–493 (1959)

Manheimer, L.H., Seligman, A.M.: Improvement in the method for the histochemical demonstration of alkaline phosphatase and its use in a study of normal and neoplastic tissues. J. Nat. Cancer Inst. *9,* 181–199 (1948)

Martin, B.F.: Histological and histochemical studies on the bladder and ureter, with particular reference to alkaline phosphatase and Golgi material. J. Anat. *42,* 286–297 (1958)

Martin, B.F.: The effect of distention of the urinary bladder on the lining epithelium and on its histochemical reaction for alkaline phosphatase. Ann. Histochem. *7,* 51–62 (1962)

Maruchi, N., Farrow, G.M., Kurland, L.T., Elveback, L.R.: Cancer of the bladder in Rochester, Minnesota. Am. J. Epidemiol. *19,* 265–272 (1974)

Massey, V.: The identity of diaphorase and lipoyldehydrogenase. Biochim. Biophys. Acta. *30,* 205–206 (1958)

Massey, V.: The identity of diaphorase and lipoyldehydrogenase. Biochim. Biophys. Acta. *37,* 314–322 (1960)

McMinn, R.M.: The cellular morphology of tissue repair. Cytology *22,* 63 (1967)

McMinn, R.M., Johnson, F.R.: Repair of artificial ulcers in the urinary bladder of the cat. Br. J. Surg. *43,* 99 (1955)

Melamed, M.R., Grabstald, H., Whitmore, W.F.: Carcinoma in situ of bladder: clinical-pathologic study of case with a suggested approach to detection. J. Urol. *96,* 466–471 (1966)

Melamed, M.R., Koss, L.G., Ricci, A., Whitmore, W.F.: Cytohistological observations on developing carcinoma of the urinary bladder in man. Cancer *13,* 67–74 (1960)

Melamed, M.R., Voutsa, N.G., Grabstald, H.: Natural history and clinical behavior of in situ carcinoma of the human urinary bladder. Cancer *17,* 1533–1545 (1964)

Melicow, M.M.: Tumours of the urinary drainage tract: urothelial tumors. J. Urol. *54,* 186–203 (1945)

Melicow, M.M.: Histological study of vesical urothelium intervening between gross neoplasms in total cystectomy. J. Urol. *68,* 261–279 (1952)

Melicow, M.M.: Tumours of the urinary bladder: a clinico-pathological analysis of over 2500 specimens and biopsies. J. Urol. *74,* 498–521 (1955)
Melicow, M.M., Hollowell, J.W.: Intraurothelial cancer, carcinoma in situ, Bowen's disease of the urinary system: discussion of thirty cases. J. Urol. *68,* 763–772 (1952)
Mende, T.J., Chambers, E.L.: Distribution of mucopolysaccharide and alkaline phosphatase in transitional epithelia. J. Histochem. Cytochem. *5,* 99–104 (1957)
Messier, B., Leblond, C.P.: Cell proliferation and migration as revealed by radioautography after injection of thymidine-^{3}H into male rats and mice. Ann. J. Anat. *106,* 247 (1960)
Meyer, J., Weinmann, J.P.: Distribution of phosphamidase activity in the male albino tract. J. Histochem. Cytochem. *5,* 354–397 (1957)
Miller, A., Mitchell, J.P., Brown, N.J.: The Bristol bladder tumour registry. Br. J. Urol. Suppl. *41,* 1–64 (1969)
Mills, K.L.G.: The clinical course of 234 neoplasms of the bladder in north-east Scotland. Br. J. Urol. *36,* 204–210 (1964)
Miyakawa, M., Yoshida, O.: DNA synthesis of the urinary bladder epithelium in rats with long-term feeding of dl-tryptophan-added and pyrodoxine-deficient diet. Gann *64,* 411–413 (1973)
Mohr, U., Althoff, J., Schmähl, D., Krüger, F.W.: The carcinogenic effect of dibutylnitrosamine in Syrian and Chinese hamsters. Z. Krebsforsch. *74,* 112–113 (1970)
Moloney, P.J., Elliot, G.B., McLaughin, M., Sinclair, A.B.: In situ transitional carcinoma and the non-specifically inflamed contracting bladder. J. Urol. *111,* 162–164 (1974)
Mostofi, F.K.: Potentialities of bladder epithelium. J. Urol. *71,* 705–714 (1954)
Mostofi, F.K.: Pathological aspects and spread of carcinoma of the bladder. Am. J. Med. Assoc. *206,* 1764–1771 (1968)
Mostofi, F.K.: Histological typing of urinary bladder tumours, No. 10. Geneva: World Health Organization 1973
Mostofi, F.K.: Histologic changes preceding carcinoma of the urinary bladder. In: Third International Symposium on Detection and Prevention of Cancer, Abs. No. 204. New York 1976
Mostofi, F.K., Morse, W.H.: Polypoid rhabdomyosarcoma (sarcoma botryoides) of bladder in children. J. Urol. *67,* 681–687 (1952)
Mostofi, F.K., Thomson, R.V., Dean, A.L.: Mucous adenocarcinoma of the urinary bladder. Cancer *8,* 741–758 (1955)
Murata, I., Kawashima, H., Mori, M.: Histochemical study on alkaline phosphatase activity in human neoplasms. Gann *57,* 513–525 (1966)
Nachlas, M.M., Seligman, A.M.: The comparative distribution of esterase in the tissues of five mammals by a histochemical technique. Anat. Rec. *105,* 677–687 (1949)
Naeim, F., Schlezinger, R.M., De la Maza, L.M.: Primary signet ring cell carcinoma of the bladder: report of a case and review of the literature. J. Urol. *108,* 274–276 (1972)
Nettesheim, P., Oehlert, W.: Die Wirkung des Wachstumshormons auf die Desoxyribonukleinsäure-Synthese in den Wechselgeweben der weißen Maus. Beitr. path. Anat. *126,* 395–412 (1962)
Nicolai, C.H., Spjut, H.J.: Primary osteogenic sarcoma of the bladder. J. Urol. *82,* 497–499 (1959)
Nodes, J.T., Reid, E.: Azo dye carcinogenesis: ribonucleotides and ribonucleases. Br. J. Cancer *17,* 745 (1963)
Oberdick, G.: Über Epithel und Drüsen der Harnblase. Dissertation, Göttingen, 1884
Okada, M., Suzuki, E.: Metabolism of butyl-(4-hydroxybutyl)nitrosamine in rats. Gann *63,* 391–392 (1972)
Okajima, E., Hiramatsu, F., Motomiya, Y., Iriya, K., Ijunin, M., Ito, N.: Effect of DL-tryptophan on tumorigenesis in the urinary bladder and liver of rats treated with N-nitrosodibutylamine. Gann *62,* 163–169 (1971)

Pang Shu-Chao: Bony and cartilaginous tumours of the urinary bladder. J. Path. Bact. *76,* 357–376 (1958)
Parker, C.: Cystitis cystica and glandularis, a study of 40 cases. Proc. Roy. Soc. Med. *63,* 239–241 (1970)
Paschkis, R.: Über Adenome der Harnblase. Z. Urol. Chir. *21,* 315–325 (1927)
Patch, F.S.: Epithelial metaplasia of the urinary tract. J. Am. Med. Assoc. *136,* 824–827 (1948)
Patch, F.S., Rhea, L.J.: Genesis and development of Brunn's nests and their relationship to cystitis cystica, cystitis glandularis and primary adenocarcinoma of the bladder. Can. Med. Assoc. J. *33,* 597–606 (1935)
Peacock, A.H., Corbett, D.G.: Colloid carcinoma of the urinary bladder. Northw. Med. (Seattle) *29,* 208–209 (1930)
Pearse, A.G.E.: Histochemistry, Vol. 2. Edinburgh, London: Churchill Livingstone 1972
Petry, G., Amon, H.: Die funktionelle Struktur des Harnblasenepithels und ihre Bedeutung für die urologische Cytodiagnostik. Klin. Wochenschr. *44,* 1371–1379 (1966a)
Petry, G., Amon, H.: Licht- und elektronenmikroskopische Studien über Struktur und Dynamik des Übergangsepithels. Z. Zellforsch. *69,* 587–612 (1966b)
Poljakoff: Grundriß der Histologie und Embryologie des Menschen und der Wirbeltiere. Charkow 1914, quoted after Danini, 1924
Pontius, E.E., Nourse, M.H., Paz, L., McCallum, D.C.: Primary malignant lymphomas of the bladder. J. Urol. *90,* 58–61 (1963)
Post, J., Hoffman, J.: The replication time and pattern of carcinogen-induced hepatoma cells. J. Cell Biol. *22,* 341–350 (1964)
Post, J., Huang, C., Hoffman, J.: The replication time and pattern of the liver cell in the growing rate. J. Cell Biol. *18,* 1–12 (1963)
Potts, I.F., Hirst, E.: Inverted papilloma of the bladder. J. Urol. *90,* 175–179 (1963)
Powers, J.H., Hawn, C.V.Z., Carter, R.D.: Osteogenic sarcoma and transitional cell carcinoma occurring simultaneously in the urinary bladder. J. Urol. *76,* 363–369 (1956)
Price, J.M.: Etiology of bladder cancer. In: Benign and Malignant Tumours of the Urinary Bladder (E. Maltry, ed.). Berne, Stuttgart, Vienna: Huber 1971
Pugh, R.C.B.: Tumors of the bladder (D.M. Wallace, ed.) Edinburgh, London: Livingstone 1959
Pyrah, L.N., Raper, F.P., Thomas, G.M.: Report of a follow-up of papillary tumours of the bladder. Brit. J. Urol. *36,* 14–25 (1964)
Rabson, S.M.: Leukoplakia and carcinoma of the urinary bladder. J. Urol. *35,* 321–341 (1936)
Radomski, J.-L., Brill, E., Glass, E.M.: Induction of bladder tumors and other malignancies in rats with 2-methoxy-3-aminodibenzofuran. J. Nat. Cancer Inst. *39,* 1069–1072 (1967)
Regele, H., Lunglmayr, G.: Zur Wachstumsdynamik des Übergangsepithels. Virchows Arch. Abt. B. Zellpath. *2,* 229–233 (1969)
Rehn, L.: Blasengeschwülste bei Fuchsin-Arbeitern. Arch. Klin. Chir. *50,* 588–600 (1895)
Reiskin, A.B., Mendelsohn, M.L.: A comparison of the cell cycle in induced carcinomas and their normal counterpart. Cancer Res. *24,* 1131–1136 (1964)
Richter, W.R., Moize, S.M.: Electron microscopic observations on the collapsed and distended mammalian urinary bladder (transitional epithelium). J. Ultrastruct. Res. *9,* 1–9 (1963)
Roe, F.J.C.: An illustrated classification of the proliferative and neoplastic changes in mouse bladder epithelium in response to prolonged irritation. Br. J. Urol. *36,* 238–254 (1964)
Rosa, C.G., Tsou, K.C.: Use of tetrazolium compounds in oxidative enzymehisto- and cytochemistry. Nature *192,* 990 (1961)

Rosas-Uribe, A., Luna, M.A.: Primary signet ring cell carcinoma of the urinary bladder. Report of two cases. Arch. Path. *88,* 294 (1969)
Rudolph, G., Klein, H.J.: Histochemische Darstellung und Verteilung der Glucose-6-phosphatdehydrogenase in normalen Rattenorganen. Histochemie *4,* 238–251 (1964)
Sandrey, J.G.: Adenocarcinoma of the bladder. Br. J. Urol. *39,*513–514 (1967)
Santana, S.: The use of rat bladder pouches to elucidate the mode of action of a chemical which induces hyperplasia in the bladder epithelium. Br. J. Cancer *17,* 715–718 (1963)
Santino, A.M., Shumaker, E.J., Garces, J.: Primary malignant lymphoma of the bladder. J. Urol. *103,* 310–313 (1970)
Saphir, O.: Signet-ring cell carcinoma of the urinary bladder. Am. J. Path. *31,* 223–228 (1955)
Saphir, O., Vass, A.: Carcinosarkoma. Am. J. Cancer *33,* 331–358 (1938)
Sarma, K.P.: Tumours of the urinary bladder. London: Butterworths 1969
Scarpelli, D.G., Hess, R., Pearse, A.G.E.: The cytochemical localization of oxidative enzymes. I. Diphosphopyridine nucleotide diaphorase and triphosphopyridine nucleotide diaphorase. J. Biophys. Biochem. Cytol. *4,* 747 (1958)
Schade, R.O.K., Swinney, J.: Pre-cancerous changes in the bladder epithelium. Lancet *1968 II,* 943–946
Schaer, J.C., Grieder, A., Heininger, H.J., Schindler, R.: Comparison of ^{3}H-Cytidine and ^{3}H-5-Uridine as precursor of RNA. Exp. Cell Res. *56,* 449–452 (1969)
Schauer, A., Kunze, E.: Enzymhistochemische und autoradiographische Untersuchungen während der Cancerisierung der Rattenleber mit Diäthylnitrosamin. Z. Krebsforsch. *70,* 252–266 (1968)
Schauer, A., Kunze, E., Krüsmann, G., Spielmann, J.: Vergleichende enzymhistochemische und autoradiographische Untersuchungen über das biologische Verhalten menschlicher und tierischer Harnblasentumoren. Verh. Dtsch. Ges. Path. *55,* 577–582 (1971)
Schlezinger, M.J.: Formation of a defective alkaline phosphatase subunit by a mutant of Escherichia coli. J. Biol. Chem. *242,* 1604–1611 (1967)
Schreiber, H., Oehlert, W., Kugler, K.: Regeneration und Proliferationskinetik des normalen und strahlengeschädigten Urothels der Ratte. Virchows Arch. Abt. B Zellpath. *4,* 30–44 (1969)
Seemayer, T.A., Knaak, J., Thelmo, W.L., Wang, N.S., Ahmed, M.N.: Further observations on carcinoma in situ of the urinary bladder: silent but extensive intraprostatic involvement. Cancer *36,* 514–520 (1975)
Seidler, E.: Charakterisierung der $NADH_2$-Lipoamid-Dehydrogenase als Tetrazoliumreduktase. Acta Histochem. *47,* 30–41 (1973)
Selberg, W.: Die Kanzerisierung des Urothels beim Harnblasenkarzinom. Verh. Dtsch. Ges. Path. *45,* 197–201 (1961)
Selberg, W.: Zur Morphologie der Harnblasencarcinome unter besonderer Berücksichtigung ihrer örtlichen Ausbreitung. Urologe *3,* 72–79 (1964)
Sen Gupta, K.P.: Hyperplasia of urinary tract epithelium induced by continuous administration of sulphonamide derivates. Br. J. Cancer *16,* 110–119 (1962)
Shaw, J.L., Gislason, G.J., Imbriglia, J.E.: Transition of cystitis glandularis to primary adenocarcinoma of the bladder. J. Urol. *79,* 815–822 (1958)
Silbar, J.D., Silbar, S.J.: Leiomyosarcoma of bladder: three case reports and a review of literature. J. Urol. *73,* 103–111 (1955)
Simon, W., Cordonnier, J.J., Snordgrass, W.T.: The pathogenesis of bladder carcinoma. J. Urol. *88,* 797–802 (1962)
Skinner, D.G., Richie, J.P., Cooper, P.H., Waisman, J., Kaufman, J.J.: The clinical significance of carcinoma in situ of the bladder and its association with overt carcinoma. J. Urol. *112,* 68–71 (1974)

So, B.T., Wynder, E.L.: Induction of hamster tumors of the urinary bladder by 3,2'-dimethyl-4-aminobiphenyl. J. Nat. Cancer Inst. *48,* 1733–1738 (1972)
Stenius, F.: Studien über Pathologie und Klinik der Papillome und Carcinome der Harnblase. Quoted after Hückel (1934)
Stiller, D., Rauscher, H.: Irreversible preneoplastic defect in alkaline phosphatase in cancerization of transitional epithelium. Exp. Path. *5,* 255–258 (1971)
Störck, O., Zuckerkandl, O.: Über Cystitis glandularis und den Drüsenkrebs der Harnblase. Z. Urol. *1,* 1–41 (1907)
Straub, F.B.: On the reoxidation of diaphorase-flavo-protein. Enzymologia *9,* 148–149 (1939)
Stutte, H.J.: Hexazotiertes Triamino-Tritolyl-Methanchlorid (Neufuchsin) als Kupplungssalz in der Fermenthistochemie. Histochemie *8,* 327–331 (1967)
Takeuchi, T.: Histochemical demonstration of branching enzyme (amylo-1,4→1,5-transglucosidase) in animal tissues. J. Histochem. Cytochem. *6,* 208–216 (1958)
Takeuchi, T., Kuriaki, H.: Histochemical detection of phosphorylase in animals tissues. J. Histochem. Cytochem. *3,* 153–160 (1955)
Temkin, J.S.: Industrial bladder carcinogenesis. Oxford, London, New York, Paris: Pergamon 1963
Thelino, W.L., Seemayer, T.A., Madarmas, P., Mount, B.M.M., McKinnon, K.J.: Carcinoma in situ of the bladder with associated prostatic involvement. J. Urol. *111,* 491–494 (1974)
Thiede, T., Christensen, B.C.: Bladder tumours induced by chlornaphazine. Acta Med. Scand. *155,* 133–137 (1969)
Thomas, D.G., Ward, A.M., Williams, J.L.: A study of 52 cases of adenocarcinoma of the bladder. Br. J. Urol. *43,* 4–11 (1971)
Thompson, I.M., Coppridge, A.J.: Bladder sarcoma. J. Urol. *82,* 239–332 (1959)
Tizzoni, G., Poggi, A.: Die Wiederherstellung der Harnblase; experimentelle Untersuchungen. Z. Chir. *15,* 921 (1888)
Trites, A.E.W.: Inverted urothelial papilloma: report of two cases. J. Urol. *101,* 216–219 (1969)
Tucci, P., Haralambidis, G.: Regeneration of the bladder: review of literature and case report. J. Urol. *90,* 193–199 (1963)
Übelhör, R.: Eine 16-Jahres-Statistik des Blasencarcinoms. Klin. Med. *20,* 480–493 (1965)
Urlesberger, H.: Quoted after Übelhör (1965)
Utz, D.C., Hanash, K.A., Farrow, G.M.: The plight of the patient with carcinoma in situ of the bladder. J. Urol. *103,* 160–164 (1970)
Vacek, Z., Schück, O.: Histology and histochemistry of the transitional epithelium of the rat bladder in response to experimental filling. Anat. Rec. *136,* 87–95 (1960)
Vahlensieck, W.: Zur sogenannten „offenen Regeneration" nach subtotaler Harnblasenresektion bzw. Zystprostatektomie. Z. Urol. *64,* 491–501 (1971)
Veenema, R.J., Fingerhut, B., Girgis, A.S.: Histochemistry: a possible guide to therapy of bladder tumors. J. Urol. *90,* 736–746 (1963)
Veenema, R.J., Fingerhut, B., Graff, S.: Nucleic acid synthesis in bladder tumours. J. Urol. *105,* 392–396 (1971)
Veenema, R.J., Fingerhut, B., Lattimer, J.K.: Experimental studies of the biological potential of bladder tumors. J. Urol. *93,* 202–211 (1965)
Walker, B.E.: Polyploidy and differentiation in transitional epithelium of mouse urinary bladder. Chromosoma *9,* 105–118 (1958)
Walker, B.E.: Electron microscopic observations on transitional epithelium of the mouse urinary bladder. J. Ultrastruct. Res. *3,* 345–361 (1960)
Walker, B.E.: Radiographic observations on regeneration of transitional epithelium. Texas Rep. Biol. Med. *17,* 375–384 (1969)
Ward, A.M.: Glandular neoplasia within the urinary tract. The etiology of adenocarcinomas of the urothelium with a review of the literature. I. Introduction: The origin

of glandular epithelium in the renal pelvis, ureter and bladder. Virchows Arch. Path. Anat. *352,* 296–311 (1971)
Wattenberg, C.A., Beare, J.B., Torney, A.R.: Exstrophy of the urinary bladder complicated by adenocarcinoma. J. Urol. *76,* 583–594 (1956)
Wheeler, J.D., Hill, W.T.: Adenocarcinoma involving the urinary bladder. Cancer *7,* 119–135 (1954)
Wood, M.: Aetiology of tumours of the urinary bladder. Induction of tumors in the urinary tract of the rabbit by aromatic amines. Path. Microbiol. *32,* 177–190 (1968)
Wood, M.: Factors influencing the induction of tumours of the urinary bladder and liver by 2-acetylaminofluorene in the mouse. Eur. J. Cancer *5,* 41–47 (1969)
Wood, M., Flaks, A., Clayson, D.B.: The carcinogenic activity of dibutylnitrosamine in IF $\times$ C_{57} mice. Eur. J. Cancer *6,* 443–440 (1970)
Yates-Bell, A.J.: Carcinoma in situ of the bladder. Br. J. Surg. *58,* 359–364 (1971)
Youngblood, V.H., Banks, R., Denney, E.E.: Rhabdomyosarcoma of the bladder. J. Urol. *67,* 957–961 (1952)
Zingg, E.J., Busser, E.: Klinik des Blasenpapilloms. Urologe *7,* 82–88 (1968)
Zuckerkandl, O.: Blasengeschwülste. Wien. med. Wochenschr. *60,* 441–448 (1910)

B-Lymphocytes in Carcinogenesis

Ch. WITTING

I. Introduction

Cancer is not a single disease entity; the term is applied to a large number of diseases in which the abnormal and continued growth of cells of a given tissue is expressed. The immunologic mechanism responsible for the rejection of solid tumors in experimental animals is generally thought to be the same as that responsible for homograft rejection, i.e., delayed hypersensivity. It has been demonstrated with the use of diffusion chambers that antibody and complement may kill some kinds of tumor cells. The cytotoxic reaction may be responsible for the destruction of tumor cells growing primarily in suspension and the delayed-type reaction may be responsible for the rejection of solid tumors. The mechanism of tumor cell destruction by specifically sensitized cells has been studied in vitro. The major mechanism of destruction is the interaction of sensitized lymphocytes with tumor cell-surface antigens. Thereby, the sensitized cell may be either activated to become a killer cell or it may synthesize and/or release mediators (lymphokines) which activate other cells, such as macrophages, to participate in target cell killing (*Sell,* 1975).

Cell-mediated immunity can be demonstrated under three general aspects:

1. Destruction of target cells by lymphocytes specifically sensitized to the target cells.

2. Production of killer cells or appropriate cell products by normal unsensitized lymphocyte populations following treatment with nonspecific lymphocyte stimulants.

3. Target cell killing by normal unsensitized lymphocytes in the presence of humoral antibodies directed against the target cell (*Sell,* 1975).

The possible situations are adumbrated in Figure 1. Direct target cell killing by specifically sensitized killer cells and mitogen-stimulated killer cells or cell products

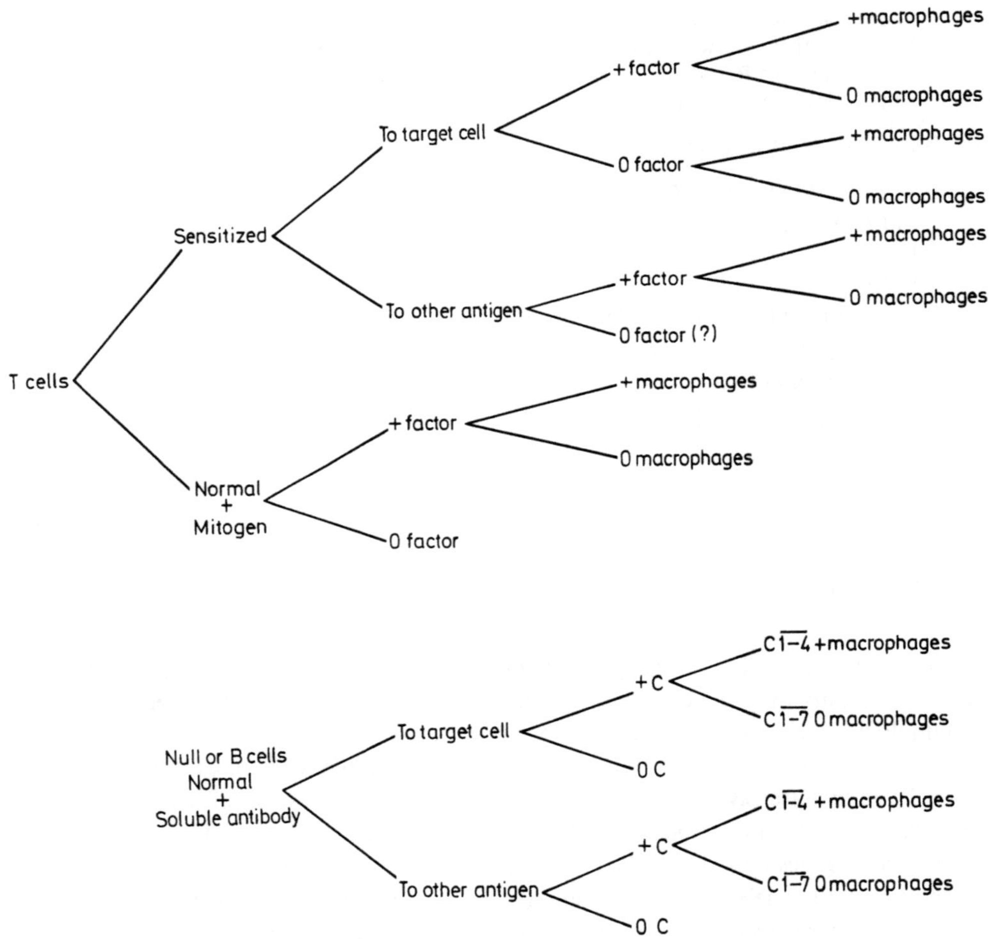

Fig. 1. Possible mechanisms of lymphoid cell-mediated cytotoxicity (from *Sell,* 1975)

is the result of T-cell activation. Antibody-dependent, cell-mediated lymphocytolysis requires Null-cells or B-cells as effectors. Sensitizing of T cells may be induced in vitro. Macrophages are required for optimal sensitization of T-cells but they do not take part in the killer cell effector stage of the reaction. On the other hand, macrophages may acquire the capacity to kill target cells by reaction with a substance produced by specifically sensitized T-cells on reaction with the target cells. Thus, macrophages may become killer cells due to the effects of activated T-cell products and so amplify cell-mediated immunity (*Sell,* 1975).

Since the time when lymphocytes were subdivided into B-cells and T-cells (*Miller* and *Mitchell,* 1969; *Raff,* 1971), most investigations of the influence of lymphocytes on tumor growth have been focused on T lymphocytes. It was found that virally or chemically induced tumors would develop more frequently in neonatally thymectomized animals, in animals pretreated with antilymphocyte serum, or in irradiated animals which are all enduring a depletion of T lymphocytes. If immune reactivity in humans is impaired by either congenital or therapy-induced immune deficiency, an increased number of tumors will develop, mainly lymphomas (vz. *Good* and *Finstad,* 1969; *Gatti* and *Good,* 1971).

In 1974 *Rygaard* and *Povlsen* showed that athymic nude mice – whose thoracic duct lymphocyte population consists purely of small B-lymphocytes – fail to get spontaneous malignant tumors in comparison with controls, as observed in approximately 45,000 months of mouse life of some 13,000 nude mice. The role of B-lymphocytes in tumor development as well as in tumor rejection has been widely discussed ever since. The role of B-lymphocytes seems to be ambivalent: sometimes they act as tumor cells and sometimes as tumor rejecting cells; it is under these aspects that its bearing on carcinogenesis shall be discussed.

II. B-Lymphocytes in Tumor Rejection

The possibility of a direct or indirect influence of B-lymphocytes and humoral antibodies on tumor growth was first suggested by certain investigations as early as 1910 (*Gaylord* et al.; *Roswing*) and subsequently reexamined and confirmed by *Hattler* and *Amos* (1966), *Old* et al. (1968), and *Smith* (1968). In these assays, cell-free sera of mice which had rejected a malignant tumor were transferred to other tumor-bearing mice. The transfer of serum was observed to inhibit tumor growth and even, in some cases, to cause destruction of the tumor and eventual curing of the animals.

These assays provided a first evidence for the potential influence of humoral antibodies on tumor growth. It is known today that humoral antibodies are produced by B-lymphocytes. Both B- and T-lymphocytes have their common origin in the bone marrow and in lymphoid tissue but acquire their specifity either in the thymus (T-cells) or in the avian Bursa of Fabricius and mammalian gastrointestinal lymphoid organs (B-cells), respectively.

Opinions differ about the origin of B-cells in man (*Stein,* 1976). In the rabbit, whose immunologic system is closely related to that of man, B-cells arise directly from the bone marrow (*Keuning,* 1972; *Nieuwenhuis* et al., 1974). The Bursa of Fabricius in chickens is known to induce an antigen-independent formation and proliferation of B-cells (*Cooper* et al., 1968). In man, however, it is the intestinal lymphoid tissue and its antigen-dependent reactions which seem to play the important role in the proliferation of B-lymphocytes (*Stein,* 1976).

After stimulation by antigens, the B-cells proliferate and differentiate into plasma cells which then synthesize and secrete antibodies (humoral immunity). T-Cells are the mediators of cellular immunity. There is, obviously, a specific cell or cell line which, upon repeated contact with the original antigen, will respond more rapidly by enhanced proliferation and differentiation (memory cell). Memory cells are found among B-cells as well as among T-cells (*Cantor* and *Asofsky,* 1970; *Tigelaar* and *Asofsky,* 1973).

Identification of B-lymphocytes is mostly carried out by means of fluorescent antisera reacting with immunoglobulins on the cell surface. In contrast, T-cells possess either very few surface immunoglobulins or none at all (*Greaves,* 1970; *Greaves* and *Hogg,* 1971). T-Lymphocytes are readily demonstrated by spontaneous rosette formation (*Jondal* et al., 1972) which is effected in human tissues by sheep erythrocytes.

Table 1. Marker from "mature" B- and T-cells (from *Stein,* 1976)

Marker	B-cell	T-cell
Ig in saline-1.-extract	↑	n or ↓
Ig in detergent-2.-extract	↑	↓
Membrane-Ig	+	–
Cytoplasmic-Ig	+ [a]	–
Complement-receptors (CR)		
C4-R, C3c-R	+	–
C3d-R	+	–
FcR		
IgG-EA	+	–
aggregated IgG	+	–
Mouse-ER	+	–
EBV-R	+	–
ER	–	+
E_NR	–	+
$E_{AET}R$	–	+
Helix promatia protectin-R	–	+
Morbilli-Virus-R	–	+
HTLA	–	+

n = Normal, ↑ = increase in number; ↓ = decrease in number; – = non present; + = present

FcR = Receptor for Fc fragment
Mouse-ER = Receptor for mouse erythrocytes
EBV-R = Receptor for Epstein-Barr-Virus
ER = Receptor for sheep erythrocytes
E_NR = Receptor for neuraminidase-treated sheep erythrocytes
$E_{AET}R$ = Receptor for AET-treated sheep erythrocytes
HTLA = Human thymus lymphocyte antigen

[a] Only secretory B-cells

B-Lymphocytes are unable to form these spontaneous rosettes. Moreover, T-cells possess a so-called surface theta-antigen that can be used for marking.

Table 1 shows the different markers for B- and T-lymphocytes. By these methods of identification it was demonstrated that human spleen, peripheral blood, and lymph nodes contain 60%–75% of T-lymphocytes and 20%–30% of B-lymphocytes (*Silveira* et al., 1972; *Ross* et al., 1973).

The specific suppressor cells of various immune reactions have been identified and characterized. There was some evidence for these cells being able to suppress the immune reaction against tumor antigens (*Gorczynski,* 1974). Consequently, suppressor cells derived from T-lymphocytes may influence the growth of B-lymphocytes and, thereby, indirectly affect the growth of a tumor. On the other hand, it appears possible that the so-called killer lymphocytes – supposedly derived from T-lymphocytes – may exert a direct influence on tumor growth.

Prompted by the investigations of *Hattler* and *Amos* (1966), *Old* et al. (1968), and *Smith* (1968), a renewed interest has focused on the possible influence of B-lymphocytes on tumor growth. The use of a diffusion chamber, permitting the flow-through of antibodies and complements but not of cells, has helped to show how antibody and complement may provoke the destruction of certain tumor cells (*Sell,* 1975).

Apparently, lymphoma and leukemia cells show a very sensitive reaction to antibodies both in vitro and in vivo whereas sarcoma and carcinoma cells, in most cases, fail to show any noticeable reaction to antibodies. *Sell* (1975) concluded that a cytotoxic activity of B-cell-derived antibodies must be responsible for the rejection of tumor cells growing preferably in suspension, while the rejection of solid tumors would fall under the influence of T-lymphocytes.

Evidence for the growing tumor being influenced by cellular and humoral immune reactions has been assembled using human material (*Eilber* and *Morton,* 1970). The study of human tumors revealed a predominant role of T-lymphocytes in tumor rejection; on the other hand, certain results pointed to a potentially important influence of humoral antibody formation on tumor rejection (*Sell,* 1975). Since then a great number of studies has been published on the subject of immuneprophylaxis and therapy of malignant diseases.

1. Direct Activity Against Tumor Development

a) Experimental Tumors

In experimentally induced benzpyrene sarcomas, high concentrations of immunoglobulins have been demonstrated, predominantly of IgG (*Witz,* 1971). These immunoglobulins are capable of dissolving and killing tumor cells in vitro (*Dmochowski* and *Bowen,* 1974). Circulating antibodies produced by B-lymphocytes and exerting a similar influence on tumor growth were also demonstrated in murine Yoshida sarcomas (*Marusic* et al., 1976). In this connection, T-lymphocytes show merely an activating influence on B-cells. The interaction serves to activate a B-cell clone with eventual formation of humoral, T-cell-independent antibodies against Yoshida tumor cells. There are, however, some reports of B-cells directly killing tumor cells. *Kilburn* et al.

(1974) demonstrated in murine malignant lymphoma that the actual rejection of the tumor was the work of B-lymphocytes.

Virally induced sarcomas in BALB/c mice are also destroyed by direct action of B-lymphocytes (*Elboim* et al., 1977). In these tumors, which are predominantly infiltrated by B-cells, it appears that the higher the concentration of B-lymphocytes within the tumor, the stronger is the T-cell-independent regression. Recently, *Niedorf* et al. (1978) emphasized the important role of B-lymphocytes in the rejection of benzpyrene-induced sarcomas in the chicken. In animals that had been hormonally bursectomized on the third day of embryonal life, sarcomas were induced after hatching. Bursectomized animals developed a significantly higher number of tumors and metastases than controls. This effect of bursectomy on tumor growth may be explained as an elimination of the "bursa inhibitor factor" (BIF). Normally, BIF mediates the suppression of T-lymphocytes; consequently, the absence of BIF results in a massed proliferation of T-cells with a subsequent potential by negative influence on tumor growth. On the other hand, it appears possible that B-lymphocytes could attack and destroy chicken sarcomas directly if they had not been eliminated primarily by way of bursectomy.

In opposition to the prevailing concept of the killer cells capable of attacking tumors having their origin directly in the T-cell line, *Haller* and *Wigzell* (1977) showed by strontium labelling in vivo that the killer cells which act against viral leukemias and lymphomas must be seen as a subpopulation of B-lymphocytes. Their results are substantiated by observations of *Burk* et al. (1977) showing that K-cells – or at least some subgroups – can be identified as a subpopulation of B-cells, possibly immature precursors. *Piguet* and *Vassalli* (1973) had already shown that under contact with tumor cells, at least in vitro, B-lymphocytes are preferably activated. Although the important role of K-cells in tumor repulsion was never refuted, these new investigations shed a better light on the role of B-cells in the defense against tumor growth.

b) Human Tumors

In human tumor pathology we have no more than indirect pointers to the possibly predominant role of B-lymphocytes in tumor defense. First evidence was collected in studies of immunoglobulin changes in tumor patients. *Takasugi* and *Hildemann* (1969) found increased levels of IgG_2 and IgM in various tumors. In contrast, breast cancer patients have shown, at all tumor stages, an increased blood level of IgA but reduced level of IgG (*Roberts* and *Bath*, 1973). In the actual tumor tissue high levels of immunoglobulins were also demonstrated: *Stuart* (1970) found a high concentration of immunoglobulins in immunoblastic sarcomas; in cervical carcinoma high concentrations of IgG were found partly in connection with IgM and complement C3 (*Vos* et al., 1972). These immunoglobulins are seen either as antibodies against cell membranes, as an antigen-antibody complex, or as intracytoplasmatic cell particles. Finally, *Stuhlmiller* and *Seigler* (1975) were able to provoke the development of antisera against human melanoma cells in monkeys; these antisera showed cytotoxic activities against tumor cells in vitro and were found to belong the IgG fraction.

2. Mediating Effect in Tumor Rejection

a) Interactions Between Lymphocytes and Macrophages

Macrophages of blood and tissue (monocytes and histiocytes) are phagocytic cells which belong to the mononuclear macrophage system. Interactions between lymphocytes and macrophages were often described; reports concern the influence of lymphocytes on macrophage activity as well as the influence of macrophages on lymphocyte activity (*Nathan* et al., 1973). Interactions of these two populations predominantly involve B-lymphocytes (*Schmidtke* and *Unanue,* 1971). The first result of macrophage action is an increased DNA synthesis in lymphocytes (*Rosenthal* et al., 1975). This primary activation is at first antigen-independent but influence in later phases depends on the lymphocyte possession of specific receptors for a macrophage-bound antigen. After contacting the antigen, immunoglobulin receptors are transferred from T-cells to macrophages (*Feldmann* and *Nossal,* 1972; *Feldmann,* 1973), thereby stimulating the B-cells. Not every B-cell-macrophage interaction would necessarily require the presence or involvement of T-cells; for a maximum formation of antibodies against several antigens in vitro, however, the presence of macrophages, B-, and T-cells is an absolute prerequisite (*Mosier* and *Coppleson,* 1968; *Mosier* et al., 1974).

The place where macrophages and lymphocytes actually start to interact has not been located anatomically with complete security. It appears possible that lymphocytes are not localized permanently in the sites of immune response but are attracted to the sites by induction of a primary antibody reaction (*Gutman* and *Weissmann,* 1972). Cellular interactions between macrophages and lymphocytes are supposed to occur frequently in the white pulp of the spleen, with dendritic macrophages playing

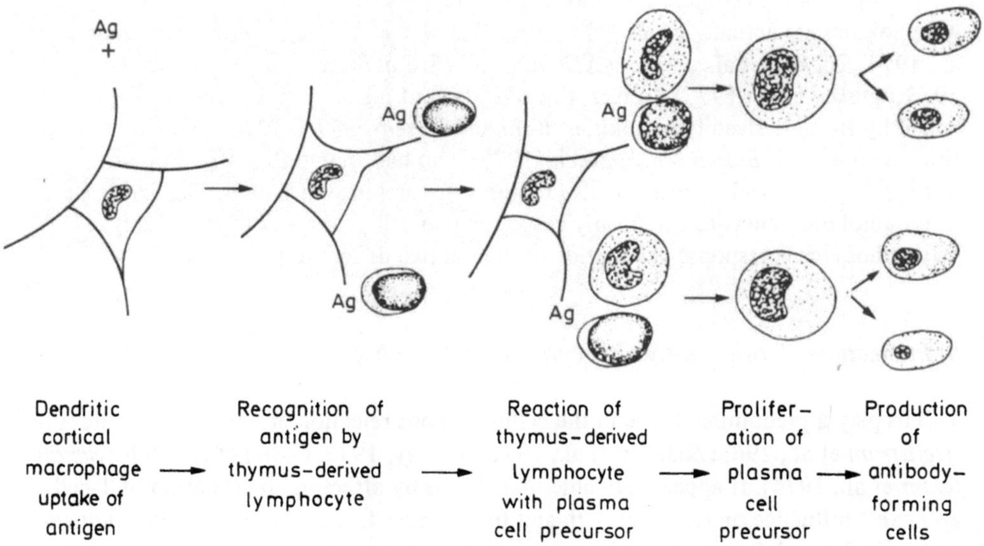

Fig. 2. Cellular interactions in induction of antibody formation (from *Sell,* 1975)

a major part in this process (*White*, 1963; *Movat* and *Fernando*, 1965). Figure 2 shows one possibility for cellular interactions in induction of antibody formation.

When lymphocytes are present, activated macrophages are capable of attacking and destroying tumor cells. The phagocytic capacity of the mononuclear macrophage system also plays a major part in the initial development of a tumor (*Keller*, 1972). The reduction of cellular immunity will increase the susceptibility of an organism for tumor development but increased phagocytic capacity will inhibit tumor growth. When activated peritoneal macrophages are transferred to an animal bearing a Walker carcinoma, tumor growth will be reduced whereas a transfer of serum to the tumor-bearing animal has no effect on tumor growth (*Keller*, 1972). On the other hand, tumor cells are capable of producing certain substances which inhibit lymphocytes and activate macrophages (*Garotta* and *Porta*, 1976). These factors preferably inhibit B-cells and activate macrophages; they are transmitted from the mother to the embryo via the placenta, thus effecting a destruction of fetal B-lymphocytes at an early stage (*Garotta* and *Porta*, 1976). Lymphocytes and macrophages are also capable of killing human tumor cells; co-operative action of lymphocytes and macrophages was found to exert a cytotoxic influence on cells of human melanoma (*Youdim* and *Sharman*, 1976). However, this influence seems to be effective only when B-cells, T-cells, and macrophages are all present together. Separation of these cellular components will abolish cytotoxicity while restoration of the trias of cell types will reanimate the cytotoxic influence (*Youdim* and *Sharman*, 1976). The actual activation of macrophages is caused by lymphokines produced by the lymphocytes after presensitization of the lymphocytes by tumor surface antigens. According to the studies of *Zbar* et al. (1970) and *Bernstein* et al. (1971) this presensitization of lymphocytes is an absolute prerequisite for starting the reaction against tumor cells. Sensitization of lymphocytes leads to lymphokine production which summons macrophages to the neighborhood of the tumor where they will eventually take up the responsibility for destroying the tumor.

In opposition to conclusions drawn from previous studies, it was established that lymphokines are actually produced by B-cells as well as by T-lymphocytes (*Cohen* et al., 1974; *Rocklin* et al., 1974; *O'Nell* et al., 1975; *Sandberg* et al., 1975; *Wahl* et al., 1975; *Jenssen* et al., 1977). In fact, the activation of macrophages seems to be provoked by B-cell-derived lymphokines. *Wahl* and *Rosenstreich* (1976) were able to confirm the results of *Bloom* and *Shevach* (1975) who had shown that MIF formation is not the work of T-cells alone but also requires the presence of B-cells. The synthesis of lymphokines seems to be an early response of B-cell precursors to an induction by T-lymphocytes, a response given prior to their actual differentiation.

b) Interactions Between B-Lymphocytes and T-Lymphocytes

T-Cells play a predominant role in the cellular tumor rejection effected by lymphocytes (*Hellström* et al., 1968; *Baldwin* et al., 1971; *Henney*, 1973; *Cossel* et al., 1974; *Schönfelder* et al., 1974). It appears possible that B-cells by affecting the function of T-cells, also exert influence on tumor growth and tumor spread. Investigations by *Perlman* and *Holm* (1970) and *Cerottini* and *Brunner* (1974) had also shown that the direct killing of target cells must be the result of T-cell activation. Previous studies proved that the tumor-destroying killer lymphocytes (K-cells) originate among the T-cell line. It was concluded that some products of activated T-cells were able to convert macrophages into K-cells which subsequently enhance cellular immune reactions (*Berke* and *Amos,* 1973; *Wagner* et al., 1973).

The significance of B-cell/T-cell interactions is stressed by the fact that neither bone marrow cells nor thymus cells are separately immune competent. A mixture of both cell types is required for an effective immune response (*Diener* and *Langman,* 1974). The interaction between them is mediated by a haptene that is initially bound to specific surface receptors of the lymphocyte. T-Cell-bound antigens are in turn capable of stimulating antibody formation in B-lymphocytes. The result is antibody production by B-cells which is faster and higher than it would be in the presence of hapten-loaded T-cells (*Mitchison,* 1969; *Dutton* et al., 1971; *Taylor* and *Iverson,* 1971; *Claman* and *Mosier,* 1972). Sometimes macrophages take part in these B-cell/T-cell interactions, but their presence is no absolute prerequisite (*Diener* and *Langman,* 1974). However, the studies of *Mosier* and *Coppleson* (1968) and *Mosier* et al. (1974) have shown that macrophages must be present for maximum formation in vitro of antibodies against several antigens. All antibodies assessed in a mixed B- and T-cell population have been produced by B-cells. Production of IgG, however, may possibly require the presence of T-cells (*Diener* and *Langman,* 1974). Consequently, T-cells may improve antibody production by B-cells against some, but not all, antigens (*Feldmann,* 1973). The surface of B-lymphocytes is equipped with acceptor molecules capable of binding T-cells or their products (*Katz* et al., 1973). On the other hand, we know about the existence of a suppressor function of T-cells against B-cells. Any depletion of T-cells, e.g., by the application of antilymphocyte serum or by thymectomy, will result in a massed increase chiefly of IgM-producing B-cells (*Feldmann* and *Nossal,* 1972; *Feldmann,* 1973). There are, however, some controversial observations of a reduced antibody production by B-cells after thymectomy or ALS application (*Kerbel* and *Eidinger,* 1971). These reactions would become manifest in alterations of the IgM blood level.

c) Interactions Between Tumor Cells and Lymphocytes

Certain interactions are known to occur between tumor cells and cells of regional lymph nodes (*Deodhar* et al., 1972). They are manifested, e.g., in a clumping of tumor cells which are subsequently dissolved by lymphocytes. Similar interactions are found in breast cancer patients without lymph node involvement. As soon as lymphnodes become involved with metastatic spread they are no longer capable of attacking the tumor cells (*Deodhar* et al., 1972). Interactions of this kind can be demonstrated in breast carcinomas of every histologic type.

The cytotoxic activity of cells from regional lymph nodes against breast tumor cells is probably initiated by macrophages, but it is essentially dependent on B-cells (*Hickok* et al., 1977). While the cells of regional nodes possess these capacities of direct attack on tumor cells, lymphocytes belonging to the peripheral blood population fail to show any influence on breast cancer cells (*Hickok* et al., 1977).

d) B-Lymphocytes in the Marginal Zone of Tumors

With reference to the studies of *Niedorf* et al. (1978) we have adopted the term "marginal zone of a tumor" for the area of peritumoral infiltration. The significance of this peritumoral inflammatory infiltration was already noticed by *Ribbert (1894). Wallbach* (1929) was the first to suspect an immune reaction of the organism against the tumor in this phenomenon. *Hackmann* (1951) and *Hamperl* (1956) have also emphasized the importance of peritumoral infiltration in tumor defense. *Grundmann* et al. (1969) described several changes in the peritumoral infiltration that were observed under therapy and treatment with antilymphocyte serum.

Within this infiltrated area, T-cells play a predominant role in tumor defense (cf. *Schönfelder* et al., 1974). *Niedorf* et al. (1978) found a substantial influence of B-lymphocytes on tumor growth in benzpyrene-induced chicken sarcoma. *Blaeser* (1975) had also emphasized the role of B-lymphocytes in the marginal zone of the tumor. He observed a great number of proliferating plasma cells in the surroundings of keratinizing squamous carcinomas of human larynx.

Burkitt lymphomas, whose tumor cells are derived from B-cell line, show a peritumoral infiltration predominantly rich in T-cells, and so do nasopharyngeal carcinomas (*Klein* et al., 1976). The problem of B-cell influence on tumor growth was further investigated in our own studies with a splenectomy model (*Witting* and *Hultsch,* 1978). When we studied the influence of splenectomy on tumor growth we came across one strain of mice whose spleens contained 80% B-lymphocytes. The strain was a hybrid of A/Jax/BOMf females and BALB/c/BOMf males. Normally, the B-cell content of mouse spleens varies between 20% (*Raff* and *Owen,* 1971) and 89% (*Suter* et al., 1972). After splenectomy at the age of 3 weeks, our animals developed significantly less tumors (benzpyrene-induced sarcomas) than the respective controls (splenectomized mice: 29%, controls: 50%). Peripheral blood counts after splenectomy showed a significant reduction of B-lymphocytes down to 11%–15% (controls: 25%–30%) and an increase in T-lymphocytes to 66%–75% (controls: 56%–65%). No comparable results after splenectomy either human or experimental have been reported until now.

T-Lymphocytes were labeled by means of a histochemical marker for unspecific esterase and by an immune adherence test. B-Lymphocytes were counted with the aid of an immune fluorescence test and an immune adherence test. Our investigations can be summarized as follows:

1. Spleens of the employed strain of animals consist of a very high percentage of B-lymphocytes.
2. After splenectomy, the number of B-lymphocytes is severely reduced but that of T-cells is increased in the peripheral blood.
3. After splenectomy, there is a significant reduction in the development of benzpyrene-induced sarcomas.
4. After splenectomy, the area of peritumoral infiltration shows a significant reduction in B-lymphocyte and an increase in T-lymphocyte populations.

One of the prerequisites for such severe alterations within the lymphocytes population seems to be an abundance of B-cells in the excised spleen. Controversial results and reports about the effect of splenectomy on tumor growth might be explained by the facts, that, firstly, several species possess very different splenic B-cell populations and that secondly, the B-cell content may vary even between animals of one species. Our results speak at least for a considerable influence of spelenctomy on the proportion of interactions between B-cells and T-cells. As yet, the changes in the individual subpopulations of both B- and T-lymphocytes after splenectomy have not been studied separately.

Obviously, the known influence of splenectomy on tumor growth, must be traced back to the change in B-cell contents. At first sight, the present results would not support an interpretation of K-cells as a subpopulation of B-cells. If that were the case, the logical inference would be that splenectomy must result in a reduction of K-cells and subsequently increased tumor incidence. On the other hand, one might presume that the B-cells settled in the spleen must be mature forms and not precursors such as the K-cells are thought to be. Consequently, it appears possible that splenectomy would remove only one group of B-lymphocytes which is not identical with K-cells. In view of the varied interactions between different subgroups of the B-cell line it appears quite plausible that the elimination of one subpopulation would enable the K-lymphocytes of the B-cell line to attack the tumor more effectively and so to reduce tumor incidence after splenectomy.

On the other hand, our studies revealed that splenectomy provoked not only an alteration in the B-cell count but also a proliferation of T-cells in the peripheral blood and in the tumor margin. One might think that murine B-cells are capable of producing a substance such as the "bursa inhibitor factor" of chickens which would able to influence the growth of T cells or their respective subgroups. If this factor were removed by splenectomy, the result would be proliferation and increase of the previously inhibited T-cells. Our experiment has shown the increase of T-cells to coincide with reduced tumor indidence, suggesting that a given T-cell population could destroy tumor cells either by producing lymphokines or by direct cellular attack. On the whole, our results speak in favor of the K-cells belongig to the T-cell line rather than to the B-cell line, always presuming that no other lymphocyte-dependent factors influence tumor growth.

III. B-Lymphocytes in Tumor Initiation

B-Lymphocytes may not only play the role of tumor-rejecting cells but also that of true tumor cells; these tumors are mostly lymphomas. The development of lymphomas was studied experimentally in NZB/NZW mice. The NZB inbred mouse strain was developed in New Zealand in the 1950s for cancer research. The response of these mice differed very much from that of other mouse strains. After immunization with a variety of exogenous antigens, NZB mice show an abnormally high humoral antibody response but a less intense delayed (cellular) hypersensivity. They also develop spontaneously a number of immunopathologic abnormalities. It was postulated that NZB mice possess a genetic abnormality of lymphoid cell control: suppressor T-cell activity becomes depleted with aging, leading to uncontrolled responses from humoral antibody-forming B-cells. A further evidence for the loss of control of lymphoid cell proliferation is the development of lymphoid cell tumors. The high incidence of lymphoid-cell-proliferative diseases speaks for an uncontrolled growth of B-cells which leads to immunoglobulin-producing tumors. In the absence of a T-cell suppressor control, an abnormal antibody response to a chronic viral infection is the most likely explanation for the immune-mediated abnormalities in NZB/NZW mice.

Even in humans, persistent antigen stimulation coinciding with disturbed antibody production is discussed as a possible cause for the development of lymphomas (*Krüger*, 1970, 1974). First, this antigen stimulation will provoke hyperplasia of lymph nodes which may subsequently lead to the development of malignant lymphomas.

1. B-Lymphocytes in Experimental Tumors

a) Chicken

Lymphatic leukemias and malignant lymphomas can be induced in chickens by certain viruses (*Cooper,* 1974). Tumor cells of a chicken lymphoid leukemia possess, in a high percentage of cases, surface IgM receptors and some intracytoplasmic deposits of IgM. No deposits of IgA or IgG were identified in the tumor cells. Tumor-bearing chickens show a high serum level of IgM, i.e., of both the low molecular and the high molecular weight IgM. The increased serum level of IgM may be plausibly traced back to increased IgM production by tumor cells (*Cooper* et al., 1974).

b) Cat

Leukemias and malignant lymphomas can be virally induced in cats (*Cockerell* et al., 1976a, b, c). Cat T-lymphocytes are readily "marked" with guinea pig erythrocytes. Thus, virally induced malignant lymphomas or lymphosarcomas are identified as T-cell sarcomas, while B-lymphocytes fail to show any remarkable response. During the later stages in feline virus leukemia, the absolute count of T-lymphocytes in the peripheral blood is increasing but, in most cases, no significant change is observed in the number of B-lymphocytes (*Cockerell* et al., 1976a, b, c).

c) Cattle

Viral induction of lymphosarcomas is also possible in the bovine species (*Takashima* et al., 1977) where these tumors are mostly B-cell sarcomas. It is generally easy to show the origin of sarcoma cells from the B-cell population by way of immune-optical demonstration of immunoglobulins. An increased percentage of B-lymphocytes can be identified in the blood of tumor-bearing cattle but the T-lymphocyte count is reduced (*Takashima* et al., 1977).

2. B-Lymphocytes in Human Tumors

a) Leukemias and Malignant Lymphomas

Changed B-lymphocyte behavior in human tumors is reported chiefly in cases of leukemia and malignant lymphoma. Studies of acute lymphatic leukemia (ALL) and chronic lymphatic leukemia (CLL) resulted in divergent findings. According to the observations of *Chin* et al. (1973), acute lymphatic leukemia is characterized by a significant increase in T-lymphocytes and reduction in B-lymphocyte number. This is contradicted by the studies of *Ross* (1977) who found a massively increased B-lymphocyte count in ALL. His observations revealed 80% of ALL to be B-cell tumors and 20% to be T-cell tumors. Accordingly, a B-cell ALL would have a much better prognosis than the T-cell variety. According to *Stein* (1976) we should distinguish three forms of ALL:

1. B-Cell type (described by *Brouet* et al., 1975)
2. T-Cell type
3. Non-B-cell, Non-T-cell type

The results in CLL are equally controversial: *Grey* et al. (1971) showed CLL to be a B-cell tumor. Based on their results, *Chin* et al. (1973) formed the opinion that ALL must be interpreted as a T-cell tumor and CLL as a B-cell tumor. In opposition, *Ross* (1977) identified ALL as a B-cell tumor. In a report about a patient with lymphosarcoma, *Hsu* et al. (1975) supported the opinion of *Chin* et al. In this patient, recorded over 8 months, the amount of peripheral B-lymphocytes rose from an initial 15% to a final 99%. Among these B-lymphocytes some 50% showed IgG receptors, 23% IgA receptors, 95% IgM receptors, 93% IgD receptors, and 28% IgE receptors. *Ross* and *Polley* (1975) identified three subtypes of CLL by their respective membrane-bound immunoglobulins:

1. Ig-positive, C3dR-positive, C3bR-negative (78%)
2. Ig-negative, C3dR-positive, C3bR-negative (11%)
3. Ig-positive, C3dR-positive, C3bR-positive (11%)

Studies of *Stein* (1976) showed CLL to be a B-cell tumor.

Studies of several malignant lymphomas were similarly divergent. *Chin* et al. (1973) demonstrated a significant increase of B-lymphocytes in the peripheral blood of patients with malignant lymphoma without any visible change in T-lymphocytes; thus, these malignant lymphomas were seen as B-cell tumors with a high percentage of IgG receptors. This findings were confirmed by *Ross* (1977) who also found an abnormal proliferation of B-cells in human malignant lymphomas. *Middelkoop* et al. (1976) arrived at a different conclusion; they found a numerical reduction of peripheral lymphocytes in their lymphoma patients, while the relative proportion of B- to T-lymphocytes remained unaltered. The tumor cells proper were not studied.

Classification of human malignant lymphomas was established chiefly by *Rappaport* (1966) and *Lennert* et al. (1975). *Stein* (1976) determined the B-cell or T-cell origin of human malignant lymphomas by morphologic and immunologic characteristics. According to him, 80% of Non-Hodgkin-lymphomas are identified as B-cell tumors, i.e., all lymphomas forming secretory Ig, all centrocytic germ cell tumors, and the majority of immunoblastic lymphomas. *Stein* defined the following malignant lymphomas in particular as B-cell tumors (excluding CLL): prolymphocytic leukemia (described by *Galton* et al., 1974), hairy cell leukemia, plasmocytoma, lympho-plasmocytoid immunocytoma (e.g., Morbus Waldenström), centroblastic-centrocytic lymphoma, centroblastic lymphoma, Burkitt lymphoma, and the majority of immunoblastic lymphomas and sarcomas.

b) Other Tumors

α) Changes in B- and T-cell populations of patients with *inoperable carcinoma* were studied by *Boh* and *Reddy* (1976); they reported a reduction of total lymphocyte count in the peripheral blood. Patients receiving radiotherapy showed even lower values than nonirradiated patients. The changes found in T-cell values were similar: decreased peripheral blood T-cells in tumor patients, lower T-cell count in irradiated than in nonirradiated tumor patients. B-Cell changes were also comparable: non-tumor-bearing controls showed the largest amount of B-cells, nonirradiated tumor patients had less, and irradiated tumor patients had the lowest values. Besides, *Goh* and *Reddy* had found an increased proportion of Null-lymphocytes in their carcinoma patients.

β) The *Sezary-syndrom* was found to be a disease of the thymus-derived lymphocytes (*Brouet* et al., 1973). The peripheral blood of these patients and of patients with mycosis fungoides had decreased T-lymphocytes and increased Null-cell counts (*Nordqvist* and *Kinney,* 1976). Predominant among the cells isolated from tumors of mycosis fungoides were T-cells (*Robinowitz* et al., 1976).

γ) Patients with *multiple myeloma* show serious abnormalities of humoral immunity and at least two types of B-cell abnormalities (*Lee,* 1977): uncontrolled proliferation of plasma cells, and a reduction in the number and functional capacity of immunoglobulin-synthesizing B-lymphocytes (*Lindstrom* et al., 1973; *Solomon*, 1975).

δ) In *Hodgkin's disease,* depressed cell-mediated immune response as an index of thymus-dependent lymphocyte dysfunction has been documented extensively (*Lee,* 1977). *Miller* (1967) postulated that Hodgkin's disease resulted from a proliferation of a thymus-dependent population of lymphocytes but results of later studies suggested a hyperactivity of B-cell population (*Lee,* 1977). It was theorized that the malignant cell in Hodgkin's disease could be a T-lymphocyte, perhaps antigenically altered and virally transformed. In 1914 *Bunting* reported the depression of blood lymphocyte count in patients with Hodgkin's disease. *Aisenberg* (1965) found that severe lymphocytopenia is seen only during the terminal months of the disease. In a retrospective and all-inclusive study of 527 patients, *Lee* et al. (1974) found the lowest survival rate in patients with lymphocyte counts below $1000/mm^3$. *Froland* (1972) reported the percentage of T- and B-lymphocytes within the normal range in five patients with Hodgkin's disease. This result resembles those of *Cohnen* et al. (1973) and *Falletta* et al. (1973). A normal amount of lymphocytes in Hodgkin's disease was also found by *Ross* (1977).

The overall lymphocyte count in the peripheral blood and the relative proportion of T-cells seem to be good indicators for the prognosis of patients with various kinds of tumors (*Lee*, 1977). For instance, patients with bone tumors, neuroblastomas, and carcinomas of breast, colon, urinary tract, protio, liver, lung, brain, and nasopharyngeal cavity have a better survival expectancy if their climax, the decrease in T-cells and increase in B-cells can be measured in the peripheral blood. In the course of adequate therapy, the lymphocyte counts will gradually return to normal. Patients who show higher lymphocyte counts due to an increase in T-cells, will have a better prognosis than patients with normal or decreased counts (*Lee,* 1977).

Besides the influence of malignant tumors on the immune situation, several congenital immune deficiencies are known. The B-cell-dependent varieties are listed in Table 2.

Table 2. B-cell dependent congenital immune deficiencies (modified after *Haferkamp,* 1974)

Origin	Immune deficiency
In stem cells	Swiss type of agammaglobulinemia
During B-cell formation from stem cells	Congenital sex-related agammaglobulinemia (Bruton)
During immune response with production of antibodies by B-lymphocytes	Wiscott-Aldrich-syndrome
During immune reaction and defense against infection	Chediak-Higashi-syndrome, lazy leucocyte syndrome myeoloperoxidase deficiency syndrome

IV. Discussion and Conclusion

Present knowledge of the role of B-lymphocytes in tumor initiation and development can be seen under two aspects: one concerns the role of B-cells as actual tumor cells, the other their role in defense against tumors.

In experimental as well as in human pathology, numerous tumors are known as "B-cell tumors." In this category are counted many of the malignant lymphomas in animals and in humans. Concepts regarding the origin of CLL and ALL are still rather controversial. Whereas CLL is generally seen as a B-cell tumor, some observations are interpreted in favour of ALL, too, being of B-cell origin; other authors have demonstrated the T-cell origin of this disease. The most plausible concept would be that there is no uniform pattern for the origin of ALL but that it may occur partly as a B-cell tumor and partly as a T-cell tumor. Some evidence has been collected that B-cell ALL would have a much better prognosis than the T-cell variety.

A very significant role is attributed to B-cells in tumor defense. Experimental pathology has collected good evidence for antibodies being formed by B-cells and being capable of destroying tumors. The immunization of an organism by a tumor or against a tumor may be interpreted as proof for the important role of B-cell-dependent humoral immunity in the rejection of, or defense against, tumors.

On the other hand, it appears possible that not every tumor cell is vulnerably to attack by antibodies. In this context, cells of leukemia or lymphoma growing in suspension, rather than in close contact, appear more susceptible to the attack of antibodies than, for example, the solid growing carcinoma cells.

By their influence on other cell systems, B-lymphocytes appear capable of indirectly affecting tumor growth. In opposition to previous studies it is now safely recognized that certain mediators are actually, or possibly, formed by B-cells. It is, however, still unclear whether these mediators exert a direct rejective effect on the tumor or are merely activating other kinds of cells that will eventually kill the tumor cells.

Interactions between B-cells and T-cells have been observed for a long time. T-Cells are known to have a suppressive effect on B-lymphocytes which, in turn, are only able to extensively proliferate after reduction of the number of T-cells. On the other hand, the "bursal inhibitor factor" (BIF) in chickens is known to attack T-lymphocytes effectively. In consequence, any elimination of this BIF will result in a proliferation of T-cells. These alternating pathways of interaction may exemplify the very intensive functional interchange between B- and T-lymphocytes.

Moreover, there are many reports about interactions between macrophages and B-cells, partly dependent, partly independent of the presence of T-cells. Mutual interactions and interchanges are at play, with macrophages influencing B-cell proliferation or B-cells influencing macrophages.

Via their effect on T-cell and macrophage functions, B-cells are certainly able to influence the growth and spread of a tumor since both macrophages and T-lymphocytes play their significant active roles in tumor defense.

Evidence is accumulating, too, for the capacity of B-cells to destroy tumor cells directly, i.e., by cell-to-cell contact. Their presence in the peritumoral zone of infiltration could be a sign similar to the cytotoxic activity of regional lymph node cells against cells from a breast carcinoma. In vivo studies of murine malignant lymphomas have safely identified as B-cells some cells that are actively destroying the tumor. Recent reports on the possible B-cell nature of killer cells (i.e., tumor destroying lymphocytes) are of increased relevance in this context. So far, these results are only taken from experimentally leukemias and lymphomas.

Despite many other studies emphasizing the predominant important of T-cells acting as killer cells in tumor defense, the present investigations have shown that B-cells, too, possess a certain capacity to directly attack and destroy a tumor.

Our presentation and discussion of results was aimed at stressing the difficulty of maintaining the rather simple classification of the lymphoid system into B- and T-cells. It may become necessary, for practical and theoretcial purposes, to reclassify the lymphoid system in terms of the functional behavior of subpopulations rather than in terms of their morphology or origin.

References

Aisenberg, A.C.: Lymphocytopenia in Hodgkin's disease. Blood *25,* 1037–1042 (1965)

Baldwin, R.W., Glaves, D., Pimm, M.V.: Embryonic and tumor antigens. Lancet *1971 I,* 767–768

Berke, G., Amos, G.B.: Mechanism of lymphocytes-mediated cytolysis: the LMC cycle and its role in transplantation immunity. Transplant. Rev. *17,* 71–107 (1973)

Bernstein, I.D., Thor, D.E., Zbar, Rapp, H.J.: Tumor immunity: tumor suppression in vivo initiated by soluble products of specifically stimulated lymphocytes. Science *172,* 729–732 (1971)

Blaeser, B.: Proliferationskinetik im peritumoralen Entzündungsfeld menschlicher Kehlkopf-Carcinome. Inaugural-Dissertation der Westf. Wilhelms-Universität Münster/Westf. 1975

Bloom, B.R., Shevach, E.: Requirement for T cells in the production of migration inhibitory factors. J. Exp. Med. *142,* 1306–1311 (1975)

Brouet, J.C., Flandrin, G., Seligmann, M.: Indications of the thymus-derived nature of the proliferating cells in six patients with Sezary's syndrome. N. Engl. J. Med. *289,* 341–344 (1973)

Brouet, J.C., Preud'Homme, J.L., Seligmann, M.: The use of B and T membrane markers in the classification of leukemia with special reference to acute lymphoblastic leukemia. Blood Cells *1,* 81–89 (1975)

Bunting, C.H.: The blood picture in Hodgkin's disease. Bull. Johns Hopkins Hosp. *25,* 173–176 (1914)

Burk, M.W., Yu, S., Burk, K.R., McKhann, C.F.: Stimulation of thymus- and bone marrow-derived lymphocytes by tumor cells in culture. Cancer Res. *37,* 603–609 (1977)

Cantor, H., Asofsky, R.: Synergy among lymphoid cells mediating the graft-versus-host syndrome. II. Synergy in g.v.h.-reactions produced by Balb/c lymphoid cells of differing anatomic origin. J. Exp. Med. *131,* 235–246 (1970)

Cerottini, J.-C., Brunner, K.T.: Cell-mediated cytotoxicity, allograft rejection and tumor immunity. Adv. Immunol. *18,* 67–132 (1974)

Chin, A.H., Saiki, J.H., Trujillo, J.M., Williams, R.C.: Peripheral blood T- and B-lymphocytes in patients with lymphoma and acute leukemia. Clin. Immunol. Immunpathol. *1,* 499–510 (1973)

Claman, H.N., Mosier, D.E.: Cell-cell interaction in antibody production. Prog. Allergy *16,* 40–80 (1972)

Cockerell, G.L., Krakowka, S., Hoover, E.A., Olsen, R.G., Yohn, D.S.: Lymphocytes mitogen reactivity in feline leukemia virus-infected cats and identification of feline T and B lymphocytes. Comp. Leukemia Res., Bibl. Haematol. *43,* 81–83 (1976a)

Cockerell, G.L., Krakowka, S., Hoover, E.A., Olsen, R.G., Yohn, D.S.: Characterization of feline T- and B-lymphocytes and identification of an experimentally induced T-cell neoplasm in the cat. J. Natl. Cancer Inst. *57,* 907–913 (1976b)

Cockerell, G.L., Hoover, E.A., Krakowka, S., Olsen, R.G., Yohn, D.S.: Lymphocytes mitogen reactivity and enumeration of circulating B- and T-cells during feline leukemia virus infection in the cat. J. Natl. Cancer Inst. *57,* 1095–1099 (1976c)

Cohen, S., Bigazzi, P.E., Yoshida, T.: Similarities of T cell function in cell-mediated immunity and antibody production. Cell. Immunol. *12,* 150–159 (1974)

Cohnen, G., Augener, W., Konig, E.: B lymphocytes in Hodgkin's disease. N. Engl. J. Med. *288,* 161–162 (1973)

Cooper, M.D., Perey, D.Y., Peterson, R.D.A., Gabrielsen, A.E., Good, R.A.: The two-component concept of the lymphoid system. In: Immunologic deficiency diseases in man. Birth defects original article series Good, R.A., Bergsma, D. (eds.), Vol. 4, pp. 7–16. New York: National Foundation Press 1968

Cooper, M.D., Purchase, H.G., Brockman, D.E., Gathings, W.E.: Studies on the nature of the abnormalitiy of B cell differentiation in avian lymphoid leukosis: production of heterogeneous IgM by tumor cells. J. Immunol. *113,* 1210–1222 (1974)
Cossel, L., Mahnke, P.F., Schwarzer, R.: "Killer"-lymphocytes in action? Light and electron microscopical findings in orthotopic liver homografts. Virchows Archiv (Pathol. Anat.) *364,* 179–190 (1974)
Deodhar, S.D., Crile, G., Esselstyn, C.B.: Study of the tumor cell-lymphocyte interaction in patients with breast cancer. Cancer *29,* 1321–1325 (1972)
Diener, E., Langman, R.E.: Antigen recognition in induction of immunity. Prog. Allergy *18,* 6–42 (1974)
Dmochowski, L., Bowen, J.M.: Current trends in basic immunology as applied to the problem of human neoplasia. Am. J. Clin. Pathol. *62,* 167–172 (1974)
Dutton, R.W., Campbell, P., Chan, E., Hirst, J., Hoffmann, M., Kettman, J., Lesley, J., McCarthy, M., Mishell, R.I., Raidt, D.J., Vann, D.: Cell cooperation during immunologic responses of isolated lymphoid cells. In: Cellular interactions in the immune responses. Cohen, S., Cudkowicz, G., McCluskey, R.T. (eds.), pp. 31–41. Basel: Karger 1971
Eilberg, F.R., Morton, D.L.: Impaired immunologic reactivity and recurrence following cancer surgery. Cancer *25,* 362–367 (1970)
Elboim, C.M., Reinisch, C.L., Schlossman, S.F.: T and B lymphocytes migration into syngeneic tumors. J. Immunol. *118,* 1042–1048 (1977)
Falletta, J.M., Ramanujam, N., Starling, K.A.: Ig-positive lymphocytes in Hodgkin's disease. N. Engl. J. Med. *288,* 581–582 (1973)
Feldmann, M.: Induction of B cell tolerance by antigen specific T cell factor. Nature New Biol. *242,* 82–84 (1973)
Feldmann, M., Nossal, G.J.V.: Tolerance, enhancement and the regulation of interactions between T cells, B cells and macrophages. Transplant. Rev. *13,* 3–34 (1972)
Froland, S.S.: Binding of sheep erythrocytes to human lymphocytes; a probable marker of T lymphocytes. Scand. J. Immunol. *1,* 269–280 (1972)
Galton, D.A.G., Goldman, J.M., Wilshaw, E., Catovsky, D., Henry, K., Goldenberg, G.J.: Prolymphocytic leukemia. Br. J. Haematol. *27,* 7–23 (1974)
Garotta, G., Porta, C.: Inhibitory tumor factors. Behavior of fetal B-lymphocytes and macrophages during cancerogenesis. In: Molecular base of malignancy. Deutsch, E. (ed.), pp. 113–119. Stuttgart: Thieme 1976
Gatti, R.A., Good, R.A.: Occurrence of malignancy in immunodeficiency diseases: a literature review. Cancer *28,* 89–98 (1971)
Gaylord, H.R., Clowes, G.H.A., Baeslack, F.W.: Contributions to the subject of immunity in cancer. In: Annual reports of the New York State Cancer Laboratory, p. 6. Albany: Lyon 1910
Gohn, K., Reddy, M.M.: B and T lymphocytes in man. II. Circulating B and T lymphocytes in cancer patients. J. Med. *7,* 297–305 (1976)
Good, R.A., Finstad, J.: Essential relationship between the lymphoid system, immunity and malignancy. Natl. Cancer Inst. Monogr. *31,* 41–58 (1969)
Gorczynski, R.M.: Immunity to murine sarcoma virus induced tumors. II. Suppression of T-cell-mediated immunity by cells from progressor animals. J. Immunol. *112,* 1826–1838 (1974)
Greaves, M.F.: Biological effects of antiimmunoglobulins: evidence for immunoglobulin receptors on "T" and "B" lymphocytes. Transplant. Rev. *5,* 45–75 (1970)
Greaves, M.F., Hogg, N.M.: Immunoglobulin determinants on the surface of antigen binding T and B lymphocytes in mice. Prog. Immunol. *1,* 111–117 (1971)
Grey, H.M., Rabellino, E., Pirofsky, B.: Immunoglobulins on the surface of lymphocytes. IV. Distribution in hypogammaglobulinemia, cellular immune deficiency, and chronic lymphatic leukemia. J. Clin. Invest. *50,* 2368–2375 (1971)

Grundmann, E., Madaus, W.-P., Hobik, H.P.: Beeinflussung der histologischen Abstoßungsreaktion gegen das Jensen-Sarkom der Ratte bei Mäusen durch heterologes Antilymphocytenserum. Beitr. Pathol. Anat. *140,* 89–109 (1969)
Gutman, G.A., Weissman, I.L.: Lymphoid tissue architecture: experimental analysis of the origin and distribution of T-cells and B-cells. Immunology *23,* 465–471 (1972)
Hackmann, Ch.: Experimentelle Studien über die Heilungsvorgänge bei bösartigen Geschwülsten. Z. Krebsforsch. *57,* 164–190 (1951)
Haferkamp, O.: Der schutzlose Organismus. Dtsch. Med. Wschr. *99,* 203–210 (1974)
Haller, O., Wigzell, H.: Suppression of natural killer cell activity with radioactive strontium: effector cells are marrow dependent. J. Immunol. *118,* 1503–1506 (1977)
Hamperl, H.: Die Morphologie der Tumoren. In: Handbuch der allgemeinen Pathologie Büchner, F. (ed.) Vol. VI/3, pp. 18–106. Berlin, Göttingen, Heidelberg: Springer 1956
Hattler, B., Amos, B.: The immunology of cancer: tumor antigens and the responsiveness of the host. Monogr. Surg. Sci. *3,* 1–34 (1966)
Hellström, J., Hellström, K.E., Pierce, G.E., Yang, J.P.S.: Cellular and humoral immunity to different types of human neoplasma. Nature *220,* 1352–1354 (1968)
Henney, C.S.: On the mechanism of T-cell mediated cytolysis. Transplant. Rev. *17,* 38–69 (1973)
Hickok, D.F., Miller, L., Harris, L.: Regional hyperplastic lymph nodes in breast cancer: the role of lymphocytes and nodal macrophages. Surgery *82,* 710–715 (1977)
Hsu, C.S., Marti, G.E., Schrek, R., Williams, R.C.: Lymphocytes bearing B- and T-cell markers in patient with lymphosarcoma cell leukemia. Clin. Immunol. Immunopathol. *3,* 385–395 (1975)
Jenssen, H.-L., Eckert, R., Werner, H., Köhler, H., Pasternak, G., Friemel, H.: Lymphokines of T and B cells. I. Demonstration that T and B cells of tumor antigensensitised mice produce different lymphokines changing surface charge of target cells. Oncology *34,* 159–163 (1977)
Jondal, M., Holm, G., Wigzell, H.: Surface markers on human T and B lymphocytes. I. A large population of lymphocytes forming non-immune rosettes with sheep red blood cells. J. Exp. Med. *136,* 207–215 (1972)
Katz, D.H., Hamaoka, T., Benacerraf, B.: Cell interactions between histoincompatible T and B lymphocyte. J. Exp. Med. *137,* 1405–1418 (1973)
Keller, R.: Beziehungen zwischen Tumorwachstum und Immunität. Schweiz. Med. Wschr. *102,* 1148–1151 (1972)
Kerbel, R.S., Eidinger, D.: Further studies of antigenic competition. 3. A model to account for the phenomenon based on a deficiency of cell-to-cell interaction in immune lymphoid cell populations. J. Exp. Med. *133,* 1043–1060 (1971)
Keuning, F.J.: Dynamics of immunoglobulin forming cells and their precursors. In: Immunoglobulins: cell bound receptors and humoral antibodies. Ballieux, R.E., Gruber, M., Seijen, H.G. (eds.), pp. 1–14. Amsterdam: North-Holland, American Elsevier 1972
Kilburn, D.G., Smith, J.B., Gorczynski, R.M.: Nonspecific suppression of T lymphocyte responses in mice carrying progressively growing tumors. Eur. J. Immunol. *4,* 784–788 (1974)
Klein, E., Becker, S., Svedmyr, E., Jondal, M., Vanky, F.: Tumor infiltrating lymphocytes. Ann. N.Y. Acad. Sci. *276,* 207–216 (1976)
Krüger, G.: Versuch einer immunologischen Deutung der Lymphomentstehung. Dtsch. Med. J. *21,* 28–34 (1970)
Krüger, G.: Lymphoreticular neoplasia in immunosuppression: facts anf fancies. Beitr. Pathol. Anat. *151,* 221–233 (1974)

Lee, Y.-T.N.: Peripheral lymphocyte count and subpopulations of T and B lymphocytes in benign and malignant diseases. Surg. Gynecol. Obstet. *144,* 435–450 (1977)

Lee, Y.N., Say, C., Hori, J.M.: Peripheral lymphocyte counts and prognosis in malignant lymphomas. Mo. Med. *71,* 69–73 (1974)

Lennert, K., Mohri, N., Stein, H., Kaiserling, E.: The histopathology of malignant lymphoma. Br. J. Haematol. (Suppl.) *31,* 193–204 (1975)

Lindstrom, F.D., Hardy, W.R., Eberle, B.J.: Multiple myeloma and benign monoclonal gammopathy; differentiation by immunofluorescence of lymphocytes. Ann. Intern. Med. *78,* 837–844 (1973)

Marusic, M., Allegretti, N., Culo, F.: Cell cooperation in abolition of tolerance to xenogeneic tumor. Cell. Immunol. *27,* 26–35 (1976)

Middelkoop, O.P., Veldhuizen, R.W., Scheper, R.J.: E and EAC rosette-forming cells in healthy donors and cancer patients. Int. Arch. Allergy Appl. Immun. *52,* 412–416 (1976)

Miller, D.G.: Immunologic deficiency and malignant lymphoma. Cancer *20,* 579–588 (1967)

Miller, J.F.A.P., Mitchell, G.F.: Thymus and antigen-reactive cells. Transplant. Rev. *1,* 3–42 (1969)

Mitchison, N.A.: Cell populations involved in immune response. In: Immunologic tolerance. Landy, M., Braun, W. (eds.), pp. 113–169). New York: Academic Press 1969

Mosier, D.E., Coppleson, L.W.: A three-cell interaction required for the induction of the primary response in vitro. Proc. Natl. Acad. Sci. USA *61,* 542–549 (1968)

Mosier, D.E., Johnson, B.M., Paul, W.E., McMaster, P.R.B.: Cellular requirements for the primary in vitro antibody response to DNP-ficoll. J. Exp. Med. *139,* 1354–1360 (1974)

Movat, H.Z., Fernando, M.V.P.: The fine structure of lymphoid tissue during antibody formation. Exp. Mol. Pathol. *4,* 155–188 (1965)

Nathan, C.F., Remold, H.G., David, J.R.: Characterization of a lymphocyte factor which alters macrophage functions. J. Exp. Med. *137,* 275–290 (1973)

Niedorf, H.R., Lusznat, A., Hultsch, E., Grundmann, E.: The influence of embryonal bursectomy on benzpyrene-induced sarcoma of the chicken. Z. Krebsforsch. *91,*323–334 (1978)

Nieuwenhuis, P., van Nouhuijs, C.E., Eggens, J.H., Keuning, F.J.: Germinal centres and the origin of the B-cell system. I. Germinal centres in the rabbit appendix. Immunol. *26,* 497–507 (1974)

Nordqvist, B.C., Kinney, J.P.: T and B cells and cell-mediated immunity in mycosis fungoides. Cancer *37,* 714–718 (1976)

Old, L.J., Boyse, E.A., Geering, G., Oettgen, H.F.: Serologic approaches to the study of cancer in animals and in man. Cancer Res. *28,*1288–1299 (1968)

O'Nell, Mackler, B.F., Wyde, P.: Complement (C3) receptor-bearing lymphocyte-mediated cytotoxicity and lymphotoxin responses. Cell Immunol. *20,* 33–41 (1975)

Payne, L.N., Rennie, M.: Sequential changes in the numbers of B and T lymphocytes and other leukocytes in the blood in Marek's disease. Int. J. Cancer *18,* 510–520 (1976)

Perlmann, P., Holm, G.: Cytotoxic effects of lymphoid cells in vitro. Adv. Immunol. *11,* 117–193 (1970)

Piguet, P.-F., Vassalli, P.: Study of the thymic-derived or independent nature of mouse spleen cells induced to proliferate in cultrue by various mitogens and antigens. Eur. J. Immunol. *3,* 477–483 (1973)

Raff, M.C.: Surface antigenic markers for distinguishing T and B lymphocytes in mice. Transplant. Rev. *6,* 52–56 (1971)

Raff, M.C., Owen, J.J.T.: Thymus-derived lymphocytes: their distribution and role in the development of peripheral lymphoid tissues of the mouse. Eur. J. Immunol. *1,* 27–30 (1971)

Rappaport, H.: Atlas of tumor pathology 3/8: Tumors of the hematopoietic system. Washington: AFIP 1966
Ribbert, H.: Beiträge zur Histogenese des Carcinomas. Virchows Arch. *135*, 433–469 (1894)
Roberts, M.M., Bath, B.M.: Local immunoglobulin production in breast cancer. Br. J. Cancer *27*, 269–275 (1973)
Robinowitz, B.N., Noguchi, S., Roenig, H.H.: Tumor cell characterization in mycosis fungoides. Cancer *37*, 1747–1753 (1976)
Rocklin, R.E., MacDermott, R.P., Chess, L., Schlossman, S.F., David, J.R.: Studies on mediator production by highly purified T and B lymphocytes. J. Exp. Med. *140*, 1303–1316 (1974)
Rosenthal, A.S., Lipsky, P.E., Shevach, E.M.: Macrophage–lymphocyte interaction and antigen recognition. Fed. Proc. *34*, 1743–1748 (1975)
Ross, G.D.: Surface markers of B and T cells. Arch. Pathol. Lab. Med. *101*, 337–341 (1977)
Ross, G.D., Polley, M.J.: Specificity of human lymphocyte complement receptors. J. Exp. Med. *141*, 1163–1180 (1975)
Ross, G.D., Rabellino, E.M., Polley, M.J., Grey, H.M.: Combined studies of complement receptor and surface immunoglobulin-bearing cells and sheep erythrocyte rosette-forming cells in normal and leukemic lymphocytes. J. Clin. Invest. *52*, 377–385 (1973)
Roswing, T.: La therapeutique nonchirurgicale du cancer. In: Travaux deuxieme Conf. Int. Cancer, Paris 1910
Rygaard, J., Povlsen, C.O.: The absence of spontaneous tumours in nude mice. In: Proceedings of the first International Workshop on Nude Mice, 1973. Rygaard, J., Povlsen, C.O. (eds.), pp. 293–297. Stuttgart: Fischer 1974
Sandberg, A.L., Wahl, S.M., Mergenhagen, S.E.: Lymphokine production by C3b-stimulated B cells. J. Immunol. *115*, 139–144 (1975)
Schmidtke, J., Unanue, E.R.: Interaction of macrophages and lymphocytes with surface immunoglobulin. Nature New Biol. *233*, 84–86 (1971)
Schönfelder, M., Wildführ, W., Gläser, A.: Zur licht- und elektronenmikroskopischen Morphologie der lymphocytären Tumorzellvernichtung in vitro. Pathol. Microbiol. (Basel) *40*, 251–258 (1974)
Sell, S.: Immunology, Immunopathology and Immunity. New York, Evanston, San Francisco, London: Harper & Row 1975
Silveira, N.P.A., Mendes, N.F., Rolnai, M.E.A.: Tissue localization of two populations of human lymphocytes distinguished by membrane receptors. J. Immunol. *108*, 1456–1460 (1972)
Smith, R.T.: Tumor-specific immune mechanisms. New Enlg. J. Med. *278*, 1207–1214 (1968)
Solomon, A.: Cellular regulation of humoral immunity. N. Engl. J. Med. *293*, 928–929 (1975)
Stein, H.: Klassifikation der malignen Non-Hodgkin-Lymphome aufgrund gemeinsamer morphologischer und immunologischer Merkmale zwischen normalen und neoplastischen lymphatischen Zellen. Immunität und Infektion *4*, 52–109 (1976)
Stuart, A.E.: Immunological aspects of reticulum cell neoplasia. Br. Med. J. *1970 IV*, 423–424
Stuhlmiller, J.M., Seigler, H.F.: Characterization of a chimpanzee antihuman melanoma antiserum. Cancer Res. *35*, 2132–2137 (1975)
Suter, E.R., Probst, H., Dukor, P.: The fine structure of complement-receptor lymphocytes in mice. Eur. J. Immunol. *2*, 189–190 (1972)
Takashima, I., Olson, C., Driscoll, D.M., Baumgartener, L.E.: B-lymphocytes and T-lymphocytes in three types of bovine lymphosarcoma. J. Natl. Cancer Inst. *59*, 1205–1209 (1977)

Takasugi, M., Hildemann, W.H.: Regulation of immunity toward allogenic tumors in mice. I. Effect of antiserum fractions on tumor growth. J. Natl. Cancer Inst. *43*, 843–856 (1969)

Taylor, R.B., Iverson, G.M.: Hapten competition and the nature of cell cooperation in the antibody response. Proc. R. Soc. Lond (Biol.)*176*, 393–418 (1971)

Tigelaar, R.E., Asofsky, R.: Synergy among lymphoid cells mediating in the graft versus host response. V. Derivation by migration in lethally irradiate recipients of two interacting subpopulations of thymus-derived cells from normal spleen. J. Exp. Med. *137*, 239–253 (1973)

Vos, G.H., Hammond, M.G., Vos, D., Grobbelaar, B.G., Auslander, H.P., Marescotti, G.: An evaluation of humoral antibody responses in patients with carcinoma of the cervix. J. Obstet. Gynecol. *79*, 1040–1046 (1972)

Wagner, H., Röllinghoff, M., Nossal, G.J.V.: T-cell-mediated immune response induced in vitro: a probe for allograft and tumor immunity. Transplant. Rev. *17*, 3–36 (1973)

Wahl, S.M., Rosenstreich, D.L.: Role of B lymphocytes in cell-mediated immunity. I. Requirement for T cells or T-cell products for antigen-induced B-cell activation. J. Exp. Med. *144*, 1175–1187 (1976)

Wahl, S.M., Wilton, J.M., Rosenstreich, D.L., Oppenheim, J.J.: The role of macrophages in the production of lymphokines by T and B lymphocytes. J. Immunol. *114*, 296–1301 (1975)

Wallbach, G.: Über das sogenannte Immunitätsgewebe transplantabler Tumoren und dessen Veränderlichkeit durch umstimmende Reize. Z. Krebsforsch. *29*, 577–622 (1929)

White, R.G.: Functional recognition of immunologically competent cells by means of fluorescent antibody technique. In: The immunologically competent cell. Wolstenholme, G.E.W., Knight, B.A. (eds.), pp. 6–19. London: Churchill 1963

Witting, Ch., Hultsch, E.: Effect of splenectomy on B and T lymphocytes and a benzpyrene-induced murine sarcoma. Z. Krebsforsch. *92*, 267–274 (1978)

Witz, I.P.: Tumor-associated immunoglobulins. Isr. J. Med. Sci. *7*, 230–238 (1971)

Youdim, S., Sharman, M.: Resistance to tumor growth mediated by listeria monocytogenes: collaborative and suppressive macrophage-lymphocyte interactions in vitro. J. Immunol. *117*, 1860–1865 (1976)

Zbar, B., Wpsic, H.T., Rapp, H.J., Steward, L.C., Borsos, T.: Two-step mechanisms of tumor graft rejection in syngeneic guinea pigs. II. Initiation of reaction by a cell reaction containing lymphocytes and neutrophils. J. Natl. Cancer Inst. *44*, 701–711 (1970)

Subject Index

The numbers set in *italics* refer to those pages on which the respective catch-word is discussed in detail

Index to Volumes 60 – 66 Current Topics in Pathology

Volume 60

Volume 61

Volume 62

Volume 63

Volume 64

Volume 65

Volume 66

MIX
Papier aus verantwortungsvollen Quellen
Paper from responsible sources
FSC® C105338

If you have any concerns about our products,
you can contact us on
ProductSafety@springernature.com

In case Publisher is established outside the EU,
the EU authorized representative is:
Springer Nature Customer Service Center GmbH
Europaplatz 3, 69115 Heidelberg, Germany

Printed by Libri Plureos GmbH
in Hamburg, Germany